SANFORD GUIDE ®

Thirty-sixth Edition

THE SANFORD GUIDE
TO ANTIMICROBIAL
THERAPY
2006

W9-AQO-233

David N. Gilbert, M.D.
Director of Medical Education & Earl A. Chiles Research Institute
Providence Portland Medical Center
Professor of Medicine
Oregon Health Sciences University
Portland, Oregon

Robert C. Moellering, Jr., M.D.
Shields Warrren-Mallinckrodt Professor of Medicine
Harvard Medical School
Boston, Massachusetts

George M. Eliopoulos, M.D.
Chief, James L. Tullis Firm, Beth Israel Deaconess Hospital
Professor of Medicine
Harvard Medical School
Boston, Massachusetts

Merle A. Sande, M.D.
Professor of Medicine
University of Washington School of Medicine
Seattle, Washington

THE SANFORD GUIDE TO ANTIMICROBIAL THERAPY 2006
36TH EDITION

Jay P. Sanford, M.D.
1928-1996

Editors

David N. Gilbert, M.D.
George M. Eliopoulos, M.D.

Robert C. Moellering, Jr., M.D.
Merle A. Sande, M.D.

The Sanford Guides are published annually by

ANTIMICROBIAL THERAPY, INC.
P.O. Box 276, 11771 Lee Hwy, Sperryville, VA 22740-0276 USA
Tel 540-987-9480 Fax 540-987-9486
Email: info@sanfordguide.com   www.sanfordguide.com

Printed in the United States of America
ISBN 1-930808-30-5
Pocket Edition (English)

PUBLISHER'S PREFACE

This edition marks the 36th revision of the SANFORD GUIDE TO ANTIMICROBIAL THERAPY. The manuscript for the first edition in 1969 was prepared by Carolyn Wickwire who was then Jay Sanford's administrative assistant. Carolyn has prepared the manuscript for every new edition that followed including this one. She retires from her service to the SANFORD GUIDE with this edition. Carolyn's remarkable tenure is not likely to be repeated. We wish her all the best in her future endeavors.

Though many readers of the SANFORD GUIDE receive their copy from a pharmaceutical company representative, please be assured that the SANFORD GUIDE has been, and continues to be, independently prepared and published since its inception in 1969. Decisions regarding the content of the SANFORD GUIDE are solely those of the editors and the publisher. We welcome your questions, comments and feedback concerning the SANFORD GUIDE. All of your feedback is reviewed and taken into account in preparing the next edition.

NOTE TO READER

Every effort is made to ensure the accuracy of the content of this guide. However, current full prescribing information available in the package insert of each drug should be consulted before prescribing any product. The editors and publisher are not responsible for errors or omissions or for any consequences from application of the information in this book and make no warranty, express or implied, with respect to the currency, accuracy, or completeness of the contents of the publication. Application of this information in a particular situation remains the professional responsibility of the practitioner.

1

—TABLE OF CONTENTS—

SUMMARY OF ABBREVIATIONS

DRUG NAME ABBREVIATIONS

Antibacterial & Antimycobacterial Drugs

AG = aminoglycoside
AMK = amikacin
AM-CL = amoxicillin-clavulanate
AM-CL-ER = amoxicillin-clavulanate extended release
Amox = amoxicillin
AMP = ampicillin
AM-SB = ampicillin-sulbactam
AP Pen = antipseudomonal penicillins
APAG = antipseudomonal aminoglycoside (tobra, gent, amikacin)
Azithro = azithromycin
BL/BLI = beta-lactam/beta-lactamase inhibitor
CARB = carbapenems (ERTA, IMP, MER)
Cefpodox = cefpodoxime proxetil
Ceftaz = ceftazidime
CFP = cefepime
Chloro = chloramphenicol
CIP = ciprofloxacin; CIP-ER = CIP extended release
Clarithro = clarithromycin; ER = extended release
Clav = clavulanate
Clinda = clindamycin
CLO = clofazimine
Dapto = daptomycin
Dirithro = dirithromycin
Doxy = doxycycline
EES = erythromycin ethyl succinate
ERTA = ertapenem
Erythro = erythromycin
ETB = ethambutol
FQ = fluoroquinolone (CIP, Oflox, Lome, Peflox, Levo, Gati, Moxi, Gemi)
Gati = gatifloxacin
Gemi = gemifloxacin
Gent = gentamicin
GNB = gram-negative bacilli
IMP = imipenem-cilastatin
INH = isoniazid
IVIG = intravenous immune globulin
Levo = levofloxacin
Lome = lomefloxacin
Macrolide = azithro, clarithro, dirithro, erythro, roxithro
MER = meropenem
Metro = metronidazole
Mino = minocycline
Moxi = moxifloxacin
NF = nitrofurantoin
O Ceph 1,2,3 = oral cephalosporins—see Table 10B
Oflox = ofloxacin

P Ceph 1,2,3,4 = parenteral cephalosporins—see Table 10B
P Ceph 3 AP = parenteral cephalosporins with antipseudomonal activity—see Table 10B
Peflox = pefloxacin
PIP-TZ = piperacillin-tazobactam
PZA = pyrazinamide
RFB = rifabutin
RFP = rifapentine
Rifamp = rifampin
SM = streptomycin
Sulb = sulbactam
Tazo = tazobactam
TC-CL = ticarcillin-clavulanate
Teico = teicoplanin
Telithro = telithromycin
Tetra = tetracycline
Ticar = ticarcillin
TMP-SMX = trimethoprim-sulfamethoxazole
Vibra = tobramycin
Vanco = vancomycin

Antifungal Drugs

Ampho B = amphotericin B
ABCC = ampho B cholesteryl complex
ABLC = ampho B lipid complex
L-AB = liposomal ampho B
Clot = clotrimazole
Flu = fluconazole
Flucyt = flucytosine
Griseo = griseofulvin
Itra = itraconazole
Keto = ketoconazole
Vori = voriconazole

Antiparasitic Drugs

AP = atovaquone proguanil
CQ = chloroquine phosphate
MQ = mefloquine

Antivirals: Anti-HIV Drugs

3TC = lamivudine
d4T = stavudine
ddC = zalcitabine
ddI = didanosine
FTC = emtricitabine
TDF = tenofovir
DLV = delavirdine
ADF = adefovir
ZDV = zidovudine
EFZ = efavirenz
NVP = nevirapine
ATV = atazanavir
FOS-APV = fos-amprenavir
IDV = indinavir
IFN = interferon

LP/R = lopinavir/ritonavir
NFR = nelfinavir
RTV = ritonavir
SQV = saquinavir
TPV = Tipranavir
ENT = enfuvirtide

PQ = primaquine
Pyri = pyrimethamine
QS = quinine sulfate

DRUG DOSAGE & DRUG ADMINISTRATION

mcg = microgram
mg = milligram
AD = after dialysis
div = divided

gm = gram
DS = double strength
bid = twice a day
tid = 3 times a day
qid = 4 times a day
BW = body weight

IP = intraperitoneal
IT = intrathecal
po = per os (by mouth)
subcut = subcutaneous
dc = discontinue
rx = treatment
DOT = directly observed therapy

DRUG-RELATED

G = generic
I = investigational
IA = injectable agent
NB = name brand
NFDA-I = not FDA-approved indication
NUS = not available in the U.S.
ASA = aspirin
NSAIDs = non-steroidal anti-inflammatory drugs

DISEASE-ASSOCIATED

ARDS = acute respiratory distress syndrome
ARF = acute rheumatic fever
CAPD = continuous ambulatory peritoneal dialysis
CAVH = continuous arteriovenous hemofiltration
CSD = cat-scratch disease
DIC = disseminated intravascular coagulation
ESRD = endstage renal disease
HEMO = hemodialysis
PEP = post-exposure prophylaxis
PTLD = post-transplant lymphoproliferative disease
RTI = respiratory tract infection
STD = sexually transmitted disease
TBc = tuberculosis
UTI = urinary tract infection

ORGANISMS

CMV = cytomegalovirus
BW group = B. distasonis, B. ovatus, B. thetaiotaomicron
DRSP = drug-resistant S. pneumoniae
EBV = Epstein-Barr virus
GC = gonorrhea
HHV = human herpesvirus
HIV = human immunodeficiency virus
HSV = herpes simplex virus
LGV = lymphogranuloma venereum
MSSA/MRSA = methicillin-sensitive/resistant S. aureus
M. Tbc = Mycobacterium tuberculosis
Rick = Rickettsia
RSV = respiratory syncytial virus
VISA = vancomycin intermediately resistant S. aureus
VZV = varicella-zoster virus

ABBREVIATIONS (2)

MISCELLANEOUS

Diagnosis
C&S = culture & sensitivity
CXR = chest x-ray
ESBLs = extended spectrum β-lactamases
ESR = erythrocyte sedimentation rate
HLR = high-level resistance
LCR = ligase chain reaction
PCR = polymerase chain reaction
TEE = transesophageal echocardiography
VL = viral load

Other
AUC = area under the curve
DBPCT = double-blind placebo-controlled trial
EDC = expected date of confinement
PRCT = Prospective randomized controlled trials
Pts = patients
R = resistant
S = potential synergy in combination with penicillin, AMP, vanco, teico
S = sensitive (susceptible)
VR = very rare

Organizations
ATS = American Thoracic Society
CDC = Centers for Disease Control
ICAAC = International Conference on Antimicrobial Agents & Chemotherapy
IDSA = Infectious Diseases Society of America
WHO = World Health Organization

ABBREVIATIONS OF JOURNAL TITLES

AAC: Antimicrobial Agents & Chemotherapy
Adv PID: Advances in Pediatric Infectious Diseases
AIDS Res Hum Retrovir: AIDS Research & Human Retroviruses
AJM: American Journal of Medicine
AJRCCM: American Journal of Respiratory Critical Care Medicine
AJTMH: American Journal of Tropical Medicine & Hygiene
Aliment Pharmacol Ther: Alimentary Pharmacology & Therapeutics
Am J Hlth Pharm: American Journal of Health-System Pharmacy
AnEM: Annals of Emergency Medicine
AnIM: Annals of Internal Medicine
AnPharmacother: Annals of Pharmacotherapy
AnSurg: Annals of Surgery
ArDerm: Archives of Dermatology
Antivir Ther: Antiviral Therapy
ArIM: Archives of Internal Medicine
ARRD: American Review of Respiratory Disease
BMJ: British Medical Journal
Brit J Derm: British Journal of Dermatology
Can JID: Canadian Journal of Infectious Diseases
CCM: Critical Care Medicine
CITD: Current Clinical Topics in Infectious Disease
CID: Clinical Infectious Diseases
Clin Micro Inf: Clinical Microbiology and Infection
Clin Micro Rev: Clinical Microbiology Reviews
COID: Current Opinion in Infectious Disease
Curr Med Res Opin: Current Medical Research and Opinion
Derm Ther: Dermatologic Therapy

Dig Dis Sci: Digestive Diseases and Sciences
DMID: Diagnostic Microbiology and Infectious Disease
EID: Emerging Infectious Diseases
EJCMID: European Journal of Clin. Micro. & Infectious Diseases
Eur J Neurol: European Journal of Neurology
Exp Mol Path: Experimental & Molecular Pathology
Gastro: Gastroenterology
Hpt: Hepatology
ICHE: Infection Control and Hospital Epidemiology
IDC No. Amer: Infectious Disease Clinics of North America
IDCP: Infectious Diseases in Clinical Practice
IJAA: International Journal of Antimicrobial Agents
Inf Med: Infections in Medicine
JAIDS: JAIDS Journal of Acquired Immune Deficiency Syndromes
AIDS & HR: Journal of AIDS and Human Retrovirology
All Clin Immun: Journal of Allergy and Clinical Immunology
J Am Ger Soc: Journal of the American Geriatrics Society
J Chemother: Journal of Chemotherapy
JCI: Journal of Clinical Investigation
J Clin Micro: Journal of Clinical Microbiology
J Clin Virol: Journal of Clinical Virology
J Derm Treat: Journal of Dermatological Treatment
J Hpt: Journal of Hepatology
J Inf: Journal of Infection
J Med Micro: Journal of Medical Microbiology
J Micro Immunol Inf: Journal of Microbiology, Immunology, & Infection
J Ped: Journal of Pediatrics

JAC: Journal of Antimicrobial Chemotherapy
JAMA: Journal of the American Medical Association
JAVMA: Journal of the Veterinary Medicine Association
JID: Journal of Infectious Diseases
JNS: Journal of Neurosurgery
JTMH: Journal of Tropical Medicine and Hygiene
J Viral Hep: Journal of Viral Hepatitis
Ln: Lancet
LnID: Lancet Infectious Disease
Mayo Clin Proc: Mayo Clinic Proceedings
Med Lett: Medical Letter
Med Mycol: Medical Mycology
MMWR: Morbidity & Mortality Weekly Report
NEJM: New England Journal of Medicine
Neph Dial Transpl: Nephrology Dialysis Transplantation
Ped Ann: Pediatric Annals
Peds: Pediatrics
Pharmacother: Pharmacotherapy
PIDJ: Pediatric Infectious Diseases Journal
QJM: Quarterly Journal of Medicine
Scand J Inf Dis: Scandinavian Journal of Infectious Diseases
Sem Resp Inf: Seminars in Respiratory Infections
SMJ: Southern Medical Journal
Surg Neurol: Surgical Neurology
Transpl: Transplantation
Transpl Inf Dis: Transplant Infectious Diseases
TRSM: Transactions of the Royal Society of Medicine
West J Med: Western Journal of Medicine

TABLE 1*

CLINICAL APPROACH TO INITIAL CHOICE OF ANTIMICROBIAL THERAPY (Abbreviations on page 2)

Treatment based on presumed site or type of infection. In selected instances, treatment and prophylaxis based on identification of pathogens

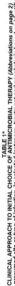

ANATOMIC SITE/DIAGNOSIS/ MODIFYING CIRCUMSTANCES	ETIOLOGIES (usual)	SUGGESTED REGIMENS*		ADJUNCT DIAGNOSTIC OR THERAPEUTIC MEASURES AND COMMENTS
		PRIMARY	ALTERNATIVE†	
ABDOMEN: See Peritonitis, pages 34–35; Gallbladder, page 13; and Pelvic Inflammatory Disease, page 19				
BONE: Osteomyelitis. Microbiologic diagnosis is essential. If blood culture negative, need culture of bone. Culture of sinus tract drainage not predictive of bone culture. Review: Ln 364:369, 2004				
Hematogenous Osteomyelitis **Empiric therapy—Collect bone and blood cultures before empiric therapy**				
Newborn (<4 mos.): See Table 16 for dose	S. aureus, Group A strep, Gm-neg. bacilli	MRSA possible: (Nafcillin or oxacillin) + P Ceph 3	MRSA possible: Vanco + P Ceph 3	Table 16 for dose. Severe allergy or toxicity: (Linezolid^MRSA 10 mg per kg IV/po q8h) + clindamycin for linezolid. Severe allergy or toxicity: clindamycin or linezolid. Dosages in Table 16. See Table 10 for adverse reactions to drugs.
Children (>4 mos.)—Adult: Osteo of extremity	S. aureus most common but Gm-neg. bacilli rare	MRSA unlikely: Nafcillin or oxacillin. MRSA possible: Vanco	MRSA unlikely: Nafcillin or oxacillin. Add P Ceph 3 if Gm-neg. bacilli on Gram stain.	Doses: Table 16.
Adult (>21 yrs) Vertebral osteo ± epidural abscess, other sites	S. aureus most common but variety other organisms. **Blood & bone cultures essential**	MRSA possible: Vanco 1 gm IV q12h	MRSA unlikely: Nafcillin or oxacillin 2 gm IV q4h	**Dx: MRI early to look for epidural abscess.** Allergy or toxicity: Clinda 600–900 mg IV q8h or TMP-SMX 8–10 mg per kg per day div. IV q8h. **If no response to clinda, check for "inducible" resistance** (CID 40:280, 2005). If susceptible in vitro: CIP 750 mg po bid or Levo 750 mg po q24h) + RIF 300 mg po bid. See Table 10 for adverse drug reactions. Linezolid rapidly penetrates & accumulates in bone (JAC 50:73 & 747, 2002). Epidural abscess ref.: AIM 164:2409, 2004
Specific therapy—Culture and in vitro susceptibility results known				
MSSA		Nafcillin or oxacillin 2 gm IV q4h or cefazolin 2 gm IV q8h	Vanco 1 gm IV q12h	Severe allergy or toxicity: Clinda 600–900 mg IV q8h or TMP-SMX 8–10 mg per kg per day div IV q8h (check for inducible resistance—CID 40:280, 2005). TMP-SMX 8–10 mg/kg/day IV. Linezolid 600 mg IV/po q12h.
MRSA	MRSA—See Table 6, page 57	Vanco 1 gm IV q12h	Linezolid 600 mg IV/po q12h	Severe allergy or toxicity: Clinda 600–900 mg IV q8h (check for inducible resistance—CID 40:280, 2005). TMP-SMX 8–10 mg/kg/day IV. Linezolid 600 mg IV/po q12h.
Hemoglobinopathy: Sickle cell/thalassemia	Salmonella, other Gm-neg. bacilli	CIP 400 mg IV q12h	Levo 750 mg IV q24h	Thalassemia: transfusion and iron chelation risk factors.
Contiguous Osteomyelitis Without Vascular Insufficiency **Empiric therapy: Get cultures**				
Foot bone osteo due to nail through tennis shoe	P. aeruginosa	CIP 750 mg po bid or Levo 750 mg po q24h	Ceftaz 2 gm IV q8h or CFP 2 gm IV q12h	See Skin—Nail puncture, page 41. Need debridement to remove foreign body.
Long bone, post-internal fixation of fracture	S. aureus, Gm-neg. bacilli (aerobic), P. aeruginosa	Vanco 1 gm IV q12h + [ceftaz or CFP [see footnote†]], See Comment	Linezolid 600 mg IV/po bid + ceftaz or CFP. See Comment	Often necessary to remove hardware to allow bone union. May need revascularization. Regimens listed are empiric. After culture data available. If susceptible Gm-neg. bacillus, CIP 750 mg po bid or Levo 750 mg po q24h.
Prosthetic joint	See Prosthetic joint, page 25			
Sternum, post-op	S. aureus, S. epidermidis	Vanco 1 gm IV q12h	Linezolid 600 mg po/IV^MRSA bid	Sternal debridement for cultures & removal of necrotic bone.
Contiguous Osteomyelitis With Vascular Insufficiency Most pts are diabetics with peripheral neuropathy & infected skin ulcers (see Diabetic foot, page 12)	Polymicrobic (Gm+ cocci [include MRSA] & Gm-neg. bacilli (aerobic & anaerobic)	Contiguous Osteomyelitis With Vascular Insufficiency Ref.: CID S115-22, 2004 Debride overlying ulcer & submit bone for histology & culture. Select antibiotic based on culture results & treat for 6 weeks. **No empiric therapy unless acutely ill—see specific suggestions, Diabetic foot, page 12.**		**Diagnosis of osteo:** Culture of biopsied bone gold standard. Marrow edema on MRI best imaging. Probe to bone has high predictive value. (2) Revascularize if possible. (3) Specific antimicrobial(s).

* **DOSAGES SUGGESTED** are for adults (unless otherwise indicated) with clinically severe (often life-threatening infections). Dosages also assume normal renal function, and not severe hepatic dysfunction. † **ALTERNATIVE THERAPY INCLUDES these considerations:** allergy, pharmacology/pharmacokinetics, compliance, costs, local resistance profiles.

† Drug dosage: **IMP** 0.5 gm IV q6h, **MER** 1 gm IV q8h, **TC-CL** 3.1 gm IV q6h, **PIP-TZ** 3.375 gm q6h or 4.5 gm q8h, **AM-SB** 3 gm IV q6h, **ceftazidime** 2 gm IV q8h, **CFP** 2 gm IV q12h, **metro** 1 gm loading dose and then 0.5 gm IV/po q6h or 1 gm IV q12h, **aztreonam** 2 gm IV q6h, **vanco** 1 gm IV q12h

TABLE 1 (2)

ANATOMIC SITE/DIAGNOSIS/ MODIFYING CIRCUMSTANCES	ETIOLOGIES (usual)	SUGGESTED REGIMENS* PRIMARY	ALTERNATIVE†	ADJUNCT DIAGNOSTIC OR THERAPEUTIC MEASURES AND COMMENTS
BONE (continued) **Chronic Osteomyelitis: Specific therapy**—implies presence of dead bone **Need valid cultures**	S. aureus, Enterobacteriaceae, P. aeruginosa	**Empiric rx not indicated.** Base systemic rx on results of culture, sensitivity testing. Do even reexamination of chronic osteo, rx as acute hematogenous osteo.		Important adjuncts: removal of orthopedic hardware, surgical debridement, revascularized muscle flaps, distraction osteogenesis (Ilizarov) techniques. Antibiotic-impregnated cement & hyperbaric oxygen adjunctive. **NOTE: RIF + (vanco or β-lactam)** effective in animal model and in a clinical trial of S. aureus chronic osteo (SMJ 79:947, 1986).
BREAST: Mastitis—Obtain culture, need to know if MRSA present. Review with definitions: Ob & Gyn Clin No Amer 29:89, 2002				
Postpartum mastitis Mastitis without abscess Ref.: JAMA 289:1609, 2003	S. aureus; less often S. pyogenes (Gp A or B), E. coli, bacteroides species, maybe Corynebacterium sp. & selected coagulase-neg. staphylococci (e.g., S. lugdunensis)	**NO MRSA: Outpatient:** Dicloxacillin 500 mg po qid or cephalexin 500 mg po qid. **Inpatient:** Nafcillin/oxacillin 2 gm IV q4h	**MRSA Possible: Outpatient:** TMP-SMX-DS po bid. **Inpatient:** Vanco 1 gm IV q12h	If no abscess, increased frequency of nursing may hasten response: no risk to infant. Corynebacterium sp. assoc. with chronic granulomatous mastitis (CID 35:1434, 2002). Bartonella henselae infection reported (Ob & Gyn 95:1027, 2000). With abscess, 1&D standard; needle aspiration reported success (Am J Surg 182:117, 2001). Resume breast feeding from affected breast as soon as pain allows.
Mastitis with abscess				
Non-puerperal mastitis with abscess	S. aureus; less often Bacteroides sp., peptostreptococcus, & selected coagulase-neg. staphylococci			**If subareolar & odoriferous**, most likely anaerobes; need to **add metro 500 mg IV/po bid.** If not subareolar, staph. Need pretreatment aerobic/anaerobic cultures. Surgical drainage for abscess.
CENTRAL NERVOUS SYSTEM Brain abscess				
Primary or contiguous source Ref.: CID 25:763, 1997	Streptococci (60–70%), bacteroides (20–40%), S. bacteroides (25–33%), S. aureus (10–15%). Rare: Nocardia (Table 11A, page 82)	**P Ceph 3 (cefotaxime 2 gm IV q12h) or ceftriaxone 2 gm IV q12h) + metro 7.5 mg per kg q6h or 15 mg/kg IV q12h** Duration rx unclear; rx until response by neuroimaging (CT/MRI)	**Pen G** 3-4 million units IV q4h + **metro** 7.5 mg per kg q6h or 15 mg per kg IV q12h	If CT scan suggests cerebritis (JINS 59:972, 1983), abscesses < 2.5 cm and pt neurologically stable and conscious. Start antibiotics and observe. Otherwise, surgical drainage necessary: Neurologic deterioration usually mandates surgery. 1st gen Ceph (cephalothin) + metro without P Ceph 3 candida and oral flora has been good. We use P Ceph 3 because of frequency of isolation of Enterobacteriaceae. **S. aureus rare without positive blood culture; if S. aureus, include vanco until susceptibility known.** Strep. milleri group esp. prone to produce abscess.
Post-surgical, post-traumatic	S. aureus, Enterobacteriaceae	**(Nafcillin or oxacillin) 2 gm IV q4h + P Ceph 3** See Table 13, page 99	**Vanco** 1 gm IV q12h + **P Ceph 3**	**If MRSA a consideration, substitute vanco for nafcillin or oxacillin.** P Ceph 3 dose as for brain abscess, primary
HIV-1 infected (AIDS)	Toxoplasma gondii			
Subdural empyema: In adult 60–90% are extension of sinusitis or otitis media. Rx same as primary brain abscess. Surgical emergency: must drain CID 20:372, 1995).				
Encephalitis/encephalopathy Ref.: Ln 359:507, 2002 (See Table 14, page 108, and for rabies, Table 20C, page 144)	Herpes simplex, arboviruses, rabies, West Nile virus, listeria, cat-scratch disease	Start IV **acyclovir** while awaiting results of CSF PCR for H. simplex.		Newly recognized strain of rabies. May not require a break in the skin. Eastern equine encephalitis caused rx local MRI changes in basal ganglia and thalamus (NEJM 336:1867, 1997). Cat-scratch ref.: PIDJ 17:1086, 1985). Ref. on West Nile & related viruses: NEJM 351:370, 2004.
Meningitis, "Aseptic": Pleocytosis of 100s of cells, CSF glucose normal, neg. culture for bacteria (see Table 14, page 106)	Enteroviruses, HSV-2, LCM, HIV, other viruses, drugs (NSAIDs, metronidazole, carbamazepine, TMP-SMX, IVIG), rarely leptospirosis	For all but leptospirosis, IV fluids and analgesics. D/C drugs that may be etiologic. For lepto: **(doxy 100 mg IV/po q12h) or (Pen G 5 million units IV q6h) or AMP 0.5–1 gm IV q6h].** Repeat LP if suspect partially-treated bacterial meningitis.		If available, PCR of CSF for enterovirus. HSV-2 unusual without concomitant genital herpes. Drug-induced aseptic meningitis. For lepto, positive epidemiologic history and concomitant hepatitis, conjunctivitis, dermatitis, nephritis.

Abbreviations on page 2.   NOTE: All dosage recommendations are for adults (unless otherwise indicated) and assume normal renal/renal function.

TABLE 1 (3)

ANATOMIC SITE/DIAGNOSIS/ MODIFYING CIRCUMSTANCES	ETIOLOGIES (usual)	SUGGESTED REGIMENS*		ADJUNCT DIAGNOSTIC OR THERAPEUTIC MEASURES AND COMMENTS
		PRIMARY	ALTERNATIVE¹	
CENTRAL NERVOUS SYSTEM *(continued)*				
Meningitis, Bacterial, Acute: Goal is empiric therapy, then CSF exam within 30 min. If focal neurologic deficit, give empiric rx, then do head CT, then do LP. NOTE: In children, treatment caused CSF cultures to turn neg. in 2 hrs with meningococci & partial response with pneumococci in 4 hrs *(Peds 108:1169, 2001)*				
Empiric Therapy—CSF Gram stain is negative–immunocompetent				
Age: Preterm to <1 month *Ln 361:2139, 2003*	Group B strep 49%, E. coli 18%, listeria 7%, misc. Gm-neg. 10%, misc. Gm-pos. 10%	**AMP + cefotaxime** Intraventricular rx not recommended. Repeat CSF exam/culture 24–36 hrs after start of rx	**AMP + gentamicin**	Primary & alternative regimens active vs Group B strep, most coliforms, & listeria. If premature infant with long nursery stay, S. aureus, enterococci, and resistant coliforms potential pathogens. Optional empiric regimens: (nafcillin + cefotaxime or cefotaxime). If high risk of MRSA, use vanco + cefotaxime. **Dexamethasone:** No data on benefit; risk of brain injury (animal data) argues against use. See Table 16
Age: 1 mo.– 50 yrs **See footnote²** for empiric treatment rationale.	S. pneumo, meningococci, H. influenzae now very rare, **listeria unlikely in young & immunocompetent** (add **ampicillin** if suspect listeria)	Adult dosage: **[Cefotaxime** 2 gm IV q4–6H OR **ceftriaxone** 2 gm IV q12h) + **dexamethasone** (see Comment) + **vanco** (see footnote⁴, vanco dose for pen/ceph allergy)] Peds: see footnote³ **Dexamethasone:** 0.15 mg per kg IV q6h times 2–4 days. **Give with or just before 1st dose of antibiotic to block TNF production** (see Comment) See footnote⁴ for rest of ped. dosage	**[(Cefotaxime 2 gm IV q4–6H OR ceftriaxone 2 gm IV q12h) + vanco dexamethasone]** + **vanco** Peds: see footnote³ For severe pen. allergy: **Dexamethasone** 0.15 mg per kg IV q6h times 2–4 days, 1st dose before or concomitant with 1st dose of antibiotic	**For pts with severe pen. allergy: Chloro** 12.5 mg per kg IV q6h (max. 4 gm per day) (for meningococcus) 3.5 mg per kg q4–6h for listeria if immunocompromised) + **vanco**. Rare meningococcal isolates chloro-resistant *(NEJM 339:868, 1998)*. The standard alternative for pts with severe pen. allergy was chloro. However, high failure rate in pts with DRSP *(Ln 339: 405, 1992; Ln 342:240, 1993)*. **So far, no vanco-resistant S. pneumo.** **Value of dexamethasone** documented in children with H. influenzae & now confirmed in adults with S. pneumo & N. meningitidis *(NEJM 347:1549 & 1613, 2002; LnID 4:139, 2004)*. **Give 1st dose 15–20 min. prior to or concomitant with 1st dose of antibiotic. Dose: 0.15 mg per kg IV q6h times 2–4 days.** For meningococcal immunization, see **Table 20, page 142.**
Age > 50 yrs or alcoholism or other debilitating associated diseases or impaired cellular immunity	S. pneumo, listeria, Gm-neg. bacilli Note absence of meningococcus	**AMP** 2 gm IV q4h) + (**cefotaxime** 2 gm IV q12h or **cefotaxime** 2 gm IV q8h) + **vanco** + **dexamethasone** For vanco dose, see footnote⁴	**MER** 2 gm IV q8h + **vanco** + **dexamethasone** 0.15 mg per kg IV q6h times 2–4 days, 1st dose before or concomitant with 1st dose of antibiotic	**Severe penicillin allergy: Vanco** 500–750 mg IV q6-8h pending culture results. Chloro has failed vs DRSP *(Ln 342:240, 1993)*.
Post-neurosurgery, post-head trauma, or post-cochlear implant *(NEJM 349:435, 2004)*	S. aureus, S. epidermidis, coliforms, esp. if CSF leak Other: S. aureus, P. aeruginosa	**Vanco** (until known not MRSA) 500–750 mg IV q6h⁴ + (**cefepime** 2 gm IV q8h or **ceftazidime** 2 gm IV q8h)(see Comment)	**MER** 2 gm IV q8h + **vanco**	**Vanco** alone not optimal for S. pneumo. If/when suscept. S. pneumo identified, quickly switch to **ceftriaxone** or **cefotaxime**. If coliform or pseudomonas meningitis, some add intrathecal gentamicin (4 mg q12h into lateral ventricles). Cure of acinetobacter meningitis with intrathecal colistin *(JAC 53:290, 2004)*.
Ventriculitis/meningitis due to infected ventriculo-peritoneal (atrial) shunt	S. epidermidis, S. aureus, coliforms, diphtheroids (rare), P. acnes	**Vanco** 500–750 mg IV q6h⁴ + (**cefepime** 2 gm IV q8h or **ceftazidime** 2 gm IV q8h)	**Vanco** 500–750 mg IV q6h⁴ + **MER** 2 gm IV q8h	Usual care: 1°: remove infected shunt & culture; external ventricular catheter for ventricular drainage + IV antibiotic; intraventricular antibiotic times10–14 days. For timing of new shunt, see CID 39:1267, 2004. If unable to remove shunt, consider intraventricular therapy; for dosages, see footnote⁴

---

¹ **Rationale**: Hard to get adequate CSF concentrations of anti-infectives, hence MIC criteria for in vitro susceptibility are lower for CSF isolates *(AIM 161:2538, 2001)*.
² Low and erratic penetration of **vanco** into the CSF *(PIDJ 16:895, 1997)*. Recommended **dosage in children** is 15 mg per kg IV q6h (double the standard adult dose).
gm/day is suggested: **500–750 mg IV q6h.**
³ **Dosage of drugs used to rx children ≥1 mo. of age:** Cefotaxime 200 mg per kg per day IV div. q6-8h; ceftriaxone 100 mg per kg per day IV div. q12h; vanco 15 mg per kg IV q6h.
⁴ **Dosages for intraventricular therapy.** The following are daily adult doses in mg: amikacin 30, gentamicin 4–8, polymyxin E (Colistin) 10, tobramycin 5–20, vanco 10–20. Ref. CID 39:1267, 2004.
NOTE: All dosage recommendations are for adults (unless otherwise indicated) and assume normal renal function.

Abbreviations on page 2

TABLE 1 (4)

ANATOMIC SITE/DIAGNOSIS/ MODIFYING CIRCUMSTANCES	ETIOLOGIES (usual)	SUGGESTED REGIMENS*		ADJUNCT DIAGNOSTIC OR THERAPEUTIC MEASURES AND COMMENTS
		PRIMARY	ALTERNATIVE†	
CENTRAL NERVOUS SYSTEM				
Meningitis, Bacterial, Acute (continued) (CID 39:1267, 2004)				
Empiric Therapy—Positive CSF Gram stain				
Gram-positive diplococci	S. pneumoniae	Either (**ceftriaxone** 2 gm IV q12h or **cefotaxime** 2 gm IV q4-6h) + **vanco** 500–750 mg IV q6h + timed **dexamethasone** 0.15 mg/kg q6h IV times 2-4 days.		**Alternatives: MER** 2 gm IV q8h or **Moxi** 400 mg IV q24h or **Gati** 400 mg IV q24h. All + **dexamethasone**.
Gram-negative diplococci	N. meningitidis	(**Cefotaxime** 2 gm IV q4-6h or **ceftriaxone** 2 gm IV q12h) + timed **dexamethasone** (dose above)		**Alternatives: Pen G** 4 mill. units IV q4h or **AMP** 2 gm q4h or **Gati/Moxi** 400 mg IV q24h or **chloro** 1 gm IV q6h
Gram-positive bacilli or coccobacilli	Listeria monocytogenes	(**AMP** 2 gm IV q4h + **gentamicin** 2 mg per kg loading dose then 1.7 mg per kg q8h		**If pen-allergic, use TMP-SMX** 5 mg per kg q6-8h or **MER** 2 gm IV q8h
Gram-negative bacilli	H. influenzae, coliforms, P. aeruginosa	(**Ceftazidime** or **cefepime** 2 gm IV q8h) + **gentamicin** 2 mg per kg q8h)		**Alternatives: CIP** 400 mg IV q8-12h; **MER** 2 gm IV q8h
Specific Therapy—Positive culture of CSF with in vitro susceptibility results available. Interest in monitoring/reducing intracranial pressure. CID 38:384, 2004				
H. influenzae	β-lactamase +	**Ceftriaxone** (peds): 50 mg per kg IV q12h		**Pen. allergic: Chloro** 12.5 mg per kg IV q6h (max. 4 gm per day.)
Listeria monocytogenes		**AMP** 2 gm IV q4h ± **gentamicin** 2 mg per kg loading dose, then 1.7 mg per kg q8h		**Pen. allergic: TMP-SMX** 20 mg per kg per day div. q6-12h. One report of greater efficacy of AMP + TMP-SMX as compared to AMP + gentamicin (JID 3:79, 1996) **Alternative: MER** 2 gm IV q8h. Success reported with **linezolid + RIF** (CID 40:908, 2005)
N. meningitidis	MIC 0.1-1 mcg per mL	**Ceftriaxone** 2 gm IV q12h times 7 days (see Comment); if pen. allergic, **chloro** 12.5 mg per kg (up to 1 gm) q6h		Rare isolates chloro-resistant (NEJM 339:868, 917, 1998) **Alternatives: MER** 2 gm IV q8h or **Gati/Moxi** 400 mg IV q8h
S. pneumoniae	Pen G MIC			
	<0.1 mcg per mL	**Pen G** 4 million units IV q4h or **AMP** 2 gm IV q4h		
	0.1-1 mcg per mL	**Ceftriaxone** 2 gm IV q12h or **cefotaxime** 2 gm IV q4-6h		**Alternatives: Cefepime** 2 gm IV q8h or **MER** 2 gm IV q8h
NOTES: 1. Assumes dexamethasone just prior to 1st dose & x4 days. 2. If MIC ≥1, repeat CSF exam can after 24-48h. 3. Treat for 10-14 days	≥2 mcg per mL	**Vanco** 500-750 mg IV q6h + (**ceftriaxone** or **cefotaxime** as above)		**Alternatives: Gati** or **Moxi** 400 mg IV q24h
	Ceftriaxone MIC ≥1 mcg per mL	**Vanco** 500-750 mg IV q6h + (**ceftriaxone** or **cefotaxime** as above)		**Alternatives: Gati** or **Moxi** 400 mg IV q24h. If MIC to ceftriaxone >2 mcg per mL, add **RIF** 600 mg once daily.
E. coli, other coliforms, or P. aeruginosa	Consultation advised—need susceptibility results	(**Ceftazidime** or **cefepime** 2 gm IV q8h) ± **gentamicin**		**Alternatives: CIP** 400 mg IV q8-12h; **MER** 2 gm IV q8h For discussion of intraventricular therapy. CID 39:1267, 2004
Prophylaxis for H. influenzae and N. meningitidis				
Haemophilus influenzae type b (Neisseria next page)		**RIF** 20 mg per kg per day (not to exceed 600 mg) times 4 doses. **Adults: RIF** 600 mg q24h times 4 days		**Household:** If there is one unvaccinated contact ≤4 yrs in the household, RIF recommended for all household contacts except pregnant women. **Child Care Facilities:** With 1 case, if attended by unvaccinated children <2 yrs, consider prophylaxis + vaccinate susceptibles. If all contacts >2 yrs: no prophylaxis. If ≥2 cases in 60 days & unvaccinated children attend, prophylaxis recommended for children & personnel. (Am Acad Ped Red Book 2003, page 2971)

Abbreviations on page 2.   NOTE: All dosage recommendations are for adults (unless otherwise indicated) and assume normal renal function.

TABLE 1 (5)

ANATOMIC SITE/DIAGNOSIS/ MODIFYING CIRCUMSTANCES	ETIOLOGIES (usual)	SUGGESTED REGIMENS*		ADJUNCT DIAGNOSTIC OR THERAPEUTIC MEASURES AND COMMENTS
		PRIMARY	ALTERNATIVE†	
CENTRAL NERVOUS SYSTEM/Meningitis, Bacterial/Prophylaxis (continued)				
Neisseria meningitidis exposure (close contact) [MMWR 46(RR-5):1, 1997] CDC recommends informing college freshmen living in dormitories & residence halls of available vaccine [MMWR 46(RR-7):1, 2000 & 50(23):487, 2001]		[RIF 600 mg po q12h times 4 doses. (Children >1 mo. age 10 mg per kg po q12h times 4 doses, <1 mo. age 5 mg per kg q12h times 4 doses)] or CIP (adults) 500 mg po single dose] or Ceftriaxone 250 mg IM times 1 dose (child <15 yrs 125 mg IM times 1)]. Spiramycin 500 mg po q6h times 5 days. Children 10 mg per kg po q6h times 5 days.		N. meningitidis spread by respiratory droplets, not aerosols, hence close contact required. ↑ risk if close contact for at least 4 hrs during week before illness onset (e.g., housemates, day care contacts, cellmates) or exposure to pt's naso-pharyngeal secretions (e.g., via kissing, mouth-to-mouth resuscitation, intubation, nasotracheal suctioning). RIF-resistant N. meningitidis documented but rare [EID 11:977, 2005]. Primary prophylactic regimen in many European countries.
Meningitis, chronic Defined as symptoms + CSF pleocytosis for 24 wks	M. tbc. 40%, cryptococcosis 7%, neoplastic 8%, Lyme, syphilis, Whipple's disease	Treatment depends on etiology. No urgent need for empiric therapy.		Long list of possibilities: bacteria, parasites, fungi, viruses, neoplasms, vasculitis, and other miscellaneous etiologies—see chapter on chronic meningitis in latest edition of Harrison's Textbook of Internal Medicine. Whipple's: JID 186:797 & 801, 2003.
Meningitis, eosinophilic AJM 114:217, 2003 (See Table 13A, page 100)	Angiostrongyliasis, gnatho-stomiasis, rarely others	Corticosteroids	Not sure antihelminthic rx works	1/3 lack peripheral eosinophilia. Need serology to confirm dx. Steroid ref. CID 31:660, 2001. Recent outbreak: NEJM 346:668, 2002.
Meningitis, HIV-1 infected (AIDS) Table 11, SANFORD GUIDE TO HIV/AIDS THERAPY	As in adults, >50 yrs: also consider cryptococci, M. tuberculosis, syphilis, HIV aseptic meningitis, Listeria monocytogenes	If etiology not identified: rx as adult >50 yrs + obtain CSF/serum cryptococcal antigen (see Comments)	For crypto rx, see Table 11A, pages 79–80	A.C: neoformans most common etiology in AIDS pts. H. influenzae, pneumococci, Tbc, syphilis, viral, histoplasma & coccidioides also need to be considered. Obtain blood cultures. L. monocytogenes risk ~60x ↑; 1% present as meningitis (CID 17:224, 1993).
EAR				
External otitis				
"Swimmer's ear" PIDJ 22:299, 2003	Pseudomonas sp., Entero-bacteriaceae, Proteus sp. (Fungi rare.) Acute infection usually 2° S. aureus	Eardrops: **Ofloxacin 0.3% soln bid** or **[(polymyxin B + neomycin + hydrocortisone) qid]** or **CIP + hydrocortisone bid]** For acute disease: **dicloxacillin** 500 mg po 4 times per day.		Rx should include gentle cleaning. Recurrences prevented (or decreased) by drying with alcohol drops (1/3 white vinegar, 2/3 rubbing alcohol) after swimming, then antibiotic drops or 2% acetic acid solution. Ointments should not be used in ear. Do not use neomycin if tympanic membrane punctured.
Chronic	Usually 2° to seborrhea	Eardrops: [(polymyxin B + neomycin + hydrocorti-sone (rd)] + selenium sulfide)		Control seborrhea with dandruff shampoo containing selenium sulfide (Selsun) or (ketoconazole shampoo) + (medium potency steroid solution, triamcinolone 0.1%).
"Malignant otitis externa" high risk groups: diabetes mellitus, AIDS, chemotherapy	Pseudomonas aeruginosa in >90%	[IMP 0.5 gm IV q6h) or (MER 1 gm IV q8h) or (CIP 400 mg IV q12h or 750 mg po q12h) or (ceftaz 2 gm IV q8h) or (CFP 2 gm q12h) or (PIP 4–6 gm IV q4–6h + tobra)] or (TC 3 gm IV q4h + tobra)		Control seborrhea with dandruff shampoo containing selenium sulfide (Selsun) or (ketoconazole shampoo) especially useful for outpatient rx with early disease. Surgical debridement usually required, but not radical excision. R/O osteomyelitis. CT or MRI scan more sensitive than x-ray. If bone involved, rx 4–6 wks. Ref: LnID 4:34, 2004

Abbreviations on page 2   NOTE: All dosage recommendations are for adults (unless otherwise indicated) and assume normal renal/renal function.

TABLE 1 (6)

ANATOMIC SITE/DIAGNOSIS/ MODIFYING CIRCUMSTANCES	ETIOLOGIES (usual)	SUGGESTED REGIMENS* PRIMARY	ALTERNATIVE§	ADJUNCT DIAGNOSTIC OR THERAPEUTIC MEASURES AND COMMENTS
EAR (continued)				

Otitis media—infants, children, adults

Acute (NEJM 347:1169, 2002; Peds 113:1451, 2004). For correlation of bacterial eradication from middle ear & clinical outcome, see LnID 2:593, 2002.

Initial empiric therapy of acute otitis media (AOM) rx children <2 yrs old [1] >2 yrs old, afebrile, no ear pain, may/questionable exam—consider analgesic treatment without anti-microbials	Overall detection in middle ear fluid: No pathogen 25% Virus 5–48% Bact. + virus 15% Bacteria only 55% Role of viruses: Clin Micro Rev 16:230, 2004 Pathogens from middle ear, 2000–2003: S. pneumo 31%, H. influenzae 56%, M. catarrhalis 11% (PIDJ 23: 829, 2004)	**If NO antibiotics in prior month:** Amox po–HD [1] For dosage, see footnotes [1] and [2]. **Duration of rx:** <2 yrs old times 10 days; ≥2 yrs old times 5–7 days. Appropriate duration unclear. 5 days may be inadequate for severe disease (NEJM 347:1169, 2002). **For adult dosages, see Sinusitis, pages 36–37, and Table 10**	**Received antibiotics in prior month:** Amox-HD [1], AM-CL HD [1] or cefdinir or cefpodoxime or cefuroxime axetil	If allergic to β-lactam drugs ? If history unclear or rash, effective oral cephs OK; or azithro or clarithro (see Comment). If penicillin-allergic (e.g., TMP-SMX po [2] or clarithro) HD, or H. influenzae OR M. catarrhalis (PIDJ 20:260, 2001). **azithro times 5 days or clarithro times 10 days** (both have ↓ activity vs DRSP). **Up to 50% S. pneumo resistant to macrolides** AM-CL superior to azithro in recent controlled trial (ICAAC Abst. 2324, 2003). Rationale & data for single dose azithro, 30 mg per kg: PIDJ 23:S102 & S108, 2004. **Spontaneous resolution:** 90% pts infected with M. catarrhalis, 50% with H. influenzae, and 10% with S. pneumoniae; overall 80% resolve within 2–14 days. Risk of DRSP ↑ if age <2 yrs, antibiotics last 3 mos., or daycare attendance. Selection of drug based on (1) effectiveness against β-lactamase producing H. influenzae & M. catarrhalis and (2) effectiveness against S. pneumo, including DRSP. **Cefaclor, loracarbef, & ceftibuten less active vs DRSP** than other agents listed. Variable acceptance of drug taste/smell by children 4–8 y.o. (PIDJ 19 [Suppl]:S174, 2000).
				Clindamycin for S. pneumo active vs H. influenzae or M. catarrhalis. S. pneumo resistant to macrolides usually also resistant to clinda (PIDJ 22:405, 2003). Definition of failure: no change in ear pain, fever, bulging TM or otorrhea after 3 days of rx. Tympanocentesis advised.
Treatment for clinical failure after 3 days rx	Drug-resistant S. pneumoniae main concern	**NO antibiotics in month prior to last 3 days:** AM-CL HD or cefdinir or cefpodoxime or cefuroxime axetil or IM ceftriaxone times 3 days.	**Antibiotics in month prior to last 3 days:** (IM ceftriaxone) and/or (tympanocentesis) See clindamycin Comments	**Newer FQs active vs DRSP, but not approved for use in children** (PIDJ 20:260, 2004) **Vanco is active vs DRSP** (PIDJ 19:1040, 2000). FDA reported successful for non-resistant S. pneumo AOM (PIDJ 20:829, 2001).
		For dosage, see footnotes [1] and [2] All doses are pediatric		
After >48 hrs of nasotracheal intubation	Pseudomonas sp., klebsiella, enterobacter	Ceftazidime or CFP or IMP or MER or TC-CL or CIP (For dosages, see Ear, malignant otitis externa, page 8)		With nasotracheal intubation >48 hrs, about ½ pts will have otitis media with effusion.
Prophylaxis: acute otitis media PIDJ 22:10, 2003	Pneumococcus, H. influenzae, M. catarrhalis, Staph. aureus, Group A strep (see Comments)	Sulfisoxazole 50 mg per kg po at bedtime or amoxicillin 20 mg per kg po q24h		**Use of antibiotics to prevent otitis media is a major contributor to emergence of antibiotic-resistant S. pneumo!** Pneumococcal protein conjugate vaccine decreases freq. AOM in general & due to vaccine serotypes. Adenoidectomy at time of tympanostomy tubes ↓ need for future hospitalization for AOM (NEJM 344:1188, 2001).

---

[1] **Amoxicillin UD or HD** = amoxicillin usual dose or high dose; **AM-CL HD** = amoxicillin-clavulanate high dose. **Dosages in footnote 2.** Data supporting amoxicillin HD: PIDJ 22:405, 2003.
[2] **Drugs & dosage suggested for acute otitis media: Amoxicillin UD** = 40 mg per kg per day div q8h or q12h; **Amoxicillin HD** = 90 mg per kg per day div q12h or q8h; **AM-CL HD** = 90 mg per kg per day of amox component. **Extra-strength AM-CL oral suspension** (Augmentin ES-600) available with 600 mg AM & 42.9 mg CL per 5 ml—dose 90/6.4 mg per kg per day bid. **Cefuroxime axetil** 30 mg per kg per day div q12h; **Ceftriaxone** 50 mg per kg IM times 3 days. **Clindamycin** 20–30 mg per kg per day div q8h.

Other drugs suitable for drug (e.g., penicillin)-sensitive S. pneumo: TMP-SMX 4 mg per kg of TMP q12h. **Erythro-sulfisoxazole** 50 mg per kg per day of erythro div q6–8h. **Clarithro** 15 mg per kg per day div q12h. **Azithro** 10 mg per kg times 1 then 5 mg per kg per day times 4 or 10 mg per kg times 3 days or 30 mg per kg times 1. **Cefprozil** 15 mg per kg per day div q12h; **cefpodoxime** 10 mg per kg per day as single dose or div q12h; **cefaclor** 40 mg per kg per day div q8h; **loracarbef** 15 mg per kg q12h; **Cefdinir** 7 mg per kg q12h or 14 mg per kg q24h.

NOTE: All dosage recommendations are for adults (unless otherwise indicated) and assume normal renal function.
Abbreviations on page 2.

TABLE 1 (7)

ANATOMIC SITE/DIAGNOSIS/ MODIFYING CIRCUMSTANCES	ETIOLOGIES (usual)	SUGGESTED REGIMENS* PRIMARY	ALTERNATIVE†	ADJUNCT DIAGNOSTIC OR THERAPEUTIC MEASURES AND COMMENTS
EAR (continued) **Mastoiditis** **Acute** Outpatient	Strep. pneumoniae 22%, S. pyogenes, S. aureus, Staph. epidermidis 7%, H. influenzae 4%, P. aeruginosa 4%, others <1%	Empirically, same as Acute otitis media, above, need **vanco** or **nafcillin/oxacillin** (if culture + for S. aureus.		Has become a rare entity, presumably as result of the aggressive rx of acute otitis media. (PIDJ 20:140, 2001)
Hospitalized		**Cefotaxime** 2 gm IV q4-8h (depends on severity) or **ceftriaxone** 2 gm IV q24h, (+ **nafcillin/oxacillin** if culture + for S. aureus.		Small % incidence in Netherlands where use of antibiotics limited to children with complicated course or high risk (PIDJ 20:140, 2001)
Chronic	Often polymicrobial; anaerobes, S. aureus, Enterobacteriaceae, P. aeruginosa	Treatment for acute exacerbations or perioperatively. Ideally, no treatment until surgical cultures obtained. Examples of empiric regimens: **IMP** 0.5 gm IV q6h, **TC-CL** 3.1 gm IV q4-6h, or **PIP-TZ** 3.375 gm IV q4-6h or 4.5 gm q8h.		May or may not be associated with chronic otitis media with drainage via ruptured tympanic membrane. Antimicrobials given in association with surgery. Mastoidectomy indications: chronic drainage and evidence of osteomyelitis by MRI or CT, evidence of spread to CNS (epidural abscess, supurative phlebitis, brain abscess)
EYE—General Reviews: CID 21:479, 1995; IDCP 7:447, 1998				
Eyelid Blepharitis	Etiol. unclear. Factors include Staph. aureus & Staph. epidermidis, seborrhea, rosacea, & dry eye	[Lid margin care with baby shampoo & warm compresses q24h. Artificial tears if assoc. dry eye (see Comment)		Usually topical ointments of no benefit. If associated rosacea, add doxy 100 mg po bid times2 wks and then q24h.
Hordeolum (Stye) External (gland of Zeis)	Staph. aureus	Hot packs only. Will drain spontaneously		Infection of superficial sebaceous gland.
Internal (Meibomian glands)	Staph. aureus	Hot packs + hot packs spontaneously		Also called acute meibomianitis. Rarely drain spontaneously
Conjunctiva: NEJM 343:345, 2000 **Conjunctivitis of the newborn (ophthalmia neonatorum)** by day of onset post-delivery—all doses pediatric				
Onset 1st day	Chemical (due to AgNO₃ prophylaxis	[None.]		Usual prophylaxis is erythro ointment; hence, AgNO₃ irritation rare.
Onset 2–4 days	N. gonorrhoeae	**Ceftriaxone** 25-50 mg per kg IV times 1 dose (see Comment), not to exceed 125 mg		Treat mother and her sexual partners. Hyperpurulent. Topical rx inadequate. **Treat neonate for concomitant Chlamydia trachomatis.**
Onset 3–10 days	Chlamydia trachomatis	**Erythro syrup** 12.5 mg per kg q6h times 14 days). No topical rx needed.		Diagnosis by antigen detection. Azithro susp 20 mg per kg q24h times 3 days reported efficacious (PIDJ 17:1049, 1998). Treat mother & sexual partner
Onset 2–16 days	Herpes simplex types 1, 2	See keratitis, next page.		Consider IV acyclovir if concomitant systemic disease.
Ophthalmia neonatorum prophylaxis: **Silver nitrate 1%** times 1 or **erythro 0.5%** ointment times 1 or **tetra** 1% ointment times 1 application				
Pink eye (viral conjunctivitis) Usually unilateral	Adenovirus (types 3 & 7 in children, 8, 11 & 19 in adults)	No treatment if symptomatic, cold artificial tears may help.		Highly contagious. Onset of ocular pain and photophobia in an adult suggests associated keratitis—rare.
Inclusion conjunctivitis (**adult**) Usually unilateral	Chlamydia trachomatis	**Doxy** 100 mg po bid times 1-3 weeks	**Erythro** 250 mg po qid times 1-3 weeks	Oculogenital disease. Diagnosis by culture or antigen detection or PCR—availability varies by region and institution. Treat sexual partner
Trachoma	Chlamydia trachomatis	**Azithro** 20 mg per kg po single dose—78% effective in children	**Doxy** 100 mg po bid times14 days or **tetracycline** 250 mg po times 14 days.	Starts in childhood and can persist for years with subsequent damage to cornea. Topical therapy of marginal benefit. Avoid doxy/tetracycline in young children. Mass treatment works (JAMA 292:721, 2004).
Suppurative conjunctivitis Non-gonococcal: non-chlamydial, no outbreak NEJM 348:1112, 2003	Staph. aureus, S. pneumoniae, H. influenzae or Moraxella sp. Outbreak due to atypical S. pneumo. Med Lett 46:25, 2004	Ophthalmic solution: Gati 0.3%, 1-2 gtts q2h while awake 1st 2 days, then q4 8h—up to 7 days.	Polymyxin B + trimethoprim 0.1% & 0.5%, or Moxi 0.5% All 1-2 gtts q3-6h times 7-10 days.	FQs best spectrum for empiric therapy but expensive: $40-50 for 5 mL. High concern over misuse of such potent drugs for minor disease when MRSA, TMP spectrum may include only Gm-neg. bacilli but no ophthal. prep of only TMP. Most S. pneumo resistant to gent & tobra.
Gonococcal (peds/adults)	N. gonorrhoeae	**Ceftriaxone 125 mg IM/IV** as one dose in children; 1 gm IM/IV as one dose in adults		

Abbreviations on page 2.   NOTE: All dosage recommendations are for adults (unless otherwise indicated) and assume normal renal function.

TABLE 1 (8)

ANATOMIC SITE/DIAGNOSIS/ MODIFYING CIRCUMSTANCES	ETIOLOGIES (usual)	SUGGESTED REGIMENS*		ADJUNCT DIAGNOSTIC OR THERAPEUTIC MEASURES AND COMMENTS
		PRIMARY	ALTERNATIVE§	
EYE (continued)				
Cornea (keratitis): Usually serious and often sight-threatening. Prompt ophthalmologic consultation essential! Herpes simplex most common etiology in developed countries; bacterial and fungal infections more common in underdeveloped countries.				
Viral				
H. simplex	H. simplex, types 1 & 2	Trifluridine, one drop qx 9 times per day for up to 21 days	Vidarabine ointment— useful in children. Use 5 times per day for up to 21 days	Fluorescein staining shows topical dendritic figures. 30–50% rate of recurrence within 2 years. 400 mg acyclovir po bid ↓ recurrences, p 0.005 (NEJM 339:300, 1998). If child fails vidarabine, try trifluridine.
Varicella-zoster ophthalmicus	Varicella-zoster virus	Famciclovir 500 mg tid or valacyclovir 1 gm po tid times 10 days	Acyclovir 800 mg po 5 times per day times 10 days	Clinical diagnosis most common: dendritic figures with fluorescein staining in patient with varicella-zoster of ophthalmic branch of trigeminal nerve.
Bacterial		*All rx listed for bacterial, fungal, & protozoan is topical*		
Contact lens users	P. aeruginosa	Tobra or gentamicin (14 mg per mL) + piperacillin or ticarcillin eye drops (6–12 mg per mL) q15–60 min. around clock times 24–72 hrs, then slow reduction	CIP 0.3% or Levo 0.5% drops q15-60 min. around clock times 24–72 hrs	Pain, photophobia, impaired vision. Recommend alginate swab for culture and sensitivity testing.
Dry cornea, diabetes, immunosuppression	Staph. aureus, S. epidermidis, S. pneumoniae, S. pyogenes, Enterobacteriaceae, listeria	Cefazolin (50 mg per mL) + gentamicin or tobra (14 mg per mL) q15-60 min. around clock times 24-72 hrs, then slow reduction	Vanco (50 mg/mL) + ceftaz-idime (50 mg/mL) q15-60 min. around clock times 24–72 hrs, then slow reduction. See Comment	Specific therapy guided by results of alginate swab culture and sensitivity. CIP 0.3% found clinically equivalent to cefazolin + tobra; only concern was efficacy of CIP vs S. pneumoniae (Ophthalmology 163:1854, 1996).
Fungal	Aspergillus, fusarium, candida. No empiric therapy—see Comment	Natamycin (5%) drops q3–4 hrs with subsequent slow reduction	Ampho B (0.05-0.15%) q3-4 hrs with subsequent slow reduction	No empiric therapy. Wait for results of Gram stain or culture in Sabouraud's medium.
Protozoan Soft contact lens users (over-night use ↑ risk 10-15 fold)	Acanthamoeba, hartmannella	Propamidine 0.1% + neomycin/gramicidin/ polymyxin	Polyhexamethylene biguanide (PHMB) 0.02% or chlorhexidine 0.02% Eyedrops q waking hour for 1 week and then slow taper	Uncommon. Trauma and soft contact lenses are risk factors. Corneal scrapings stained with calcofluor white show characteristic cysts with fluorescent microscopy. PHMB source: Leiter's Park Ave. Pharm., 800-292-6773. Ref.: CID 35:434, 2002.
Lacrimal apparatus				
Canaliculitis	Actinomyces most common. Rarely, Arachnia, fusobacterium, nocardia, candida	Remove granules & irri-gate with pen G (100,000 approx. 5 mcg per mL) + gtt tid If fungi, irrigate with nystatin (1 gtt tid)		Digital pressure produces exudate at punctum; Gram stain confirms diagnosis. Hot packs to punctal area qid.
Dacryocystitis (lacrimal sac)	S. pneumo, S. aureus, H. influenzae, S. pyogenes, P. aeruginosa	Child: AM-CL or O Ceph 2		Need ophthalmologic consultation. Can be acute or chronic.
		Often consequence of obstruction of lacrimal duct. Empiric rx based on Gram stain of aspirate—see Comment.		Culture to detect MRSA.
Endophthalmitis For post-op endophthalmitis, see CID 38:542, 2004				
Bacterial: Haziness of the vitreous is key to diagnosis. Needle aspirate of both vitreous and aqueous humor for culture prior to therapy. Intravitreal administration of antimicrobials essential				
Postop, acute onset (incidence 0.05%) Early, acute onset	S. epidermidis 60%, Staph. aureus, streptococci & enterococci each 5-10%, Gm-neg. bacilli 6%	Immediate ophthal. consult. If only light perception or worse, immediate vitrectomy + intravitreal vanco 1 mg & intravitreal ceftazidime 2.25 mg. No clear data on intravitreal steroid. May need to repeat intravitreal antibiotics in 2–3 days. Can usually leave lens in.		
Low grade, chronic	Propionibacterium acnes, S. epidermidis, S. aureus (rare)	May require removal of lens material. Intraocular vanco ± vitrectomy.		

Abbreviations on page 2.   NOTE: *All dosage recommendations are for adults (unless otherwise indicated) and assume normal renal/renal function.*

TABLE 1 (9)

ANATOMIC SITE/DIAGNOSIS/ MODIFYING CIRCUMSTANCES	ETIOLOGIES (usual)	SUGGESTED REGIMENS* PRIMARY	ALTERNATIVE[1]	ADJUNCT DIAGNOSTIC OR THERAPEUTIC MEASURES AND COMMENTS
EYE / Endophthalmitis (Bacterial) *(continued)*				
Post filtering blebs for glaucoma	Strep. species (viridans & others), H. influenzae	Intravitreal agent and topical agent and consider systemic **AM-CL, AM-SB** or **P Ceph 2**		
Post-penetrating trauma	Bacillus sp., S. epiderm.	Intravitreal agent as above + systemic **clinda** or **vanco**. Use topical antibiotics (tobra & ceftazidin drops).		
None, suspect hematogenous	S. pneumoniae, N. meningitidis, Staph. aureus	**P Ceph 3** (**cefotaxime** 2 gm IV q4h or **ceftriaxone** 2 gm IV q24h) + **vanco** 1 gm IV q12h pending cultures. Intravitreal antibiotics as with early post-operative.		
IV heroin abuse	Bacillus cereus, Candida sp.	Intravitreal agent + (systemic **clinda** or **vanco**)		
Mycotic (fungal)	Candida albicans	Intravitreal **ampho B** 0.005–0.01 mg in 0.1 mL. Also see Table 11, pages 76-78 for concomitant systemic therapy. See Comment.		With moderate/marked vitritis, options include systemic rx + vitrectomy ± intravitreal ampho B *(CID 27:1130 & 1134, 1998)*. Report of failure of ampho B lipid complex *(CID 28:1177, 1999)*.
Broad-spectrum antibiotics, often corticosteroids, indwelling venous catheters	Candida sp., Aspergillus sp.			
Retinitis				
Acute retinal necrosis	Varicella zoster, Herpes simplex	IV **acyclovir** 10–12 mg per kg IV q8h times 5–7 days, then 800 mg po 5 times per day times 6 wks. See Table 14, page 108		Strong association of VZ virus with atypical necrotizing herpetic retinopathy *(CID 24:603, 1997)*.
HIV+ (AIDS) CD4 usually <100 per mm³	Cytomegalovirus			Occurs in 5–10% of AIDS patients
Orbital cellulitis (see page 39 for erysipelas, facial)	S. pneumoniae, H. influenzae, M. catarrhalis, S. aureus, anaerobes; group A strep. occ. Gm-neg. bacilli post-trauma	**Nafcillin** 2 gm IV q4h (or if MRSA-**vanco** 1 gm IV q12h) + **ceftriaxone** 2 gm IV q24h + **metro** IV q12h		**if penicillin/ceph allergy: Vanco + levo** 750 mg IV once daily + **metro** IV. Problem is frequent inability to make microbiologic diagnosis. Image orbit (CT or MRI). Risk of cavernous sinus thrombosis.
FOOT				
"Diabetic"—Empiric therapy. Refs.: *CID 39:885, 2004; NEJM 351:48, 2004*		See Table 11, page 80, fungal infections		**General:**
Ulcer without inflammation	Colonizing skin flora	No antibacterial therapy		1. Disease control, no weight-bearing
Ulcer with <2 cm of superficial inflammation	S. aureus (assume MRSA), S. agalactiae (Gp B), S. pyogenes predominate	**Oral therapy: (TMP-SMX-DS** or **minocycline)** plus (**Pen VK** or selected **FQ**) *Dosages in footnote³*		2. Assess for peripheral vascular disease—very common *(CID 39:437, 2004)* **Principles of empiric antibacterial therapy:** 1. Include drug predictably active vs MRSA. If outpatient, can assume community-acquired MRSA (CA-MRSA) until culture results available.
Ulcer with ≥2 cm of inflammation with extension to fascia	As above, plus coliforms	**Oral therapy: (AM-CL-ER** plus **TMP-SMX-DS)** or (**CIP** or **Levo** plus **linezolid**) *Dosages in footnote³*		2. As culture results dominated by S. aureus & Streptococcus species. empiric drug regimens should include strep & staph. Role of enterococci uncertain
Extensive local inflammation plus systemic toxicity	As above, plus anaerobic bacteria	**Parenteral therapy: (Vanco** plus β-lactam/β-lactamase inhibitor)** or (**vanco** plus **carbapenem**)** Other alternatives: 1. **CIP** or **Levo** plus **linezolid** or 2. (**Dapto** or **linezolid**) plus metronidazole plus β-lactam/β-lactamase inhibitor *Dosages in footnote³*		3. Severe limb &/or life-threatening infections require initial parenteral therapy with predictable activity vs Gm-positive cocci, coliforms & other aerobic Gm-neg. rods, & anaerobic Gm-neg. bacilli. **NOTE:** The regimens listed are suggestions consistent with above principles. Other alternatives exist & may be appropriate for individual patients.
Onychomycosis. See Table 11, page 80, fungal infections				
Puncture wound: Nail/Toothpick	P. aeruginosa	Cleanse. Tetanus booster. Observe.		Tetanus booster. Observe. Other organisms if toothpick injury *(PID 23:60, 2004)*, evolve to osteomyelitis.

¹ **Vanco** 1 gm IV q12h, **parenteral β-lactam/β-lactamase inhibitors: PIP-TZ** 3.375 gm IV q6h or 4.5 gm IV q8h; **TC-CL** 3.1 gm IV q6h; **carbapenems: ERTA** 1 gm IV q24h, **IMP** 0.5 gm IV q6h; **MER** 1 gm IV q8h; **daptomycin** 6 mg per kg IV q24h; **linezolid** 600 mg IV q12h. **CIP** and **Levo** dosages in footnotes 2 and 3, **metro** 1 gm IV loading dose & then 0.5 gm IV q6h or 1 gm IV q12h.
² **CIP** 400 mg IV q12h, **minocycline** 100 mg po bid, **Pen VK** 500 mg po qid, **cefprozil** 500 mg po q12h, **cefuroxime axetil** 500 mg po q12h, **cefdinir** 300 mg po q12h or 600 mg po q24h.
³ **cefpodoxime** 200 mg po q12h, **CIP** 750 mg po q12h, **Levo** 750 mg po q24h
AM-CL-ER 2000/125 po bid, **TMP-SMX-DS** 2 tabs po bid, **Levo** 750 mg po bid, **CIP** 750 mg po bid. NOTE: All dosage recommendations are for adults (unless otherwise indicated) and assume normal renal function.
Abbreviations on page 2.

TABLE 1 (10)

ANATOMIC SITE/DIAGNOSIS/ MODIFYING CIRCUMSTANCES	ETIOLOGIES (usual)	SUGGESTED REGIMENS*		ADJUNCT DIAGNOSTIC OR THERAPEUTIC MEASURES AND COMMENTS
		PRIMARY	ALTERNATIVE†	
GALLBLADDER				
Cholecystitis, cholangitis, biliary sepsis, or common duct obstruction (partial: 2° to tumor, stones, stricture)	Enterobacteriaceae 68%, enterococci 14%, bacteroides 10%, Clostridium sp. 7%, rarely candida	**PIP-TZ** or **AM-SB** or **TC-CL** or **ERTA** or **IMP** if life-threatening	**P Ceph 3 + metro** OR **Aztreonam + metro** OR **CIP + metro**	For severely ill pts, antibiotic rx is complementary to adequate biliary drainage. 15–30% pts will require decompression: surgical, percutaneous or ERCP-placed stent. Whether empirical rx should always cover pseudomonas & anaerobes is uncertain (CID 19:279, 1994). Ceftriaxone associated with biliary sludge (by ultrasound 50%, symptomatic 9%, NEJM 322:1821, 1990), clinical relevance still unclear but has led to surgery (MMWR 42:39, 1993).
			Dosages in footnote 1, previous page	
GASTROINTESTINAL				
Gastroenteritis—Empiric Therapy (laboratory studies not performed or culture, microscopy, toxin results NOT AVAILABLE)** (Ref. NEJM 350:38, 2004)**				
Premature infant with intestinal necrotizing enterocolitis	Associated with intestinal flora		Treatment and rationale as for diverticulitis/peritonitis, pages 16–17. See Table 16, page 133 for pediatric dosages.	Pneumatosis intestinalis on x-ray confirms dx. Bacteremia-peritonitis in 30–50%. If Staph. epidermidis isolated, add vanco (IV).
Mild diarrhea (≤3 unformed stools per day, minimal associated symptomatology)	Bacterial (see Severe, below), viral, parasitic. Viral usually causes mild to moderate disease. For traveler's diarrhea, see page 15	Fluids only + lactose-free diet, avoid caffeine		
Moderate diarrhea (≥4 unformed stools per day and/or systemic symptoms)		Antimotility agents (see Comments) + fluids		**Rehydration: For po fluid replacement, see Cholera, page 15.** **Antimotility:** Loperamide (Imodium) 4 mg po, then 2 mg after each loose stool to max. 16 mg per day, Bismuth subsalicylate (Pepto-Bismol) 2 tablets (262 mg) po qid. Do not use if suspect hemolytic uremic syndrome. **Hemolytic uremic syndrome (HUS):** Risk in **children** infected with E. coli O157:H7 is 8–10%. Early treatment with TMP-SMX or FQs ↑ risk of HUS (NEJM 342:1930 & JWD 170:272, 2000). Controversial meta-analysis: JAMA 288:996 & 3111, 2002.
Severe diarrhea (≥6 unformed stools per day, and/or temperature ≥101°F, tenesmus, blood, or fecal leukocytes) **NOTE: Severe afebrile non-bloody diarrhea should suggest suspicion of E. coli O157:H7 infection**—in U.S. only 1–3% all cases diarrhea but 6 to 36% cases of bloody diarrhea (CID 32:573, 2001)	Shigella, salmonella, C. jejuni, E. coli O157:H7, C. difficile, E. histolytica. For typhoid fever, see page 44	**FQ** (CIP 500 mg po q12h or **Levo** 500 mg po q24h) times 3–5 days	**TMP-SMX-DS** po bid times 3–5 days. Campylobacter resistance to TMP-SMX common in tropics.	**Other potential etiologies:** Cryptosporidia—no treatment in immunocompetent host (see Table 13A & JID 170:272, 1994). Cyclospora—usually chronic diarrhea, responds to TMP-SMX (see Table 12A & AIM 123:409, 1995). **Severe diarrhea** treated with CIP 500 mg po bid decreases duration of diarrhea and other symptoms without changing duration of fecal carriage. Increasing resistance of campylobacter to FQs.
		Metro 500 mg po tid times 10–14 days	**Vanco** 125 mg po qid times 10–14 days	
Gastroenteritis—Specific Therapy (results of culture, microscopy, toxin assay AVAILABLE). Ref. NEJM 350:38, 2004				
If culture negative, probably **Norovirus** (Norwalk) or rarely (in adults) **Rotavirus** see Table 14A, page 112	Aeromonas/Plesiomonas	**CIP** 500 mg po bid times 3 days.	**TMP-SMX-DS** po bid times 3 days.	Although no absolute proof, increasing evidence as cause of diarrheal illness.
NOTE: In 60 hospital pts with unexplained WBCs ≥15,000, 35% had C. difficile toxin present (AJM 115:543, 2003; CID 34:1585, 2002)	Amebiasis (Entamoeba histolytica, Cyclospora, Cryptosporidia and Giardia), see Table 13A	**Azithro** 500 mg po q24h times 3 days or **CIP** 500 mg po bid (See Comment)	**Erythro stearate** 500 mg po qid times 5 days	**↑ worldwide resistance to FQs** varies by region from 10% (USA) to 84% (Thailand) (AAC 47:2358, 2003). Erythro resistance rarely reported (CID 37:131, 2003). **Post-Campylobacter Guillain-Barré** assoc.: 15% of cases (CID 39:307, 2003). Assoc. with small bowel lymphoproliferative disease, may respond to antimicrobials (NEJM 350:239, 2003). **Reactive arthritis** another potential sequelae.
	Campylobacter jejuni CAUTION: See Comment re FQ resistance. H₂O¹ positive, WBCs, H₂O¹ bloody stools 37%			

¹ **H/O** = history of

Abbreviations on page 2

NOTE: All dosage recommendations are for adults (unless otherwise indicated) and assume normal renal function.

TABLE 1 (11)

ANATOMIC SITE/DIAGNOSIS/ MODIFYING CIRCUMSTANCES	ETIOLOGIES (usual)	SUGGESTED REGIMENS*		ADJUNCT DIAGNOSTIC OR THERAPEUTIC MEASURES AND COMMENTS
		PRIMARY	ALTERNATIVE†	
Gastrointestinal/Gastroenteritis—(continued from above)	**Specific Therapy** (continued) **C. difficile toxin positive** antibiotic-associated colitis (Ref.: LnID 5:549, 2005) **Remember: Contact isolation indicated** Fever in 28%. Diagnosis: Tissue culture—detects toxin A&B, most sensitive. Takes 48 hrs. Rapid immunoassays. Less sens., detect toxin A, B, or both. 10-20% false-neg. rate.	**Metro** 500 mg po tid or 250 mg qid times 10-14 days. If severe, use **vanco** (AAC 46:1647, 2002; CID 40:1586 & 1591 & 1598, 2005)	**Vanco** 125 mg po qid or **bacitracin** 25,000 units po qid; or (**cholestyramine** 4 gm po tid times 10-14 days. **Teicoplanin**[NUS] 400 mg po bid times 10 days	**DC antibiotic if possible; avoid antimotility agents; hydration; enteric isolation.** **Relapse occurs in 10-20%.** First, re-treat with **metro**. For refractory disease, **vanco** po + **RIF** po reported effective (JCHE 16:459, 1995). **Metro + RIF** should work but not published data. **Other relapse rx regimens: Metro** times 10 days, then (**cholestyramine** 4 gm po tid + **lactobacillus** 1 gm (qid) times 4 wks **OR vanco** 125 mg po every other day times 4 wks **OR vanco taper**, all doses 125 mg po: week 1—qid, week 2— bid, week 3—q24h, week 4—every other day, weeks 5 and 6 q3 days. **When po rx not possible**, use IV **metro + vanco**. 500 mg (per L saline via small bowel tube and/or via pigtail catheter in cecum (in severe/refractory pts). or nasal-small bowel tube, per min. to q24h max. of 2 gm (CID 35:690, 2004). **NOTE: IV vanco not effective.** Unclear how much IV metro gets to colonic mucosa & colonic content; hence combination of IV metro and po (via tube) vanco.
	E. coli O157:H7 H/O° bloody stools 63%	**NO TREATMENT** with antimicrobials or anti-motility drugs, may enhance toxin release and ↑ risk of hemolytic uremic syndrome (HUS) (NEJM 342:1930 & 1990, 2000). Hydration important (Ln 365:1073, 2005).		NOTE: 5-10% of pts develop HUS (approx. 10% with HUS die or have permanent renal failure; 50% HUS pts have some degree of renal impairment (CID 38:1298, 2004).
	Listeria monocytogenes	**AMP** 50 mg per kg IV q6h	**TMP-SMX** 20 mg per kg per day IV div. q6-8h	Recently recognized cause of food poisoning, manifest as febrile gastroenteritis. Percentage with complicating bacteremia/meningitis unknown. Not detected in standard stool culture (NEJM 336:100 & 130, 1997).
	Salmonella, non-typhi—For typhoid fever, see page 44 Fever in 71-91%, H/O° bloody stools in 34%	If no asymptomatic or illness mild, antimicrobial therapy not indicated. Treat if < 1 yr old or > 50 yrs old, if immunocompromised, if vascular graft or prosthetic joints (see typhoid fever, page 44). **CIP** 500 mg po bid times 5-7 days. Resistance↑ (Ln 353:1590, 1999)	**Azithro** 1 gm po once, then 500 mg q24h times 6 days (AAC 43:1441, 1999)	If resistance to TMP-SMX and chloro. Ceftriaxone or chloro. Ceftriaxone usually active (see footnote, page 19, for dosage); ceftriaxone & FQ resistance in SE Asia (CID 40:1315, 2005; Ln 363:1285, 2004). Primary treatment of enteritis is fluid and electrolyte replacement. No adverse effects from FQs in children (CID 38:1596, 1996). If immunocompromised, rx 14 days.
	Shigella Fever 58%, H/O° bloody stools 51%	**FQs** po (**CIP** 500 mg bid or **Levo** 500 mg q24h)—times 3 days.	**TMP-SMX-DS** po bid times 3 days, or **azithro** 500 mg po times 3 days.	Peds doses: TMP-SMX 5/25 mg per kg po times 3 days. For severe disease, ceftriaxone 50 mg per kg per day (max 2 gm) times 2-5 days. For susp. or ceftriaxone 10 mg per kg times 5 days. CIP superior to or ceftriaxone in children (LnID 3:537, 2003) **Immunocompromised children & adults: Treat for 7-10 days.**
		See Comment for peds doses		Azithro superior to cefixime in trial in children (PIDJ 22:374, 2003).
	Staphylococcus aureus See Comment	**Vanco** 1 gm IV q12h + 125 mg po qid reasonable	**TMP-SMX-DS** po bid times 4 days	Case reports of toxin-mediated pseudomembranous enteritis/colitis (pseudomembranous colitis in small bowel) (CID 38:9747, 2004). **Clinda** to stop toxin production reasonable in suspected cases febrile.
	Spirochetosis (Brachyspira pilosicoli)	Benefit of treatment unclear. Susceptible to **metro**, ceftriaxone, and **Moxi** (AAC 47:2354, 2003)		Anaerobic intestinal spirochete that colonizes colon of domestic & wild animals plus humans. Case reports of diarrhea with large numbers of the organism (AAC 39:347, 2001; Am J Clin Path 120:828, 2003).

† **H/O** = history of
Abbreviations on page 2.

NOTE: All dosage recommendations are for adults (unless otherwise indicated) and assume normal renal function.

TABLE 1 (12)

ANATOMIC SITE/DIAGNOSIS/ MODIFYING CIRCUMSTANCES	ETIOLOGIES (usual)	SUGGESTED REGIMENS[*] PRIMARY	ALTERNATIVE[1]	ADJUNCT DIAGNOSTIC OR THERAPEUTIC MEASURES AND COMMENTS
Gastrointestinal/Gastroenteritis—Specific Therapy *(continued)*				
Treatment decreases duration of disease, vol. losses, and duration of excretion *C/D 37:272, 2003; Ln 363:223, 2004*		**CIP** 1 gm po times 1 + fluids. **Primary rx is hydration** (see *Comment*)	**Doxy** 300 mg po times 1 + fluids (see *Comment*). For children < 8 yrs & in pregnancy: **TMP-SMX-DS**, one bid po times 3 days or for Peds alternative **azithro** or CIP times 1—see *doses in Comment*	Primary rx is fluid **IV** use (per liter): 4 gm NaCl, 1 gm lactate, 8 gm glucose. **PO** use (per liter potable water): 1 level teaspoon table salt + 4 heaping teaspoons sugar *(JTMH 84:73, 1981)*. Add orange juice or 2 bananas for K⁺. Volume given = fluid loss. Mild dehydration, give 5% body weight; for moderate, 7% body weight. (Refs. *CID 20:1485, 1995; PIDM 89:103, 1995*). Peds azithro: 20 mg per kg (to 1 gm max.) times 1 *(Ln 360:1722, 2002)*; CIP 20 mg per kg *(Ln 366:1085, 2005)*.
Vibrio parahaemolyticus		Antimicrobial rx does not shorten course. Hydration.		Shellfish exposure common. Treat severe disease: **FQ, doxy, P Ceph 3**
Vibrio vulnificus		Usual presentation is skin lesions & bacteremia, *see page 40*.		Treat early: **ceftaz ± doxy**—*see page 40*.
Yersinia enterocolitica Fever in 68%, bloody stools in 26%		No treatment unless severe. If severe, combine **doxy** 100 mg IV bid + (**tobra** or **genta** 5 mg per kg per day once q24h). **TMP-SMX** or **FQs** are alternatives.		Mesenteric adenitis pain can mimic acute appendicitis. Lab diagnosis difficult: requires "cold enrichment" and/or yersinia selective agar. Desferrioxamine rx ↑ severity, discontinue if pt on it. Iron overload states predispose to yersinia *(CID 21:1362 & 1367, 1998)*.
Gastroenteritis—Specific Risk Groups—Empiric Therapy				
Anoreceptive intercourse Proctitis (distal 15 cm only)	Herpes viruses, gonococci, chlamydia, syphilis. *See Genital Tract, page 18*			
Colitis	*Shigella, salmonella, campylobacter, E. histolytica (see Table 13A)*	**FQ** (e.g. **CIP** 500 mg po) q12h times 3 days.		
HIV-1 infected (AIDS): >10 day diarrhea				
Acid-fast organisms	*Cryptosporidium parvum, Cyclospora cayetanensis*		See Table 13A	For influenze of highly active antiretroviral therapy, *see CID 28:701, 1999*
Other	[G. lamblia]		See Table 13A	
Neutropenic enterocolitis or "typhlitis" *(CID 27:695 & 700, 1998)*	Mucosal invasion by *Clostridium septicum*. Occasionally caused by C. sordelli or P. aeruginosa	As for empiric regimen that includes drug active vs Clostridia species; e.g. **pen G**, **AMP** also **clinda** (see *Comment re: resistance*). Empiric regimen should warrant activity vs P. aerugi-nosa also.		Primary right lower quadrant. Surgical resection controversial but may be necessary. **NOTE:** Resistance of clostridia to clindamycin reported.
Traveler's diarrhea, self-medication. Patient usually afebrile. *(LnID 5:349, 2005)*	**Acute** 60% due to toxigenic E. coli; shigella, salmonella, or campylobacter. C. difficile, amebiasis (see *Table 13*). **If chronic**: cyclospora, cryptosporidia, giardia, isospora	**Levo** 500 mg po times 1 dose. Alternative **CIP** or **Ofox** 400 mg po bid times 3 days. **Imodium** optional: 4 mg times 1, then 2 mg after each loose stool to max 16 mg per day.	**Azithro** 1 gm po times 1 dose or **rifaximin** 200 mg po bid times 3 days.	Treatment based on randomized trial *(CID 37:1165, 2003)*. Peds & pregnancy: Avoid FQs. Azithro peds dose: 5–10 mg per kg times 1 dose. Rifaximin approved for age 12 or older. Adverse effects similar to placebo.
Prevention	Not routinely indicated. Current recommendation is to take **FQ + imodium** with 1st loose stool		**Alternative** during 1st 3 weeks & only if activities are essential: **Rifaximin** 200 mg po bid times 1.	No loperamide if fever or blood in stool.
Gastrointestinal Infections by Anatomic Site: Esophagus to Rectum				
Esophagitis	*Candida albicans, HSV, CMV*	[See SANFORD GUIDE TO HIV/AIDS THERAPY]		

[*] **FQ** dosage po for self-rx traveler's diarrhea—mild disease: **CIP** 750 mg times 1; severe: 500 mg times 3 days. **Levo** 500 mg times 3 days. **Oflox** 300 mg po bid times 3 days. Once q24h times 3 days: **Gati** or **Moxi**, 400 mg po q24h would work but not FDA-approved indication.

[1] NOTE: All dosage recommendations are for adults (unless otherwise indicated) and assume normal renal function.

Abbreviations on page 2

TABLE 1 (13)

ANATOMIC SITE/DIAGNOSIS/ MODIFYING CIRCUMSTANCES	ETIOLOGIES (usual)	SUGGESTED REGIMENS* PRIMARY	SUGGESTED REGIMENS* ALTERNATIVE†	ADJUNCT DIAGNOSTIC OR THERAPEUTIC MEASURES AND COMMENTS
Gastrointestinal Infections by Anatomic Site: Esophagus to Rectum *(continued)*				
Duodenal/Gastric ulcer; gastric cancer, MALT lymphomas (not 2° NSADs) [NEJM 347:1175, 2002; Can J Gastro 17:25B, 2003]	**Helicobacter pylori** See Comment Prevalence of pretreatment resistance increasing	Rx q12h po for 14 days: **(Omeprazole 20 mg)1 or rabeprazole 20 mg)1 + amox 1 gm + clarithro 500 mg.** Efficacy 80-95%	Rx po for 14 days: **Bismuth** (see footnote²) bismuth subsalicylate 2 tabs qid + **tetracycline** 500 mg qid + metro 250 mg qid or **omeprazole** 20 mg bid. Efficacy 90-99%	**Dx: Stool antigen—>90% sens. & specific. Cheap & practical. Rare false-pos. due to other Helicobacter species [BMJ 320:148, 2000]. Other tests: Urea breath test, if endoscopic, rapid urease &/or histology &/or culture. Antimicrobial resistance: Predicts rx failure [AnIM 139:463, 2003]. Geographic differences but overall resistance: amox & tetra uncommon, clarithro 10%, metro 35-50%. Treatment success: Correlates with active drugs & pt compliance. Suggested rx duration varies between 7-14 days; we suggest last regimen times 14 days to ↑ compliance & hopefully efficacy (7-9% ↑ cures with 14 days) [Aliment Pharmacol Ther 14:603, 2000]. Test of cure: Repeat stool antigen >8 wks post-treatment.**
Small intestine: Whipple's disease [CID 32:457, 2001; Ln 363:654, 2004] See Infective endocarditis, culture-negative, page 23	Tropheryma whipplei	**Initial 10-14 days (Pen G-24 million units IV q24h + streptomycin 1 gm IM/IV q24h) OR ceftriaxone 2 gm IV q24h Then, for approx. 1 year TMP-SMX-DS 1 tab po bid**	TMP-SMX-DS 1 tab po bid **Doxy** 100 mg po bid) + **(Pen VK** 500 mg po qid)	Rx regimen based on empiricism and retrospective analyses. TMP-SMX relapses during TMP-SMX rx reported. Interesting in vitro susceptibility study: combination of doxy & hydroxychloroquine bactericidal [AAC 48:747, 2004]. Cultivated from CSF in pts with intestinal disease and no neurologic findings [JID 188:797 & 801, 2003]
Inflammatory bowel disease: Ulcerative colitis, Crohn's disease Mild to moderate Ref. Ln 359:331, 2002	Unknown	**Sulfasalazine** 1 gm po q6h or **mesalamine (5ASA)** 1 gm po q6h	**Coated mesalamine** (Asacol) 800 mg bid or qid **Corticosteroid enemas** [Gastro 123:33, 2002]	Check stool for E. histolytica. Try aminosalicylates 1st in mild/mod. disease. See review article for more aggressive therapy
In randomized controlled trial		Etanercept	Infliximab/adalimumab	*
Severe Crohn's	Unknown			
Diverticulitis, perirectal abscess, peritonitis Also see Peritonitis, page 34 CID (in press)	Enterobacteriaceae, occ. P. aeruginosa, Bacteroides sp., enterococci	**Outpatient rx—mild diverticulitis, drained perirectal abscess:** (**TMP-SMX-DS** bid or **CIP** 750 mg bid or **Levo** 750 mg q24h) + **metro** 500 mg q6h. All po times 7-10 days.	**AM-CL-ER** 1000/62.5 mg 2 tabs po bid times 7-10 days	Screen for latent TB: before blocking TNF [MMWR 53:683, 2004]. Delay anti-TNF drugs until TB prophylaxis complete. For other anti-TNF risks: NEJM 351:42, 2004. Must "cover" both aerobic/anaerobic Gm-neg. & anaerobic bacteria. **Drugs active only vs anaerobic Gm-neg. bacilli:** clinda, metro. **Drugs active only vs aerobic Gm-neg. bacilli:** APAG³, Ceph 2/3/4, aztreonam, AP Pen, Gti. Levo,Gati. **Drugs active vs both aerobic & anaerobic Gm-neg. bacteria:** cefoxitin, cefotetan, TC-CL, PIP-TZ, AM-SB, ERTA, IMP, MER, & Moxi, tigecycline. Increasing resistance to metro, TC-CL, & clinda of Bacteroides species. Cefoxitin Cefotetan Clindamycin % Resistant: 4-25 16-44 17-87 Resistance to metro, PIP-TZ rare [CID 35(Suppl.1):S126, 2002]. Few case *(continued on next page)*

---

1. Can substitute other **proton pump inhibitors** for omeprazole or rabeprazole—all bid esomeprazole 20 mg (FDA-approved), lansoprazole 30 mg (FDA-approved), pantoprazole 40 mg (not FDA-approved for this indication).

2. **bismuth preparations:** (1) In U.S., **bismuth subsalicylate** (Pepto-Bismol) 262 mg tabs; adult dose for helicobacter is 2 tabs (524 mg) qid (2) Outside U.S., colloidal bismuth subcitrate (De-Nol) 120 mg chewable tablets; dose is 1 tablet qid (3) Another treatment option: Ranitidine bismuth citrate 400 mg bid po with metro 500 mg and clarithro 500 mg—all bid times 7 days. Worked despite metro/clarithro resistance [Gastro 114:A323, 1998).

3. **APAG = antipseudomonal aminoglycoside**, e.g., **amikacin, gentamicin, tobramycin**

Abbreviations on page 2. NOTE: All dosage recommendations are for adults (unless otherwise indicated) and assume normal renal function.

TABLE 1 (14)

ANATOMIC SITE/DIAGNOSIS/ MODIFYING CIRCUMSTANCES	ETIOLOGIES (usual)	SUGGESTED REGIMENS* PRIMARY	ALTERNATIVE†	ADJUNCT DIAGNOSTIC OR THERAPEUTIC MEASURES AND COMMENTS
Gastrointestinal Infections by Anatomic Site: Esophagus to Rectum (continued)				(continued from previous page)
Diverticulitis, perirectal abscess, peritonitis (continued)				reports of metro resistance (CID 40:e67, 2005; J Clin Micro 42:4127, 2004). Resistance mechanisms reviewed: CID 39:92, 2004). Penicillin/Acinetobacter more active vs cloxacillin. Check sample; for IMP or MER.
				Concomitant surgical management important, esp. with moderate-severe disease. **Role of enterococci remains debatable**. Probably pathogenic in infections of biliary tract. Probably need drugs active vs enterococci in pts with valvular heart disease.
		Rectum (continued) **Mild-moderate disease**—Diverticulitis, focal peri-appendiceal peritonitis, peri-diverticular abscess, endomyometritis) **P-Tz** 3.375 gm IV q6h or AM-SB 3 gm IV q6h, or AM-CL 3.1 gm IV q6h or TC-CL 3.1 gm IV q6h or **ERTA** 1 gm IV q24h	**CIP** 400 mg IV q12h or (**Levo** 750 mg IV q24h]) + (**metro** 500 mg IV q6h or 1 gm IV q12h **OR** **tigecycline** 100 mg IV 1ˢᵗ dose & then 50 mg IV q12h	
		Severe life-threatening disease, ICU patient: **IMP** 500 mg IV q6h or **MER** 1 gm IV q8h	**AMP + metro + CIP** 400 mg IV q12h or (**Levo** 750 mg IV q24h) **OR** [**AMP** 2 gm IV q6h + **metro** 500 mg IV q6h + **APAG** (see *Table 10D, page 74*)]	**Severe penicillin/cephalosporin allergy:** (**aztreonam** 2 gm IV q6h) + (**metro** 500 mg IV q6h or (1 gm IV q12h)) **OR** [(**CIP** 400 mg IV q12h or (**Levo** 750 mg IV q24h) + **metro**]. Based on in vitro data, could sub **Gati/Moxi** for **CIP/Levo**, but insufficient clinical data.
GENITAL TRACT: Mixture of empiric & specific treatment. Divided by sex of pt. For sexual assault (rape), see *Table 15A, page 124*. See Guidelines for Dx of Sexually Transmitted Diseases, *MMWR 51(RR-6), 2002 or CID 35(Suppl.2):S135, 2002*.				
Both Women & Men:				
Chancroid Ref: *CID 28(Suppl 1):S14, 1999*	H. ducreyi	**Ceftriaxone** 250 mg IM single dose or **azithro** 1 gm po single dose	**CIP** 500 mg bid po times 3 days **OR erythro base** 500 mg po qid times 7 days.	In HIV+ pts, failures reported with single dose azithro (*CID 21:409, 1995*).
Chlamydia, et al. non-gonococcal or post-gonococcal urethritis, cervicitis **NOTE: Assume concomitant N. gonorrhoeae** Chlamydia conjunctivitis, see *page 70*	Chlamydia 50%, Myco-plasma hominis. Other known etiologies (10–15%): Ureaplasma, trichomonas, herpes simplex virus. Myco-plasma genitalium. Chlamydia ref.: *NEJM 349:2424, 2003*	**Doxy** 100 mg po bid times 7 days or **azithro** 1 gm po as single dose. Evaluate & rx sex partner	(**Erythro base** 500 mg po times 7 days) or (**Ofloxa** 300 mg q12h po times 7 days) or (**Levo** 500 mg po qid times 7 days).	**Diagnosis:** Nucleic acid amplification tests for C. trachomatis & N. gonorrhoeae on urine specimens or swab of cervix or urethra specimens (*AnIM 142:914, 2005*). **For recurrent or persistent disease:** either metro (2 gm po x1) or erythro base 500 mg po qid times 7 days or erythro ethylsuccinate 800 mg po qid times 7 days. **Evaluate & treat sex partners.**
Recurrent/persistent urethritis	Occult trichomonas, tetra-resistant U. urealyticum	**Metro** 2 gm po x1 + **erythro base** 500 mg po qid times 7 days.	**Erythro ethylsuccinate** 800 mg po qid times 7 days	In men with NGU, 20% infected with trichomonas (*JID 188:465, 2003*).
Gonorrhea (*MMWR 51(RR-6), 2002 or CID 35 (Suppl.2):S135, 2002*) **Conjunctivitis** (adult)	N. gonorrhoeae	**Ceftriaxone** 1 gm IM or IV times one dose	**Spectinomycin** 2 gm IM q12h	Consider saline lavage of eye times 1
Disseminated gonococcal infection (DGI, dermatitis-arthritis syndrome)	N. gonorrhoeae	**Ceftriaxone** 1 gm IV q24h) or (**cefotaxime** 1 gm IV q8h) or (**ceftizox-ime** 1 gm q8h IV)—see Comment	(**Spectinomycin** 2 gm IM q12h or **CIP** 400 mg IV q12h or **Ofloxa** 400 mg IV q12h or **Levo** 250 mg IV q24h)—see Comment	Continue IM or IV regimen for 24 hrs after symptoms ↓; reliable pts may be dis-charged 24 hrs after sx resolve to complete 7 days rx with **cefixime** 400 mg po bid or CIP 500 mg po bid or Ofloxa 400 mg po bid or Levo 500 mg po q24h. R/O meningitis/ endocarditis. **Treat presumptively for concomitant C. trachomatis.**
Endocarditis	N. gonorrhoeae	**Ceftriaxone** 1–2 gm IV q12h		
Pharyngitis	N. gonorrhoeae	**Ceftriaxone** 125 mg IM times 1	**CIP** 500 mg po times 1 or **Levo** 250 mg po times 1.	If chlamydia not ruled out: Azithro 1 gm po times 1 or doxy 100 mg po times 7 days. Some suggest test of culture after 1 week. Spectinomycin not effective for pharyngitis due to N. gonorrhoeae.

Abbreviations on page 2.   *NOTE: All dosage recommendations are for adults (unless otherwise indicated) and assume normal renal function.*

TABLE 1 (15)

ANATOMIC SITE/DIAGNOSIS/ MODIFYING CIRCUMSTANCES	ETIOLOGIES (usual)	SUGGESTED REGIMENS*		ADJUNCT DIAGNOSTIC OR THERAPEUTIC MEASURES AND COMMENTS
		PRIMARY	ALTERNATIVE†	
GENITAL TRACT/Both Women & Men/Gonorrhea (MMWR 51(RR-6), 2002) (continued)				
Urethritis, cervicitis, proctitis (uncomplicated) For prostatitis, see page 20. **Diagnosis:** Nucleic acid amplification test on urine or urethral swab—see MMWR 51 (RR-15), 2002	N. gonorrhoeae (50% of pts with urethritis, cervicitis concomitant C. trachomatis —**treat for both**)	[[**Ceftriaxone** 125 mg IM times 1) or (**cefixime** 400 mg po times 1) or (**cefpodoxime** 400 mg po times 1) or (**CIP** 500 mg po times 1) or (**Oflox** 400 mg po times 1) or (**Levo** 250 mg po times 1)] **PLUS** [(**Azithro** 1 gm po times 1) or (**doxy** 100 mg po q12h times 7 days)] **NOTE:** Due to resistance of approx .5%, do not use FQs to treat (1) men who have sex with men or (2) GC acquired in Hawaii, other Pacific Islands, West Coast of U.S., or England.	**Spectinomycin** 2 gm IM times 1 Other single-dose cephalosporins: ceftizoxime 500 mg IM, cefoxitin 2 gm IM + probenecid 1 gm po, and cefotaxime 500 mg IM, cefotaxime 1 gm po x1 effective for chlamydia but need 2 gm po for GC; not recommended for GC due to GI side-effects and expense.	Treat for both GC and C. trachomatis. Screen for syphilis. Other alternatives for GC: FQ resistance refs. MMWR 53:335, 2004; CID 38:849, 2004; EID 11:1009, 2005
Granuloma inguinale (Donovanosis)	Calymmatobacterium granulomatis	**Doxy** 100 mg po bid times 3-4 wks OR **TMP-SMX-DS** q12h times 3 weeks	**Erythro** 500 mg po qid times 3 weeks OR **CIP** 750 mg po times 3 weeks OR **azithro** 1 gm po q wk times 3 weeks	Clinical response usually seen in 1 week. Rx until all lesions healed; may take 4 weeks. Treatment failures & recurrence seen with doxy and TMP-SMX. Report of FQ resistance with FQ and chloro. Ref. CID 25:24, 1997
Herpes simplex virus	See Table 14, page 110			Dx based on serology; biopsy contraindicated because sinus tracts develop.
Lymphogranuloma venereum serovars. L1, L2, L3	Chlamydia trachomatis.	**Doxy** 100 mg po bid times 21 days	**Erythro** 0.5 gm po qid times 21 days	Nucleic acid ampli tests in development
Phthirus pubis (pubic lice, "crabs") & scabies	See Table 14, page 110	See Table 13, page 103		
Syphilis & HIV: LnID 4:456, 2004; MMWR 53:RR-15, 2004				
Syphilis Early, primary, secondary, or latent < 1 year	T. pallidum	**Benzathine pen G (Bicillin L-A)** 2.4 million units IM times 1	**Doxy** 100 mg po bid times 14 days or **(tetracycline** 500 mg po qid times 14 days) or (**ceftriaxone** 1 gm IM/IV q24h times 8–10 days). Follow-up mandatory.	If early or congenital syphilis, **quantitate VDRL at** 0, 3, 6, 12 & 24 months after rx. If 1° or 2° syphilis, VDRL should ↓ 2 tubes at 6 months, 3 tubes 12 months, & 4 tubes 24 months. Early failure & reinfection with ↓ or no ↑ titers: 50% with one RPR seronegative at 12 months; 24% neg FTA/ABS at 2-3 yrs (AJM 114:1005, 1991). **Azithro-resistant syphilis** documented in California, Ireland, & elsewhere (NEJM 351:122 & 154, 2004).
More than 1 yr's duration (latent of indeterminate duration, cardiovascular, late benign)		**Benzathine pen G (Bicillin L-A)** 2.4 million units IM q wk times 3 = 7.2 million units total.	**Doxy** 100 mg po bid times 28 days or **tetracycline** 500 mg po qid times 28 days	No published data on efficacy of alternatives. The value of routine lumbar puncture in asymptomatic late syphilis is being questioned in the U.S., i.e., no LP, rx all patients as primary recommendation. AJM 145:465, 1985. **Indications for LP (CDC): neurologic symptoms, treatment failure, serum non-treponemal antibody titer ≥1:32, other evidence of active syphilis (aortitis, gumma, iritis), non-penicillin rx, + HIV test.**
Neurosyphilis—Very difficult to treat. Includes ocular (retrobulbar neuritis) syphilis The MEDICAL LETTER on Drugs & Therapeutics & refs. in Comments		**Pen G** 3-4 million units IV q4h times 10-14 days. Treatment same as HIV negative. Recommend CSF exam of all syphilis of stage	**(Procaine pen G** 2.4 million units IM q24h + **probenecid** 0.5 gm po qid) both times 10–14 days—See Comment	**Ceftriaxone** 2 gm (IV or IM) q24h times 14 days. 23% failure rate reported (AJM 93:481, 1992). For penicillin allergy: either desensitize to penicillin or obtain infectious diseases consultation. **Serologic criteria for response to rx: 4-fold or greater ↓ in VDRL titer over 6–12 mos.** (CID 28 [Suppl 1]:S21, 1999). HIV + pts: RPR at 3, 6, 9, 12, & 24 mo. rx increases risk of neurosyphilis nearly 19-fold. HIV infection plus RPR ≥1:32 CSF & CD4 count ≤350 per mm3 increases likely of neurosyphilis. CID 38:1001, 2004. Reviews of syphilis & HIV: LnID 4:456, 2004; MMWR 53:RR-15, 2004
Pregnancy and syphilis		Same as for non-pregnant, some recommend 2nd dose (2.4 million units) **benzathine pen G** 1 wk after initial dose esp. in 3rd trimester or with 2° syphilis	Skin test for penicillin allergy. **Desensitize** if necessary.	Monthly quantitative VDRL or equivalent. If 4-fold ↑, re-treat. Doxy, tetracycline contraindicated. Erythro not recommended because of high risk of failure to cure fetus.

Abbreviations on page 2.   NOTE: All dosage recommendations are for adults (unless otherwise indicated) and assume normal renal function.

TABLE 1 (1/6)

ANATOMIC SITE/DIAGNOSIS/ MODIFYING CIRCUMSTANCES	ETIOLOGIES (usual)	SUGGESTED REGIMENS*		ADJUNCT DIAGNOSTIC OR THERAPEUTIC MEASURES AND COMMENTS
		PRIMARY	ALTERNATIVE†	
GENITAL TRACT/Both Women and Men/Syphilis (continued)				
Congenital syphilis	T. pallidum	**Aqueous crystalline pen G** 50,000 units per kg per day...	**Procaine pen G** 50,000 units per kg IM q24h for 10–14 days	Another alternative: Ceftriaxone ≤30 days old, 75 mg per kg IV/IM q24h; or >30 days old 100 mg per kg IV/IM q24h. Treat 10–14 days. If symptomatic, ophthalmologic exam indicated. If more than 1 day of tx is missed, restart entire course. **Need serologic follow-up!**
Warts, anogenital		*See Table 14, page 112*		
Women:				
Amnionitis, septic abortion	Bacteroides, esp. Prevotella bivius; Group B, A streptococci; Enterobacteriaceae; C. trachomatis	[(Cefoxitin or TC-CL or IMP or MER or AM-SB or PIP-TZ) + doxy] OR [Clinda + (APAG or P Ceph 3)] *Dosage: see footnote¹*		D&C of uterus. **In septic abortion,** Clostridium perfringens may cause fulminant intravascular hemolysis. **In postpartum patients** with enigmatic fever and/or pulmonary emboli, **consider septic pelvic vein thrombophlebitis** (see *Vascular, septic pelvic vein thrombophlebitis, page 47*). After discharge: doxy or continue clinda. **NOTE:** IV clinda effective for C. trachomatis, no data on po clinda (*CID 19:720, 1994*).
Cervicitis, mucopurulent	N. gonorrhoeae; Chlamydia trachomatis	Treat to gonorrhoeae, page 18; Treat for non-gonococcal urethritis, page 17		Criteria for dx: yellow or green pus on cervical swab, >10 WBC/oil field. Gram stain for GC. If negative rx for C. trachomatis. If in doubt, send swab or urine for culture, EIA or nucleic acid amplification test and rx for both.
Endomyometritis/septic pelvic phlebitis; Early postpartum (1°–48 hrs) (usually after C-section)	Bacteroides, esp. Prevotella bivius; Group B, A streptococci; Enterobacteriaceae; C. trachomatis	[(Cefoxitin or TC-CL or ERTA or IMP or MER or AM-SB or PIP-TZ) + doxy] OR [Clinda + (APAG or P Ceph 3)] *Dosage: see footnote¹*		See Comments under *Amnionitis, septic abortion,* above
Late postpartum (48 hrs to 6 wks) (usually after vaginal delivery)	Chlamydia trachomatis; M. hominis	Doxy 100 mg IV or po q12h times 14 days		Tetracyclines not recommended in nursing mothers; discontinue nursing. M. hominis sensitive to tetra, clinda, not erythro (*CCTID 17:5200, 1993*).
Fitzhugh-Curtis syndrome	C. trachomatis, N. gonorrhoeae	Treat as for pelvic inflammatory disease		Perihepatitis (violin-string adhesions)
Pelvic inflammatory disease (PID), salpingitis, tubo-ovarian abscess — *MMWR 51(RR-6), 2002* Outpatient rx: limit to pts with temp <38°C, WBC <11,000 per mm³, minimal evidence of peritonitis, active bowel sounds & able to tolerate oral nourishment	N. gonorrhoeae, chlamydia, bacteroides, Enterobacteriaceae, streptococci	**Outpatient rx:** [(Ofloxacin 400 mg bid or Levo 500 mg q24h) ± (metro 500 mg po bid times 14 days)] OR [(ceftriaxone 250 mg IM or IV times 1) + (doxy 100 mg po bid times 14 days) ± (metro 500 mg po bid times 14 days)]	**Inpatient regimens:** [(Cefotetan 2 gm IV q12h or cefoxitin 2 gm IV q8h) + (doxy 100 mg IV/po q12h)]. OR [(Clinda 900 mg IV q8h) + (gentamicin 2 mg per kg loading dose, then 1.5 mg per kg q8h or 4.5 mg per kg once per day), then doxy 100 mg po times 14 days]	Alternative parenteral regimens: 1. [(Ofloxacin 2 gm IV q12h or Levo 500 mg IV q24h) + metro 500 mg IV q8h] 2. AM-SB 3 gm IV q6h + doxy 100 mg IV/po q12h + Levo Remember: Evaluate and treat sex partner
Vaginitis—*MMWR 51(RR-6), 2002*				*See Table 11A, page 78*
Candidiasis; Pruritus, thick cheesy discharge, pH 4.4–5; *See Table 11A, page 78*	Candida albicans 80–90%; C. glabrata, C. tropicalis may be increasing; they are less susceptible to azoles.	**Oral azoles:** Fluconazole 150 mg po times 1 OR Itraconazole 200 mg po bid times 1 day	**Intravaginal azoles:** variety of strengths—from 1 dose to 7–14 days. Drugs available (all end in -azole): butoconazole, clotrim, micon, ticon, tercon (doses: *Table 11A, footnote⁸*)	Nystatin vag. tabs times 14 days less effective. Other rx for azole-resistant strains: If recurrent candidiasis (4 or more episodes per yr): 6 mos. suppression with: fluconazole 150 mg po q week or itraconazole 100 mg po q week or clotrimazole vag. suppositories 500 mg q week.

¹ **P Ceph 2** (cefotetan 2 gm IV q6-8h, **clinda** 450–900 mg IV q8h; **APAG gentamicin**, see *Table 10D, page 74*) **P Ceph 3** (**cefotaxime** 750 mg IV q12h; **TC-CL** 3.1 gm IV q4-6h; **AM-SB** 3 gm IV q6h; **PIP-TZ** 3.375 gm IV q6h or for nosocomial pneumonia: 4.5 gm IV q6h; **doxy** 100 mg IV/po q12h; **cefoxitin** 2 gm IV q8h; **cefotetan** 2 gm IV q12h; see *Table 10D, page 74*); **P Ceph 3** (**cefotaxime** 2 gm IV q8h; **ceftriaxone** 2 gm IV q24h); **ertapenem** 1 gm IV q24h); **IMP** 0.5 gm IV q6h; **MER** 1 gm IV q8h; **linezolid** 600 mg IV q12h. NOTE: All dosage recommendations are for adults (unless otherwise indicated) and assume normal renal/renal function. *Abbreviations on page 2*

TABLE 1 (17)

ANATOMIC SITE/DIAGNOSIS/ MODIFYING CIRCUMSTANCES	ETIOLOGIES (usual)	SUGGESTED REGIMENS*		ADJUNCT DIAGNOSTIC OR THERAPEUTIC MEASURES AND COMMENTS
		PRIMARY	ALTERNATIVE†	
GENITAL TRACT, Women/Vaginitis (continued)				
Trichomoniasis Copious foamy discharge, pH >4.5 Treat sexual partners—see Comment	Trichomonas vaginalis	**Metro** 2 gm as single dose or 500 mg po bid times 7 days **OR Tinidazole** 2 gm po single dose **Pregnancy:** See Comment	**For rx failure:** Re-treat with metro 500 mg po bid times 7 days; if 2nd failure: metro 2 gm po q24h times 3–5 days If still failure, suggest ID consultation and/or contact CDC: 770-488-4115 or www.cdc.gov/std.	Treat sexual partners (2 gm metronidazole as single dose). Nearly 20% men with NGU are infected with trichomonas (JID 188:465, 2003). Another option if metro-resistant: **Tinidazole** 500 mg po qid + intravaginal 500 mg po bid times 14 days. Ref.: CID 33:1341, 2001. **Pregnancy:** No data indicating metro teratogenic or mutagenic [MMWR 51(RR-6), 2002].
Bacterial vaginosis Malodorous vaginal discharge, pH >4.5	Polymicrobic: associated with Gardnerella vaginalis, bacteroides non-fragilis, mobiluncus, peptococci, Mycoplasma hominis	**Metro** 0.5 gm po bid times 7 days or **metro vaginal gel** (1 applicator intravaginally) 1 time per day times 5 days.	**Clinda** 0.3 gm po bid times 7 days or **clinda vaginal cream** 2 gm intravaginally at bedtime times 7 days or **clinda ovules** 100 mg intravaginally at bedtime times 3 days.	Rx of male sex partner **not indicated** unless balanitis present. **Metro 2 gm po times 1 not as effective as 5–7 day course** (JAMA 268:92, 1992). Metro extended release tabs 750 mg q24h times 7 days available; no published data. **Pregnancy:** Rx same as non-pregnancy, except avoid clindamych cream (↑ risk premature birth). Treatment of asymptomatic pts with oral clinda ↓ premature birth (Ln 361:983, 2003).
Men:				
Balanitis	Candida 40%, Group B strep, gardnerella	Oral **azoles** as for vaginitis		Occurs in ¼ of male sex partners of women infected with candida. Exclude circinate balanitis (Reiter's syndrome). Plasma cell balanitis (non-infectious) responds to hydrocortisone cream.
Epididymo-orchitis Age <35 years	N. gonorrhoeae, Chlamydia trachomatis	**Ceftriaxone** 250 mg IM times 1 + **doxy** 100 mg po bid times 10 days or **Oflox** 300 mg po bid times 10 days.		Also: bedrest, scrotal elevation, and analgesics.
Age >35 years or homosexual men (insertive partners in anal intercourse)	Enterobacteriaceae (coliforms)	**FQ: CIP-ER** 500 mg po 1 time per day or **CIP** 400 mg IV bid or **Levo** 750 mg IV po 1 time per day, times 10–14 days.		Midstream pyuria and scrotal pain and edema. Also: bedrest, scrotal elevation, and analgesics.
Prostatitis—Review: AJM 106:327, 1999				
Acute ≤35 years of age	N. gonorrhoeae, C. trachomatis	**Oflox** 400 mg po times 1 then 300 mg po bid times 10 days or **ceftriaxone** 250 mg IM times 1 then **doxy** 100 mg po bid times 10 days		Oflox effective vs gonococci & C. trachomatis and penetrates prostate. In AIDS pts, prostate may be focus of Cryptococcus neoformans.
≥35 years of age	Enterobacteriaceae (coliforms)	**FQ** (Dosage: see Epididymo-orchitis, ≥35 yrs, above) or **TMP-SMX** 1 DS tablet (160 mg TMP) po bid times 10–14 days		Treat as acute urinary infection, 14 days (not single dose regimen). Some authorities recommend 3–4 week rx (IDCP 4:325, 1995).
Chronic bacterial	Enterobacteriaceae 80%, enterococci 15%, P. aeruginosa	**FQ** (CIP 500 mg po bid times 4 weeks, **Levo** 500 mg po q24h times 4 weeks—see Comment	**TMP-SMX-DS** 1 tab po bid times 1–3 mos.	With rx failures consider infected prostatic calculi.
Chronic prostatitis/chronic pelvic pain syndrome (New NIH classification, JAMA 282:236, 1999)	The most common prostatitis syndrome. Etiology is unknown, molecular probe data suggest infectious etiology (Clin Micro Rev 11, 604, 1998).	**α-adrenergic blocking agents** (α-adrenergic blockade) controversial (AHM 133:367, 2000).		Pt has ⊕ of prostatitis but negative cultures and no cells in prostatic secretions. Rev. JAMA 282: 467, 2000). In another controlled double-blind study, CIP and an alphablocker of no benefit (AnIM 141:581 & 639, 2004).

---

¹ 1 applicator contains 5 gm of gel with 37.5 mg metronidazole

* The dosage recommendations are for adults (unless otherwise indicated) and assume normal renal function

NOTE: All dosage recommendations are for adults (unless otherwise indicated) and assume normal renal function

Abbreviations on page 2

TABLE 1 (18)

ANATOMIC SITE/DIAGNOSIS/ MODIFYING CIRCUMSTANCES	ETIOLOGIES (usual)	SUGGESTED REGIMENS* PRIMARY	ALTERNATIVE†	ADJUNCT DIAGNOSTIC OR THERAPEUTIC MEASURES AND COMMENTS
HAND (Bites: See Skin)				
Paronychia				
Nail biting, manicuring	Staph. aureus (maybe MRSA)	I&D or culture	TMP-SMX-DS 2 tabs po bid while waiting for culture result. See Table 6 for alternatives	
Contact with oral mucosa— dentists, anesthesiologists, wrestlers	Herpes simplex (Whitlow)	Acyclovir 400 mg po times 10 days	Famciclovir or valacyclovir should work, see Comment	Gram stain and routine culture negative. Famciclovir/valacyclovir doses used for primary genital herpes; see Table 14, page 170
Dishwasher (prolonged water immersion)	Candida sp.	Clotrimazole (topical)		Avoid immersion of hands in water as much as possible
HEART				
Atherosclerotic coronary artery disease	Chlamydia pneumoniae	New name: Chlamydophila pneumoniae. Ref: JAMA 290:1459 & 1515, 2003		
Infective endocarditis—Native valve—empirical rx awaiting cultures—"culture negative"	NOTE: Diagnostic criteria include evidence of continuous bacteremia (multiple positive blood cultures), new murmur (worsening of old murmur) of valvular insufficiency, definite emboli, and echocardiographic (transthoracic or transesophageal) evidence of valvular vegetations. Refs.: Circulation 111:3167, 2005; Ln 363:139, 2004			
Valvular or congenital heart disease including bicuspid valve prolapse with no modifying circumstances See Table 15C, page 127 for prophylaxis	Viridans strep 30–40%, "other" strep 15–25%, enterococci 5–18%, staphylococci 20–35%	(Pen G 20 million units IV q24h), or (ampicillin 12 gm IV q24h), either continuous or div (q4h) + (AMP 12 gm IV q24h, continuous or div q4h) + (nafcillin or oxacillin 2 gm IV q24h) + gentamicin 1 mg per kg IM or IV (q8h) [see Comment]	Vanco 15 mg per kg¹ IV q12h (not to exceed 2 gm q24h unless serum levels monitored) + gentamicin 1 mg per kg IM or IV q8h	If patient not acutely ill and not in heart failure, we prefer to wait for blood culture results. If initial 3 blood cultures neg. after 24–48 hrs, obtain 2–3 more blood cultures before empiric rx started. Nafcillin/oxacillin + gentamicin may not be adequate coverage of enterococci, hence addition of penicillin G pending cultures. When blood cultures +, modify regimen from empiric to specific based on organism, in vitro susceptibilities, clinical experience. Gentamicin used for synergy; peak levels need not exceed 4 mcg per mL.
Infective endocarditis—Native valve—IV illicit drug use ± evidence rt-sided endocarditis—empiric rx	S. aureus. All others rare	Vanco 1 gm IV q12h	Dapto 6 mg per kg q24h (not FDA-approved indication; 9/04)	Dapto clinical trials for bacteremia/endocarditis in progress. Quinupristin-dalfo-pristin (Cidal vs S. aureus if both constituents active.
Infective endocarditis—Native valve—culture positive (JAMA 274:1706, 1995; NEJM 345:1318, 2001; CID 36:615, 2003; JAC 54:971, 2004⁴)				
Viridans strep, S. bovis with penicillin G MIC ≤0.1 mcg per mL	Viridans strep, S. bovis	(Pen G 12–18 million units per day IV, continuous or q4h) times 2 wks) PLUS gentamicin 1 mg per kg q8h times 2 wks] OR Pen G 12–18 million units per day IV (continuous or q4h) times 4 wks OR (ceftriaxone 2 gm IV q24h) times 4 wks	(Ceftriaxone 2 gm IV q24h + gentamicin 1 mg per kg IV) (q8h both times 2 wks. If allergy pen G or ceftriax. use vanco 15 mg per kg IV q12h to 2 gm per day unless serum levels measured) times 4 wks	Also effective: (ceftriaxone 2 gm IV q24h) + (netilmicin^NUS 4 mg per kg q24h) times 2 wks (CID 21:1406, 1995). Target peak levels: peak 3 mcg per mL, trough <1 mcg per mL. If very obese pt, recommend consultation for dosage adjustment. Infuse vanco over ≥1 hr to avoid "red man" syndrome. S. bovis associated with occult bowel pathology (new name: S. gallolyticus). Since relapse rate may be greater in pts ill for >3 mos. prior to start of rx, the penicillin-gentamicin synergism theoretically may be needed in this group.
Viridans strep, S. bovis, nutritionally variant strep³	Viridans strep, S. bovis, nutritionally variant streptococci, tolerant strep³	Pen G 18 million units per day IV (continuous or q4h) times 4 wks PLUS gentamicin 1 mg per kg IV q8h times 2 wks NOTE: Low dose of gentamicin	Vanco 15 mg per kg¹ IV q12h to max. 2 gm per day unless vanco levels documented times 4 wks	Can use cefazolin for pen G in pt with allergy that is not IgE-mediated (e.g., anaphylaxis). Alternatively, can use vanco. (See Comment above on gent and vanco) NOTE: If necessary to remove infected valve & valve culture neg., 2 weeks antibiotic treatment post-op sufficient (CID 41:187, 2005).
Viridans strep, S. bovis (S. gallolyticus) with penicillin G MIC >0.1 to <0.5 mcg per mL				

¹ Assumes estimated creatinine clearance ≥80 mL per min., see Table 17.
² Ref. for Guidelines of British Soc. for Antimicrob. Chemother. Includes drugs not available in U.S.: flucloxacillin IV, teicoplanin IV
³ Tolerant streptococcus = MBC 32-fold greater than MIC

NOTE: All dosage recommendations are for adults (unless otherwise indicated) and assume normal renal function.

Abbreviations on page 2.

TABLE 1 (19)

ANATOMIC SITE/DIAGNOSIS/MODIFYING CIRCUMSTANCES	ETIOLOGIES (usual)	SUGGESTED REGIMENS* PRIMARY	ALTERNATIVE†	ADJUNCT DIAGNOSTIC OR THERAPEUTIC MEASURES AND COMMENTS
HEART/Infective endocarditis—Native valve—culture positive (continued)				
For viridans strep or S. bovis with **pen G MIC ≤0.5 and** enterococci susceptible to AMP/pen G, vanco, gentamicin NOTE: Inf. Dis. consultation suggested	"Susceptible" enterococci, viridans strep, S. bovis, nutritionally variant streptococci (new names are: Abiotrophia sp. & Granulicatella sp.)	(Pen G) 18–30 million units per 24h IV, either q4h times 4–6 wks) PLUS gentamicin 1–1.5 mg per kg q8h IV times 4–6 wks **OR** (AMP 12 gm per day IV, continuous or q4h + gent as above times 4–6 wks)	Vanco 15 mg per kg IV q12h to max 2 gm per day unless serum levels measured PLUS gentamicin 1–1.5 mg per kg q8h IV times 4–6 wks NOTE: Low dose of gent	**4 wks of rx if symptoms <3 mos.; 6 wks of rx if symptoms >3 mos.** Vanco for pen-allergic pts; do not use cephalosporins. Do not give gent once-q24h for enterococcal endocarditis. Target gentamicin peak: 3 mcg per mL, trough <1 mcg per mL. Vanco target serum levels: peak 20–50 mcg per mL, trough 5–12 mcg per mL. NOTE: Because of ↑ frequency of resistance (see below), all enterococci causing endocarditis should be tested in vitro for susceptibility to penicillin, β-lactamase production, gent susceptibility and vanco susceptibility.
Enterococci: MIC streptomycin >2000 mcg per mL, MIC gentamicin >500–2000 mcg per mL, no resistance to penicillin	Enterococci, high-level aminoglycoside resistance	Pen G or AMP IV as above times 8–12 wks (approx. 50% cure)		10–25% E. faecalis and 45–50% E. faecium resistant to high gent levels. May be sensitive to streptomycin, check MIC. Case report of success with combination of AMP, IMP, and vanco (Scand J Inf Dis 29:628, 1997).
Enterococci: β-lactamase production test is **positive** and **no** gentamicin resistance	Enterococci, penicillin resistance	AM-SB 3 gm IV q6h PLUS gentamicin 1–1.5 mg per kg q8h IV times 4–6 wks. Low dose of gent	AM-SB 3 gm IV q6h PLUS vanco 15 mg per kg IV q12h (check levels if >2 gm) times 4–6 wks	β-lactamase not detected by MIC tests with standard inocula. Detection requires testing with the chromogenic cephalosporin nitrocefin. **Once-q24h gentamicin rx not** efficacious in animal model of E. faecalis endocarditis (JAC 49:437, 2002).
Enterococci: β-lactamase test neg., pen G/AMP resistance	Enterococci, intrinsic pen G/AMP resistance	Vanco 15 mg per kg IV q12h (check levels if >2 gm) PLUS gent 1–1.5 mg per kg q8h IV times 4–6 wks (see Comment)		Desired vanco serum levels: peak 20–50 mcg per mL, trough 5–12 mcg per mL. Gentamicin used for synergy; peak levels need not exceed 4 mcg per mL.
Enterococci: Pen/AMP resistant + high-level gent/strep resistant + vanco resistant, usually VRE **No reliable cidal regimen suggested**	Enterococci, vanco-resistant, usually E. faecium	No reliable effective rx. Can try quinupristin-dalfopristin (Synercid) or linezolid—see Comment, footnote1, and Table 6	Teicoplanin active against a subset of vanco-resistant enterococcus. Teicoplanin is not available in U.S.	Synercid activity limited to E. faecium and is usually bacteriostatic, therefore expect high relapse rate. Dose: 7.5 mg per kg IV (via central line) q8h. Linezolid active most enterococci, but bacteriostatic. Dose: 600 mg IV or q12h times 4–6 wks. Linezolid failed in all of E. faecalis endocarditis (CID 37:e29, 2003).
Staphylococcal endocarditis Aortic and/or mitral valve infection—MSSA	Staph. aureus, methicillin sensitive	Nafcillin (oxacillin) 2 gm IV q4h times 4–6 wks PLUS gentamicin 1 mg per kg IV q8h times 3–5 days	(Cefazolin 2 gm IV q8h times 4–6 wks) PLUS gentamicin 1 mg per kg IV q8h times 3–5 days) Low dose of gent	If IgE-mediated penicillin allergy; 10% cross-reactivity to cephalosporins (AnIM 141:16, 2004). Cefazolin failures reported (CID 37:1194, 2003). No definitive data, pro or con, on once-q24h gentamicin for S. aureus endocarditis. May need TEE to detect endocarditis. 23% of S. aureus bacteremia in association with IV catheter had endocarditis (CID 115:106 & 115, 1999). If TEE neg., may only need 2 wks of therapy.
Aortic and/or mitral valve—MRSA	Staph. aureus, methicillin resistant	Vanco 15 mg IV q12h times 4–6 wks	Dapto 6 mg per kg IV q24h times 4–6 wks	Quinupristin-dalfopristin cidal if both components active (both active if S. aureus sensitive to erythro in vitro). Other alternatives less desirable because bacteriostatic, e.g., TMP-SMX, clinda, linezolid. See Table 6.
Tricuspid valve infection (usually IVDUs): MSSA *(MRSA, next page)*	Staph. aureus, methicillin sensitive	Nafcillin (oxacillin) 2 gm IV q4h PLUS gentamicin 1 mg per kg IV q8h times 2 wks. NOTE: low dose of gent	If penicillin allergy: Not clear. High failure rate with 2-week regimen of vanco + gentamicin (CID 33:120, 2001). Can try longer duration rx if sensitive) **OR RIF** (if sensitive)	**For left-sided MRSA recommended rx if metastatic infection (e.g., osteo) or left-sided endocarditis.** 2 reports of success with **4-week oral** regimen: CIP 750 mg bid + RIF 300 mg bid. Less than 10% pts had MRSA (Ln 2:1071, 1989; AJM 101:68, 1996).

---

¹ Three interesting trend reports: (1) Successful rx of vanco-resistant E. faecium prosthetic valve endocarditis (CID 25:163, 1997), (2) resistance to Synercid emerged during therapy of E. faecium (CID 24:90, 1997), and (3) super-infection with E. faecalis occurred during Synercid rx of E. faecium (CID 24:91, 1997).
† NOTE: Alt. regimens are for adults (unless otherwise indicated) and assume normal renal function.

Abbreviations on page 2

TABLE 1 (20)

ANATOMIC SITE/DIAGNOSIS/MODIFYING CIRCUMSTANCES	ETIOLOGIES (usual)	SUGGESTED REGIMENS*		ADJUNCT DIAGNOSTIC OR THERAPEUTIC MEASURES AND COMMENTS
		PRIMARY	ALTERNATIVE†	
HEART, Infective endocarditis-Native valve-culture positive/Staphylococcal endocarditis/Tricuspid valve infection *(continued)*				
Methicillin resistant (MRSA)	Staph. aureus, methicillin-resistant	**Vanco** 15 mg per kg IV q12h (check levels if >2 gm per day) **times 4-6 wks**	Fails/intolerant to vanco, can try daptomycin, quinu-gm dalfo, or linezolid	For MRSA, no difference in duration of bacteremia or fever between pts with vanco or **vanco + RIF** (AnIM 115:674, 1991). **Daptomycin:** Endocarditis studies in progress. **Linezolid** Bacteriostatic. See Table 6.
Slow-growing fastidious Gm-neg. bacilli	HACEK group (see Comments) (change to HACEK if add Bartonella)	**Ceftriaxone 2 gm IV q24h times 4 wks**	**AMP** 12 gm/24h (continuous or div q4h) **times 4 wks + gentamicin** 1 mg per kg IV/IM q8h **times 4 wks**	**HACEK:** Haemophilus parainfluenzae, **H. aphrophilus, Actinobacillus, Cardiobacterium, Eikenella, Kingella).** H. aphrophilus resistant to vanco, clinda and methicillin. Penicillinase-positive HACEK organisms should be susceptible to AM-SB + gentamicin. For haemophilus, see CID 24:1087, 1997.
Bartonella species (for bacteremia, see page 43 — Urban trench fever) AAC 48:1921, 2004	B. henselae, B. quintana	Optimal rx evolving. Retrospective & open prospective trials support **gentamicin** 3 mg per kg IV once q24h times 14 days + **doxy** 100 mg po bid times 4-6 wks		**Dx:** Immunofluorescent antibody titer ≥1:800; blood cultures only occ. positive, or PCR of tissue from surgery. **Surgery:** Over ½ pts require valve surgery: relation to cure unclear. B. quintana transmitted by body lice among homeless; asymptomatic colonization of RBCs described (Ln 360:226, 2002)
Infective endocarditis—"culture negative" Fever, valvular disease, and ECHO vegetations ± embolic and neg. cultures. Rev. Medicine 84:162, 2005	Etiology in 348 cases identified by serology, culture, histopath, & molecular detection: C. burnetti 48%, Bartonella sp. 28%, and rarely (Abiotrophia elegans, Mycoplasma hominis, Legionella pneumophila, Tropheryma whipplei—together 1%), & rest without etiology identified (most on antibiotic).			Early surgical consultation advised. Watch for evidence of heart failure.
Infective endocarditis—Prosthetic valve—empiric therapy (cultures pending)				
Early (<2 months post-op)	S. epidermidis, S. aureus. Rarely, Enterobacteriaceae, diphtheroids, fungi	**Vanco** 15 mg per kg IV q12h **+ gentamicin** 1 mg per kg IV q8h **+ RIF** 600 mg po q24h		If S. epidermidis is susceptible to nafcillin/oxacillin, then substitute nafcillin (or oxacillin) for vanco.
Late (>2 months post-op)	S. epidermidis, viridans strep, enterococci, S. aureus			
Infective endocarditis—Prosthetic valve—positive blood cultures	Staph. epidermidis	(**Vanco** 15 mg per kg IV q12h **times 6 wks + gentamicin** 1 mg per kg IV q8h **times 14 days**		
	Staph. aureus	Methicillin sensitive: (**Nafcillin** 2 gm IV q4h + **RIF** 300 mg q8h) **times 6 wks + gentamicin** 1 mg per kg IV q8h **times 14 days.** Methicillin resistant: (**Vanco** 1 gm IV q12h + **RIF** 300 mg po q8h) **times 6 wks + gentamicin** 1 mg per kg IV q8h **times 14 days.**		In theory, could substitute CIP for APAG, but no clinical data.
	Viridans strep, enterococci	See infective endocarditis, native valve, culture positive, pages 21–23		
	Enterobacteriaceae or P. aeruginosa	**Aminoglycoside** (tobra IV Table 11) **+ P or AP Ceph 3** AP or P Ceph f		*(Table 11, page 77)*
	Candida, aspergillus	**Ampho B** ± **an azole** e.g. fluconazole (Table 11, page 77)		High mortality. Valve replacement plus antifungal therapy standard therapy but some success with antifungal therapy alone (CID 22:262, 1996).
Infective endocarditis—Q fever LnID 3:709, 2003	Coxiella burnetii	**Doxy** 100 mg po bid **+ hydroxychloroquine** 600 mg per day times 1.5-3 yrs (J Infection 45:127, 2002)		**Dx:** Complement-fix IgG antibody of 1:40 to phase II diagnostic of acute Q fever. IgG C-F antibody of 1:200 to phase I antigen diagnostic of chronic Q fever (LnID 3:709, 2003). Want doxy serum conc. >5 mcg per mL (JID 188:1322, 2003).
Intracardiac-device related infections: Pacemaker/defibrillator, left ventricular assist device LnID 3:709, 2003	S. aureus, S. epidermidis, rarely others	**Device removal + vanco** 1 gm IV q12h + **RIF** 300 mg po bid	**Device removal + dapto** 6 mg per kg IV q24h[MSSA & MR] + **RIF** (no data)	**Duration of rx after device removal:** For "pocket" or subcutaneous infection, 10-14 days. If lead-assoc. endocarditis, 4-6 wks depending on organism. Refs.: Circulation 108:2015, 2003; NEJM 350:1422, 2004.

† **Daptomycin** 6 mg per kg IV q24h; **Linezolid** 600 mg IV or po q12h. **Quinupristin/dalfopristin** (Synercid) 7.5 mg per kg IV q8h.   NOTE: *All dosage recommendations are for adults (unless otherwise indicated) and assume normal renal function.*

Abbreviations on page 2.

TABLE 1 (21)

ANATOMIC SITE/DIAGNOSIS/ MODIFYING CIRCUMSTANCES	ETIOLOGIES (usual)	SUGGESTED REGIMENS* PRIMARY	ALTERNATIVE†	ADJUNCT DIAGNOSTIC OR THERAPEUTIC MEASURES AND COMMENTS
HEART (continued)				
Pericarditis, purulent—empiric rx *Rev. Medicine pg. 385, 2003*	Staph. aureus, Strep. pneumoniae, Group A strep, Enterobacteriaceae	**Vanco + CIP** (Dosage, see footnote*)	**Vanco + CFP** (see footnote*)	Drainage required if signs of tamponade. Forced to use empiric vanco due to high prevalence of MRSA.
Rheumatic fever with carditis *Ref.: Ln 366:155, 2005* *For acute rheumatic fever, see page 44; reactive arthritis, below*	Post-infectious sequelae of Group A strep infection (usually pharyngitis)	ASA, and usually prednisone for symptomatic treatment of fever, arthritis, arthralgia. May not influence carditis.		Clinical features: Carditis, polyarthritis, chorea, subcutaneous nodules, erythema marginatum. For Jones criteria: see page 44. Prophylaxis: see page 44
JOINT—Also see Lyme Disease, page 42				
Reactive arthritis Reiter's syndrome (See Comment for definition)	Occurs wks after infection with C. trachomatis, Campylobacter jejuni, Yersinia enterocolitica, Shigella/Salmonella sp.	Only treatment is non-steroidal anti-inflammatory drugs		Definition: Urethritis, conjunctivitis, arthritis, and sometimes uveitis and rash. Arthritis: asymmetrical oligoarthritis of ankles, knees, feet, sacroiliitis. Rash: palms and soles—keratoderma blennorrhagica, circinate balanitis of glans penis. HLA-B27 positive predisposes to Reiter's.
Post-streptococcal reactive arthritis (See Rheumatic fever, above)	Immunologic reaction after strep pharyngitis: (1) arthritis onset in <10 days, (2) lasts months, (3) unresponsive to ASA	Treat strep pharyngitis and then NSAIDs (prednisone needed in some pts)		A reactive arthritis after a β-hemolytic strep infection in absence of sufficient Jones criteria for acute rheumatic fever. Ref.: Mayo Clin Proc 75:144, 2000.
Septic arthritis: Treatment requires both adequate drainage of purulent joint fluid and appropriate antimicrobial therapy. Review Gram stain of joint fluid. For full differential, see LN 357:1998. **Infants <3 months (neonate)**	Staph. aureus, Enterobacteriaceae, Group B strep, N. gonorrhoeae	**If MRSA no concern: (Nafcillin or oxacillin) + P Ceph 3** (Dosage, see Table 16, page 133)	**If MRSA concern: Vanco + P Ceph 3**	There is no need to inject antimicrobials into joints. Empiric therapy after collection of blood and joint fluid for culture. Adjacent bone involved in 2/3 pts. Group B strep and gonococcus most common community-acquired etiologies.
Children (3 months–14 years) See Table 16 for dosage	Staph. aureus 27%, S. pyogenes & S. pneumo 14%, H. influenzae, Gm-neg bacilli 6%, other (GC, N. meningitidis) 14%, unknown 36%	**Vanco + P Ceph 3** until culture results available See Table 16 for dosage Steroids ?—see Comment		Marked ↓ in H. influenzae since use of conjugate vaccine. NOTE: Septic arthritis due to salmonella has no association with sickle cell disease, unlike salmonella osteomyelitis. Duration of treatment varies with specific microbial etiology. Short-course steroid: Benefit reported (PIDJ 22:883, 2003).
Adults (review Gram stain)				
Acute monoarticular At risk for sexually-transmitted disease	N. gonorrhoeae (see page 17), S. aureus, streptococci, rarely aerobic Gm-neg. bacilli	**Gram stain negative: Ceftriaxone** 1 gm IV q24h or **cefotaxime** 1 gm IV q8h or **ceftizoxime** 1 gm IV q8h	**If Gram stain shows Gm-+ cocci in clusters—add vanco** 1 gm IV q12h	For GC comments, see Disseminated GC, page 17
Not at risk for sexually-transmitted disease	S. aureus, streptococci, Gm-neg. bacilli	**All empiric choices guided by Gram stain: Vanco + P Ceph 3** For treatment duration, see Tables 2, 11, & 12	**Vanco + (CIP or Levo)** For dosage, see footnote page 25	Differential includes gout and chondrocalcinosis (pseudogout). Look for crystals in joint fluid. NOTE: See Table 6 for MRSA treatment.
Chronic monoarticular	Brucella, nocardia, mycobacteria, fungi			
Polyarticular, usually acute	Gonococci, B. burgdorferi, acute rheumatic fever, viruses, e.g., hepatitis B, rubella (vaccine), parvo B19	**Gonococci:** Gram stain usually negative for GC. If sexually active, culture urethra, cervix, anal canal, throat, blood, joint fluid, and then **ceftriaxone** 1 gm IV q24h	See Tables 2, 11, & 12	If GC, usually associated petechiae and/or pustular skin lesions and tenosynovitis. Consider Lyme disease if exposure areas known to harbor infected ticks. See page 42. Expanded differential includes gout, pseudogout, reactive arthritis (HLA-B27 pos.).

* **APAG** (see Table 10D, page 74), **IMP** 0.5 gm IV q6h, **MER** 1 gm IV q8h, **nafcillin** or **oxacillin** 2 gm IV q4h, **TC-CL** 3.1 gm IV q6h or 4.5 gm q8h, **AM-SB** 3 gm IV q6h, **P Ceph 1** (**cephalothin** 2 gm IV q4h or **cefazolin** 2 gm IV q8h), **CIP** 750 mg po bid or 400 mg IV q8h, **vanco** 1 gm IV q12h, **PIP-TZ** 3.375 gm IV q6h or 4.5 gm q8h, **RIF** 600 mg po q24h, **aztreonam** 2 gm IV q8h, **CFP** 2 gm IV q12h
NOTE: All dosage recommendations are for adults (unless otherwise indicated) and assume normal renal function.

Abbreviations on page 2

ANATOMIC SITE/DIAGNOSIS/MODIFYING CIRCUMSTANCES	ETIOLOGIES (usual)	SUGGESTED REGIMENS*		ADJUNCT DIAGNOSTIC OR THERAPEUTIC MEASURES AND COMMENTS
		PRIMARY	ALTERNATIVE†	
JOINT (continued)				
Septic arthritis, post intra-articular injection	MSSE/MRSE 40%, MSSA/MRSA 20%, P. aeruginosa, Propionibacteria	**NO empiric therapy.** Arthroscopy for culture/sensitivity, crystals.		Treat based on culture results x14 days (assumes no foreign body present).
Infected prosthetic joint *CID 36:1157, 2003; JAC 53:127, 2004; NEJM 351:1645, 2004*	See below	**No empiric therapy.** Need culture & sens. results. Surgical options in Comment.		**Surgical options: 1. 2-stage:** Remove infected prosthesis, then new prosthesis. Highest cure rate **2. 1-stage: Remove infected prosthesis, debride, new prosthesis, then antimicrobics. 3. Extensive debridement & leave prosthesis in place.** Antimicrobic therapy:
	S. pyogenes; Gps A, G, or B; S. viridans strep	Debridement & prosthesis retention; **Pen G** or **ceftriax** IV times 4 wks. Last 17/19 pts *(CID 36:847, 2003)*		Other: retain prosthesis & treat ± bone fusion of joint. Last: Chronic oral suppression
See surgical options in Comments	MSSE/MSSA	**Nafcillin/oxacillin** IV + (**RIF** po) times 6 wks	(**Vanco** IV + **RIF** po) times 6 wks	**RIF**-based therapy only in chronic oral suppression
Drug dosages in footnote¹	MRSE/MRSA	(**Vanco** IV + **RIF** po) times 6 wks	(**CIP** or **Levo** - if susceptible-po) + (**RIF** po) **OR** (**linezolid** po) times 6 wks	**RIF** bactericidal vs surface-adhering, slow-growing, & biofilm-producing bacteria. Never use RIF alone due to rapid development of resistance. Limited linezolid experience favorable *(JAC 55:387, 2005).* Watch for toxicity. Table 10C, page 70.
	P. aeruginosa	**Ceftaz** IV + (**CIP** or **Levo** po)		*AAC 39:2423, 1995*
Rheumatoid arthritis	TNF inhibitors (adalimumab, etanercept, infliximab)	↑ risk of TBc, fungal infection *(CID 38:1261, 2004).* Treat latent TBc: first *(MMWR 53:683, 2004)*		
Septic bursitis; Olecranon bursitis; prepatellar bursitis	Staph. aureus >80%, M. tuberculosis (rare), M. marinum (rare)	(**Nafcillin** or **oxacillin** 2 gm IV q4h or **dicloxacillin** 500 mg po qid) if MSSA	(**Vanco** 1 gm IV q12h or **linezolid** 600 mg po bid) if MRSA	**Initially aspirate q24h and treat for a minimum of 2-3 weeks.** If recurrence, surgical excision of bursa—should not be necessary often if treated for at least 3 weeks.¹ Ref.: *Semin Arth & Rheum 24:391, 1995*
KIDNEY, BLADDER AND PROSTATE *[For review, see AJM 113(Suppl 1A):1S, 2002 & NEJM 349:259, 2003]*			*Other doses, see footnote page 26*	
Acute uncomplicated urinary tract infection (cystitis-urethritis) in females [NOTE: Routine urine culture not necessary, self-rx works *(AnIM 135:9, 2001)*]. Try to spare FQs *(CID 39:75, 2004)*	Enterobacteriaceae (E. coli), Staph. saprophyticus, enterococci	**TMP-SMX-DS** bid times 3 days; if sulfa allergy, **NF** times 7 days or **fosfomycin** single dose	Local IL. coli resistant to TMP-SMX <20%, use sulfonamides. Local IL. coli resistant to TMP-SMX >20%, use FQ. If sulfa allergy, then 3 days of **CIP** 250 mg, **CIP-ER** 500 mg q24h, **Gati** 200 mg q24h, **Levo** 250 mg q24h. **Do not use Moxi or Gemi.**	1-day rx recommended (discontinue or do not use sulfonamides (TMP-SMX) or nitrofurantoin (NF)) because of potential ↑ in kernicterus). If failure on 3-day course, culture and rx 2 weeks. **Fosfomycin** *(CID 39:66, 1997).* Fosfo active vs E. faecalis; poor activity vs other coliforms *(Med Lett 39:66, 1997).* **Moxifloxacin & gemifloxacin:** Neither approved for UTIs. Do not use; inadequate urine concentration. **Phenazopyridine (Pyridium)**—non-prescription;—may relieve dysuria. 200 mg po tid times 2 days. Hemolysis if G6PD deficient.
Risk factors for STD: Dipstick: positive leukocyte esterase or hemoglobin, neg. Gram stain	C. trachomatis	**Doxy** 100 mg po bid times 7 days	**Azithro** 1 gm po single dose	Pelvic exam for vaginitis & herpes simplex, urine LCR/PCR for GC and C. trachomatis.
Recurrent (3 or more episodes/year) in young women	Any of the above bacteria	Eradicate infection, then **TMP-SMX-DS** tab po q24h long term	**TMP-SMX** 1 single-strength tab po q24h	A cost-effective alternative to continuous prophylaxis is self-administered single dose rx (TMP-SMX DS, 2 tabs, 320/1600 mg) at symptom onset. Another alternative: 1 DS tablet TMP-SMX post-coitus.
Child: ≤5 yrs old and grade 3-4 reflux	Coliforms	**TMP-SMX** (2 mg TMP/10 mg SMX) per kg po q24h	**nitrofurantoin** 2 mg per kg po q24h	CIP approved as alternative drug ages 1–17 yrs.
Recurrent UTI in postmenopausal women *See JAGS 30:152, 2000*	E. coli & other Enterobacteriaceae, enterococci, S. saprophyticus	Evaluate for potentially correctable urologic factors—see **Comment**		Definition: ≥3 culture + symptomatic UTIs in 1 yr or 2 UTIs in 6 months. Urologic factors: (1) cystocele, (2) incontinence, (3) ↑ residual urine volume (≥50 mL). NF more effective than vaginal cream in decreasing frequency, but Editors worry about pulmonary fibrosis with long-term NF rx *(CID 36:1362, 2003).*

¹ **Aqueous Pen G** 2 million units IV q4h; **ceftriaxone** 2 gm IV q24h, **nafcillin** or **oxacillin** 2 gm IV q4h, **vancomycin** 1 gm IV q12h, **RIF** 300 mg IV/po bid, **CIP** 400 mg IV/po q12h, **Levo** 750 mg IV/po q24h, **ceftazidime** 2 gm IV q8h

Abbreviations on page 2.

NOTE: All dosage recommendations are for adults (unless otherwise indicated) and assume normal renal function.

TABLE 1 (23)

ANATOMIC SITE/DIAGNOSIS/ MODIFYING CIRCUMSTANCES	ETIOLOGIES (usual)	SUGGESTED REGIMENS* PRIMARY	ALTERNATIVE†	ADJUNCT DIAGNOSTIC OR THERAPEUTIC MEASURES AND COMMENTS
KIDNEY, BLADDER AND PROSTATE (continued)				
Acute uncomplicated pyelonephritis, usually in women 18–40 yrs. temperature >102°F, definite costovertebral tenderness). Report of involving urinary syndrome or as result of conditions producing Gm+. E. coli (NEJM 335:465, 1996). **If male, look for obstructive uropathy or other complicating pathology.**				
Moderately ill (outpatient)	Enterobacteriaceae (most likely E. coli), enterococci (Gram stain of **uncentrifuged urine** may allow identification of Gm+/neg. bacilli vs Gm+ cocci)	An FQ po times 7 days: CIP 500 mg bid or CIP-ER 1000 mg po q24h. **Gati** 400 mg q24h, **Levo** 250 mg q24h, **Ofloxa** 400 mg bid	AM-CL, O Ceph. or TMP-SMX-DS Treat for 14 days.	In randomized double-blind trial, bacteriologic and **clinical success higher for 7 days of CIP than for 14 days TMP-SMX**; failures correlated with in vitro resistance to TMP-SMX. (JAMA 283:1583, 2000). Since CIP worked with 7-day rx, suspect other FQs effective with 7 d. of rx. Do not use Moxi or Gemi due to low urine concentrations.
NOTE: Increasing resistance of E. coli to both TMP-SMX & FQs is a concern				
Hospitalized	E. coli most common, enterococci 2° in frequency	FQ (IV) or (AMP + gentamicin) or P Ceph 3 or AP Pen. Treat for 14 days. Do not use cephalosporins for suspect or proven enterococcal infection	TC-CL or AM-SB or PIP-TZ or ERTA. Treat for 14 days. Dosages in footnotes¹ For dosages, see footnote¹	Treat IV until pt afebrile 24–48 hrs, then complete 2-wk course with oral drugs (as Moderately ill, above). If no clinical improvement in 3 days, we recommend imaging. On CT if single focal lesion avg. response requires 6 d., if lesions diffuse avg. response 13 days. (AJM 93:289, 1992). **If pt hypotensive, prompt imaging (Echo or CT) is recommended to ensure absence of obstructive uropathy.** **NOTE: Cephalosporins & ertapenem not active vs enterococci.**
Complicated UTI/catheters Obstruction, reflux, azotemia, transplant, Foley catheter-related	Enterobacteriaceae, P. aeruginosa, enterococci	Switch to po FQ or TMP-SMX when possible		Rule out obstruction. Watch out for enterococci and P. aeruginosa—not all listed drugs have predictable activity. CIP-ER oral dose: 1000 mg po q24h
Asymptomatic bacteriuria. IDSA Guidelines: CID 40:643, 2005				
Preschool children		Base regimen on C&S, not empirical		Diagnosis requires ≥10^5 CFU per mL urine of same bacterial species in 2 specimens obtained 3–7 days apart.
Pregnancy	Aerobic Gm-neg. bacilli & Staph. hemolyticus	Screen 1st trimester. If positive, rx 3 days with **amox**, **NF**, O Ceph. **TMP-SMX**, or **TMP** alone		Screen monthly for recurrence. Some authorities treat continuously until delivery (stop TMP-SMX 2 wks before EDC). ↑ resistance of E. coli to TMP-SMX.
Before and after invasive urologic intervention, e.g., Foley catheter	Aerobic Gm-neg. bacilli	Obtain urine culture and then rx 3 days with TMP-SMX DS		In one study, single dose 2-TMP-SMX 80% effective (AnIM 114:713, 1991). Use of silver-alloy Foley catheter may ↓ risk of clinically significant bacteriuria (AJM 105:236, 1998; AJM 160:3294, 2000).
Neurogenic bladder		No rx in asymptomatic; intermittent catheterization if possible		Ref. AJM 113(1A):67S, 2002—Bacteriuria in spinal cord injured patient.
Asymptomatic, advanced age, male or female		No rx indicated unless in conjunction with surgery to correct obstructive uropathy		Chronic pyelo with abnormal inflammatory response. See CID 29:444, 1999
Malacoplakia	E. coli	Bethanechol chloride + (CIP or TMP-SMX)		
Perinephric abscess				
Associated with staphylococcal bacteremia	Staph. aureus	Nafcillin/oxacillin or P Ceph 1 (Oxa- + Vanco if cillin, see footnote page 24)	MSSA MRSA	Drainage, surgical or image-guided aspiration
Associated with pyelonephritis	Enterobacteriaceae	See pyelonephritis, complicated UTI, above		Drainage, surgical or image-guided aspiration
Prostatitis		See prostatitis, page 23		
Spinal cord injury pts with UTI	E. coli, Klebsiella sp., enterococcus	CIP 250 mg po bid times 14 days		Suspect assoc. pyelonephritis, in RDBPC* trial microbiologic cure greater after 14 vs 3 days of CIP (CID 39:658 & 665, 2004)

¹ **NOTE:** bid = twice a day, tid = 3 times a day, qid = 4 times a day   * RDBPC = Randomized double-blind placebo-controlled

AM-CL: 875/125 mg q12h or 500/125 mg po tid or 2000/125 mg po q12h; **aztreonam** 2 gm IV q8h; **Gati** 400 mg q24h; **Levo** (250 mg po q24h for mild uncomplicated disease, 500 mg IV q24h for hospital pt), **cefotaxim** 2.0 gm IV q8h, **P Ceph 3 [cefotaxime** 1 gm IV q12h for uncomplicated infections, up to 2 gm IV q4h for life-threatening infections; **ceftriaxone** 1 gm IV q24h (use 2 gm q24h for meningitis)], **AP Pen [PIP** 3 gm IV q6h], **AM-SB** 3 gm IV q6h, **PIP-TZ** 3.375 gm IV q6h or for nosocomial pneumonia 4.5 gm IV q6h; **gentamicin** (see page 65), **O Ceph [cefpodoxime** 200 mg po q12h; **cefdinir** 300 mg po q12h; **cefpodoxime** 100 mg po q12h], **TMP-SMX-DS** (160/800 mg po q12h), **Ceph 4, P Ceph 3, AP Pen] O oral cephalosporin** dosages; see Table 10C, page 69. **Metronidazole** 500 mg po q6h or 15 mg per kg IV q12h (max. 4 gm per **Nafcillin or oxacillin** 2 gm IV q4h; **Dicloxacillin** 500 mg po q6h times 14 days day); **Vanco** 1 gm IV q12h, **linezolid** 600 mg IV/po q12h.

TABLE 1 (24)

ANATOMIC SITE/DIAGNOSIS/ MODIFYING CIRCUMSTANCES	ETIOLOGIES (usual)	SUGGESTED REGIMENS* PRIMARY	ALTERNATIVE†	ADJUNCT DIAGNOSTIC OR THERAPEUTIC MEASURES AND COMMENTS
LIVER (for spontaneous bacterial peritonitis, see page 34)				
Cholangitis		See Gallbladder, page 13		
Hepatic abscess Pyogenic abscess ref. CID 39:7654, 2004	Enterobacteriaceae (esp. Klebsiella sp.), bacteroides, enterococci, Entamoeba histolytica, Yersinia enterocolitica (rare) For echinococcus, see Table 13, page 102. For cat-scratch disease (CSD), see pages 55.	**Metro + (P Ceph 3 or cefoxitin or TC-CL or PIP-TZ or AM-SB or FQ)** or **AMP + APAG + metro** traditional & effective but AMP-resistant Gm-neg. bacilli increasing.	**Metro** (for amoeba) + either **IMP or MER** (Dosage, see footnote page 26)	Serological tests for amebiasis should be done on all patients; if neg. surgical drainage or percutaneous aspiration. In pyogenic abscess, if one identifiable GI source or underlying biliary tract disease. If amoeba serology positive, treat with metro alone without surgery. Metro included for both E. histolytica & pyogenic liver abscess (CID 18:938, 1994); regimens listed are effective for yersinia. **Hepatomatosis** associated with Yersinia enterocolitica liver abscess (CID 18:938, 1994); regimens listed are effective for yersinia.
Leptospirosis	Leptospirosis, see page 43			
Peliosis hepatis in AIDS pts	Bartonella henselae and B. quintana			Leptospirosis, see page 43
Post-transplant biloma (CID 39:517, 2004)	Enterococci (incl. VRE), candida, Gm-neg. bacilli (P. aeruginosa 8%), anaerobes	**Linezolid** 600 mg IV bid + **CIP** 400 mg IV q24h + **fluconazole** 400 mg IV q24h	**Dapto** 6 mg per kg per day + **Levo** 750 mg IV q24h + **fluconazole** 400 mg IV q24h	Suspect if fever & abdominal pain post-transplant. Exclude hepatic artery thrombosis. Presence of candida and/or VRE bad prognosticators.
UGI bleeding & cirrhosis		**CIP** 500 mg IV/po bid times 7 days. Cautious support from recent meta-analysis: Cochrane Database 2002 (2): CD002907.		
Viral hepatitis	Hepatitis A, B, C, D, E, G	See Table 14		
LUNG/Bronchi				
Bronchiolitis/wheezy bronchitis (respiratory wheezing) Infants/children (≤ age 5) See RSV, Table 14B(3)	Respiratory syncytial virus (RSV) 50%, parainfluenza 25%, other viruses 20%	Antibiotics not useful, mainstay of rx is oxygen. Ribavirin of no benefit (AJRCCM 160:829, 1999). 2 products available for treatment: RSV-immune globulin and a humanized monoclonal antibody, palivizumab. See Table 14, page 113		RSV most important. Rapid dx with antigen detection methods. Ribavirin: No data on IV ribavirin but little enthusiasm. Emphasis now on vaccine development and preventive modulation with immunoglobulins. Reviews: PIDJ 18:773, 2000; Red Book of Peds 2003, 26th Ed.
Bronchitis				
Infants/children (≤ age 5)	< Age 2: Adenovirus; age 2-5: Respiratory syncytial virus, parainfluenza 3 virus	Antibiotics indicated only with associated sinusitis or heavy growth on throat culture for S. pneumo, Group A strep, H. influenzae or no improvement in 1 week. Otherwise rx is symptomatic.		
Adolescents and adults with acute tracheobronchitis (Acute bronchitis)	Usually viral. M. pneumoniae 5%, C. pneumoniae 5%. See Persistent cough below.	Antibiotics not indicated. Antitussive ± inhaled bronchodilator.		Purulent sputum alone not an indication for antibiotic rx. Azithro was no better than low-dose vitamin C in a controlled trial (Ln 359:1648, 2002). Expect cough to last 2 weeks. If fever/rigors, get chest x-ray.
Persistent cough (>14 d.), afebrile during community outbreak: Pertussis (whooping cough) 10-25% adults with cough >14 d. have pertussis (CID 32:1691, 2001). Rev: LnID 2:744, 2002	Bordetella pertussis & occ. Bordetella parapertussis. Also consider asthma, gastroesophageal reflux, post-nasal drip	**Peds doses: Azithro**-**clarithro** (dose in footnote¹) OR **erythro esto-late** 40 mg per kg per day po q6-8h times 14 days OR **erythro base** po 40 mg per kg per day div 4x. **See footnote¹**	**Adult doses: Azithro** 500 mg day 1, 1,250 mg q24h times 2-5 OR **erythro esto-late** 500 mg po qid times 14 days OR **TMP-SMX-DS** tab po bid times14 days OR **clarithro** 500 mg po bid or **div** q12h times 14 days. **See footnote¹**	**M. pneumoniae & C. pneumoniae rare (LnID 1:334, 2001. Rare pt with true C. pneumo infection may require 6 wks of clarithro to clear organism (J Med Micro 52:265, 2003).** **3 stages of illness**: catarrhal (1-2 wks), paroxysmal coughing (2-4 wks), and convalescence (1-2 wks). Treatment may abort or eliminate pertussis in catarrhal stage, but does not shorten paroxysmal stage. Diagnosis: PCR on nasopharyngeal secretions or (pertussis immune)PCR. **Rx aimed at eradication of NP carriage.** Azithro works fastest (PIDJ 22:847, 2003). Hypertrophic pyloric stenosis reported in infants under 6 wks of age given erythro (MMWR 48:1117, 1999).
Prophylaxis of household contacts		**Erythromycin—Children: clarithro** 7.5 mg per kg po q12h times 14 days. **Alternative: clarithro** 7.5 mg per kg po q12h times 14 days. **Adults: clarithro** 500 mg po q6h times 14 days. **See footnote²**		Recommended by Am. Acad. Ped. Red Book 2003 for all household or close contacts. community-wide prophylaxis not recommended.

¹ Peds doses: azithro 10 mg per kg per day on day 1, then 5 mg per kg per day times 4 days (PIDJ 22:847, 2003) or clarithro 7.5 mg per kg po q12h times 5-7 days.
² Peds doses: azithro 10 mg per kg per day on day 1, then 5 mg per kg per day times 4 days or clarithro 7.5 mg per kg po q12h times 5-7 days.

Compliance with erythro hard due to nausea/vomiting, clarithro costs more but compliance should be better.

Abbreviations on page 2.   NOTE: All dosage recommendations are for adults (unless otherwise indicated) and assume normal renal function.

TABLE 1 (25)

ANATOMIC SITE/DIAGNOSIS/ MODIFYING CIRCUMSTANCES	ETIOLOGIES (usual)	SUGGESTED REGIMENS* PRIMARY	ALTERNATIVE[1]	ADJUNCT DIAGNOSTIC OR THERAPEUTIC MEASURES AND COMMENTS
LUNG/Bronchi/Bronchitis (continued) **Acute bacterial exacerbation of chronic bronchitis (ABECB), adults (almost always smokers with COPD)** Pertinent refs.: Chest 118: 193, 2000; NEJM 347:465, 2002; CID 26:809; 987; 2004; AJM 165:891, 2005	Viruses 20-50%, C. pneumoniae <1%; role of S. pneumo, H. influenzae & M. catarrhalis controversial. Tobacco use, air pollution contribute.	**Severe ABECB** = ↑ dyspnea, ↑ sputum viscosity/purulence, ↑ sputum volume. Severe low O₂ sat: (2) Inhaled anticholinergic bronchodilator, (3) Inhaled positive pressure ventilation amox, doxy, TMP-SMX, or O Ceph. **For severe disease,** AM-CL, azithro/clarithro, or O Ceph or telithro or FQs with enhanced activity vs drug-resistant S. pneumo (Gati, Gemi, Levo, or Moxi). **Drugs & doses:** See Comment and Table 10C. Placebo-controlled studies: Pul Pharm & Therap 14:449, 2001; Ln 358:2020, 2001		**Severe ABECB** (1) consider chest x-ray, esp. if febrile (3) oral corticosteroid; taper over 2 wks, (4) D/C tobacco use; (5) non-invasive positive pressure ventilation **For mild or moderate disease,** no antimicrobial treatment or maybe O Ceph or telithro or FQs with enhanced activity vs drug-resistant S. pneumoniae. Ref. PIDJ 22(Suppl):S150-S167, 2003.
Pneumonia **Neonatal: Birth to 1 month**	**Viruses:** CMV, rubella, H. simplex **Bacteria:** Group B strep, listeria, coliforms, S. aureus, P. aeruginosa **Other:** Chlamydia trachomatis, syphilis	**AMP + gentamicin ± cefotaxime.** Add **vanco** if MRSA a concern. For chlamydia rx, **erythro** 12.5 mg per kg po or IV qid times 14 days.		Blood cultures indicated. Consider C. trachomatis if afebrile pneumonia, staccato cough. IgM >1:8, rx with erythro or sulfisoxazole. If MRSA documented, **vanco. TMP-SMX, & linezolid** alternatives. **Linezolid** dosage birth to age 11 yrs is **10 mg per kg q8h.** Ref. PIDJ 22(Suppl):S150-S167, 2003.
CONSIDER TUBERCULOSIS IN ALL PATIENTS: ISOLATE ALL SUSPECT PATIENTS				
Age 1-3 months (Adapted from NEJM 346:429, 2002) Usually afebrile	C. trachomatis, RSV, parainfluenza virus 3, Bordetella, S. pneumoniae, S. aureus (rare)	**Outpatient: po erythro** 10 mg per kg q6h or **azithro** 10 mg per kg times 1 dose, then 5 mg per kg times 4 days.	**Inpatient: If afebrile erythro** 10 mg per kg IV q6h or **azithro** 2.5 mg per kg IV q12h (see Comment). **If febrile,** add **cefotaxime** 200 mg per kg per day div q8h **For RSV:** see bronchiolitis, page 27	Pneumonitis syndrome: cough, tachypnea, dyspnea, diffuse infiltrates, afebrile. Usually requires hospital care. Reports of hypertrophic pyloric stenosis after erythro use age 6 wks; not sure about azithro; but azithro dosing theoretically might ↑ risk of hypertrophic pyloric stenosis. If lobar pneumonia, give AMP 200-300 mg per kg per day div q6h for S. pneumoniae. No empiric coverage for S. aureus, as it is rare etiology.
Age 4 months-5 years Pneumonia syndrome. Usually afebrile Refs.: NEJM 346:429, 2002; Ln 364:1141, 2004	RSV, other resp. viruses, S. pneumo, H. flu, Mycoplasma, S. aureus (rare)	**Outpatient: Amox** 100 mg per kg per day div q8h **Inpatient (not ICU): Cefotaxime** 200 mg per kg per day IV or q8h or **ceftriaxone** 50-75 mg per kg per day IV once	**Inpatient (ICU):** (**Amox** 100 mg per kg per day) + (**azithro** 10 mg per kg IV q24h) **OR erythro** 500 mg per kg per day (Peds dose: <5 yrs old) **For RSV:** see bronchiolitis, page 27	Common "other" viruses: rhinovirus, influenza, parainfluenza, adenovirus (PIDJ 19: 293, 2000). Often of mild to moderate severity. S. pneumo, non-type B H. flu in 4-20%. Treat times 10-14 days. See footnote[1], footnote[3] page 27, footnote 2 page 29, and Table 5, page 56, for rx of drug-resistant S. pneumo.
Age 5-15 years, immunocompetent NEJM 346:429, 2002; PIDJ 21:592, 2002	Mycoplasma, Chlamydophila pneumoniae, S. pneumoniae, Mycobacterium tuberculosis Respiratory viruses: mixed, e.g., influenza. Bacterial/viral infection in 23% (Peds 113:701, 2004)	(**Amox** 100 mg per kg per day) + (**Clarithro** 500 mg po bid or 1 gm ER q24h. Peds dose: 7.5 mg per kg (q12h)) **OR** (**azithro** 0.5 gm po times 1, then 0.25 gm per day. Peds dose: 10 mg per kg times 1 day, then 5 mg per kg per day to day 5, max. 250 mg)	**Inpatient (not ICU):** No antibiotic if not afebrile. **Inpatient (ICU):** (**Amox** 100 mg per kg per day) + (**azithro** 10 mg per kg IV q24h po bid) if pt >8 yrs old) or **erythro** 500 mg per kg per day (Peds dose: <5 yrs old)	If otherwise healthy and not concomitant with (or post-) influenza. TB pneumonia is key, as it is uncommon in this subset; suspect S. pneumo if sudden onset and large amount of purulent sputum. **Macrolide-resistant S. pneumo** an issue. Higher prevalence of macrolide-resistant S. pneumo in pts <5 yrs old (JAMA 286:1857, 2001). Mycoplasma PCR/viral culture usually not done for outpatients. Erythro times 2-3 wks or AM-C. Pneumonian up to 6 wks. (LnID 1:334, 2001; J Med Micro 52:265, 2003). Linezolid approved for peds for pen-susceptible S. pneumo (including bacteremia) & methicillin-sensitive S. aureus.

See Comment regarding macrolide resistance

NOTE: bid = twice q24h; tid = 3 times a day; qid = 4 times a day

---

[1] **TMP-SMX** (standard double-strength tab (160 mg TMP) po bid, **doxy** 100 mg po bid; **amox** 500 mg po tid or 2000/125 mg po bid, adult dose of **O Ceph** (**cefaclor** 500 mg q8h or 500 mg **CD** (extended release) po q12h; **cefditoren** 200 mg tabs—2 tabs po bid, **cefixime** 400 mg po q24h, **cefpodoxime proxetil** 200 mg po q12h, **cefprozil** 500 mg po q12h, **loracarbef** 400 mg po q12h, **cefuroxime axetil** 250 or 500 mg po q12h, **cefdinir** 300 mg q12h or 600 mg q24h, **azithro** 500 mg po initial dose then 250 mg q24h times 4, or 500 mg po q24h times 3 days, **clarithro** 500 mg po q12h or **clarithro ER** 1000 mg po q24h times 7 days, **dirithromycin** 500 mg po q24h, **Oflox** 400 mg po q24h, **CIP** 750 mg po q24h times 5 days, **Gati** 400 mg po q24h, **Gemi** 320 mg po q24h, **Levo** 500 mg po q24h times 7 days. **Ketolide: Telithromycin** 800 mg po q24h times 5 days.
NOTE: CIP and telithro have relatively low in vitro activity vs S. pneumo.
NOTE: All dosage recommendations are for adults (unless otherwise indicated) and assume normal renal function.

Abbreviations on page 2

TABLE 1 (26)

ANATOMIC SITE/DIAGNOSIS/ MODIFYING CIRCUMSTANCES	ETIOLOGIES (usual)	SUGGESTED REGIMENS* PRIMARY	ALTERNATIVE†	ADJUNCT DIAGNOSTIC OR THERAPEUTIC MEASURES AND COMMENTS
LUNG/Pneumonia *(continued)* **Children, hospitalized, immunocompetent—2–18 yrs**	S. pneumoniae, viruses, mycoplasma, consider S. aureus with clinical setting.	**Ceftriaxone** 50 mg per kg per day IV (to max. 2 gm) per day OR 100 mg/kg/day (to 4 gm/day) IV q12–24h + **azithro** 10 mg per kg per day IV to 500 mg IV div q12h. Add anti-staph drug if evidence of lung necrosis		**Alternatives are a problem in children:** If proven S. pneumo resistant to azithro & cefotaxime or severe ceftriaxone allergy.) IV vanco; linezolid, or off-label respiratory FQ. No adq under age 8. Linezolid reported efficacious in children *(PIDJ 21:677, 2003)*. Cefuroxime failures vs drug-resistant S. pneumo *(CID 29:462, 1999)*.
Adults (over age 18)—See IDSA Guidelines *(CID 37:1405, 2003; Chest 125:1888 & 1913, 2004; AJM 117(3A):39S, 2004; Thorax 56(Suppl):1, 2001)* **Community-acquired, not hospitalized** Guidelines reflect variable approaches. **1.** Focus on S. pneumo, ignore atypicals, & emphasize **high dose amox** or **AM-CL**. **2.** If no co-morbidity, focus on atypicals & emphasize **macrolides** that are still active vs majority of S. pneumo **3.** Focus on both S. pneumo & atypicals by combining (**high dose amox** or **AM-CL**) with a **macrolide** OR suggesting a **respiratory FQ** OR **telithromycin**	**No co-morbidity:** S. pneumo, Mycoplasma pneumo, C. pneumo, H. influenzae, viral **Co-morbidity:** Alcoholism: S. pneumo, anaerobes, coliforms Bronchiectasis, e.g. Cystic fibrosis, page 32 COPD: H. influenzae, M. catarrhalis, S. pneumo IVDU: Hematogenous S. aureus Post-CVA aspiration: Oral flora, incl. S. pneumo Post-obstruction—e.g. S. pneumo, anaerobes Post-viral: e.g., influenza	**No co-morbidity present:** **Azithro** 0.5 gm po times 1, then 0.25 gm po qd x 4 days or **azithro-ER** 2 gm times 1 OR **clarithro** 500 mg po bid or **clarithro-ER** 1 gm po qd OR **doxy** 100 mg po bid **Co-morbidity:** (**azithro** or **clarithro**) + (**high dose amox** or **high dose AM-CL**) OR **cefdinir** or **cefpodoxime** or **cefprozil**) OR **telithromycin** **Duration of rx:** S. pneumo—Not bacteremic: until afebrile 3 days —Bacteremic: 10–14 days C. pneumoniae—Unclear. Some reports suggest 21 days. Some bronchitis pts required 5–6 wks of clarithro *(J Med Micro 52:265, 2003)* Legionella—10–21 days	(see footnote³) **Respiratory FQ present:** Gemi 320 mg po q24h, Gati 400 mg po q24h, Levo 750 mg po q24h x 5 days, Moxi 400 mg po q24h OR **azithro** + (**high dose amox-CL**, high dose AM-CL, **cefdinir** or **cefpodoxime** or **cefprozil**) OR telithromycin Doses in footnote²	**Azithro:** Pro: appropriate spectrum of action; more in vitro resistance than clinical failure *(CID 34(Suppl 1):S4, 2002)*. Con: Overall ≤ 30% S. pneumo resistance in vitro to 20–30% *(CID 34(Suppl 1):S4, 2002)*. In pt G resist. S. pneumo, up to 50%+ resistance. Breakthrough infections reported *(NEJM 346:630, 2002; CID 35:556, 2002)* **Amoxicillin:** Pro: Active vs 90–95% S. pneumo at 3–4 gm per day Con: Need high dose. No activity atypicals or β-lactamase + bacteria. **Cephalosporins**—See footnote³. Pro: spectrum includes β-lactamase + H. influenzae, M. catarrhalis, MSSA, & Bacteroides sp. Con: No activity atypicals Pro: Active 75–85% S. pneumo & H. influenzae. Cefuroxime least active & higher mortality rate when S. pneumo resistant *(CID 37:230, 2003)*. Con: Inactive vs atypicals **Doxycycline:** Pro: Active vs S. pneumo *(DMID 49:147, 2004)* but resistance may be increasing. Active vs H. influenzae, atypicals, & bioterrorism agents (anthrax, plague, tularemia). Con: Resistance of S. pneumo 18–20% *(CID 35:633, 2002)*. Sparse clinical data *(AIM 159: 266, 1999; CID 37:870, 2003)* **FQs—Respiratory FQs:** Pro: In vitro & clinically effective vs pen-resistant S. pneumo. **NOTE: dose of Levo is 750 mg q24h.** Q24h dosing. Gemi only available po. Con: Geographic pockets of resistance with clinical failure *(NEJM 346:747, 2002)*. Drug-drug interactions (see Table 22A, page 147). Unique reversible rash in young females given Gemi. **Telithromycin:** Pro: Active vs atypical pathogens, active vs macrolide-resistant S. pneumo. Con: Virtually no resistance to date. Transient reversible blurry vision due to paralysis of lens accommodation; avoid in myasthenia gravis pts.
Community-acquired, hospitalized—NOT in the ICU **Empiric therapy** Pneumo resistance data (TRUST6-2003–2004) Penicillin—high level 18.6 Azithro/Erythro 26	Etiology by co-morbidity & risk factors as above. Culture sputum & blood. S. pneumo, M. catarrhalis, M. pneumoniae urine antigen helpful. Legionella urine antigen helpful.	**Ceftriaxone** 2 gm IV q24h or gm IV q24h + **azithro** 500 mg IV q24h	**Gati** 400 mg IV q24h or **Levo** 750 mg IV q24h or **Moxi** 400 mg IV q24h	**Ceftriaxone/cefotaxime:** Pro: Drugs of choice for pen-resistant S. pneumo, active H. influenzae, MSSA Con: No active atypicals or drug-resistant pathogens. Add macrolide for atypicals.

NOTE: q24h = once q24h; bid = twice q24h; tid = 3 times a day; qid = 4 times a day.

¹ Atypical pathogens: Chlamydophila pneumoniae, C. psittaci, Legionella sp., M. pneumoniae, C. burnetii (Q fever) (Q fever rate).
² Respiratory FQs with enhanced activity vs S. pneumo with HLR to penicillin: **Gati** 400 mg IV/po q24h, **Levo** 320 mg po q24h, **Gemi** 320 mg po q24h, **Moxi** 400 mg IV/po q24h. Ketolide: **telithro** 800 mg po qd.
³ **Oral cephalosporin dosage:** **Cefdinir** 300 mg po q12h, **cefditoren pivoxil** 200 mg, 2 tabs po bid, **cefpodoxime proxetil** 200 mg po q12h, **high dose amox** 1 gm po tid, **high dose AM-CL—use AM-CL-ER** 1000/62.5 mg, 2 tabs po bid, **telithromycin** 800 mg po q24h times 7–10 days.
NOTE: All dosage recommendations are for adults (unless otherwise indicated) and assume normal renal function.
Abbreviations on page 2.

TABLE 1 (27)

ANATOMIC SITE/DIAGNOSIS/ MODIFYING CIRCUMSTANCES	ETIOLOGIES (usual)	SUGGESTED REGIMENS*		ADJUNCT DIAGNOSTIC OR THERAPEUTIC MEASURES AND COMMENTS
		PRIMARY	ALTERNATIVE†	
LUNG/Pneumonia/Adults (continued)				
Community-acquired, hospitalized—IN ICU Empiric therapy	Severe COPD, S. pneumo, H. influ, M. catarrhalis Legionella Post-influenza, S. aureus Coliforms + P. aeruginosa rare unless bronchiectasis (see below)	Aggressive attempts at microbiol. diagnosis justified: Culture sputum, blood, maybe pleural fluid. Urine antigen tests for both legionella & S. pneumoniae. Empiric rx therapy must be active vs S. pneumo & Legionella. **Gati** 400 mg IV q24h or **Levo** 750 mg IV q24h or **Moxi** 400 mg IV q24h	**Ceftriaxone** 2 gm IV q24h (1 gm IV q24h – age 65) + **azithro** 500 mg IV q24h) or **ERTA** 1 gm IV q24h + **azithro** 500 mg IV q24h (see Comment)	Various studies indicate improved outcome when azithro added to a β-lactam (CID 36:389 & 1239, 2003; AJM 164:1837, 2001 & 159:2562, 1999). Similar results in prospective study of critically ill pts with pneumococcal bacteremia (AJRCCM 170:440, 2004). Ceftriaxone could substitute for ceftriaxone but limited clinical experience. Need azithro to cover atypical pathogens. Do not use if suspect P. aeruginosa. Not all Legionella species detected by urine antigen; if suspicious culture or PCR on airway secretions.
Hospital-acquired— usually with mechanical ventilation (ventilator-associated pneumonia) Diagnosis confirmed by quantitative cultures (see Comment) Guidelines: AJRCCM 171:388, 2005	Highly variable depending on clinical setting: S. pneumo, S. aureus, Legionella, stenotropho- monas, P. aeruginosa, stenotrophomonas, acinetobacter, anaerobes all possible	**IMP** 0.5 gm IV q6h or **MER** 1 gm IV q8h) plus, if suspect legionella or bioterrorism, **respiratory FQ (Gati, Levo or Moxi)** NOTE: Regimen not active vs **MRSA**—see specific rx below. See Comment regarding diagnosis. Dosages: See footnotes pages 19, 26, 28, & 29	**Cefepime or high-dose PIP-TZ**²) + **tobra**. Add active vs resp. P. aeruginosa if suspect legionella or bioterrorism.	Dx of ventilator-associated pneumonia: Fever & lung infiltrates often **not** pneumonia (Chest 106:221, 1994). Quantitative cultures helpful. 1 bronchoalveolar lavage (>10⁴ per mL pos.) or protect. spec. brush (>10³ per mL pos.) Ref.: AJRCCM 165:867, 2002. Microbial etiology: No empiric regimen covers all possibilities. Regimens listed active vs most of S. pneumo legionella & **most coliforms**. Regimens not active vs MRSA, Stenotrophomonas & others; see below. Specific rx when culture results known. Ventilator-associated pneumonia—Prevention: If possible, keep head of bed elevated 30° or more. Remove N.G. endotracheal tubes as soon as possible. If available, continuous subglottic suctioning. Limit stress ulcer prophylaxis. Refs.: NEJM 340:627, 1999, CCM 31:1560, 2003.
Hospital- or community-acquired, neutropenic pt (<500 neutrophils per mm³)	Any of organisms listed under community-acquired + fungi (aspergillus) See Table 11	See Hospital-acquired, immediately above. Vanco not included See Comment in initial rx unless high suspicion of infected IV access or drug-resistant S. pneumo. Ampho not used unless still febrile after 3 days or high clinical likelihood. See Comment		See Table 11 documents document on management of febrile neutropenic pt. 34:730, 2002.
Adults—Selected specific rx when culture results (sputum, blood, pleural fluid, etc.), page 49				
Burkholderia (Pseudomonas) pseudomallei (etiology of melioidosis) Ref.: Ln 361:1715, 2003	Gram-negative	Initial parenteral rx: **Ceftazidime** 30-50 mg per kg IV q8h or **IMP 20** mg per kg IV q6h (for children). **Chloro** 10 mg per kg q6h x 8 wks.; then po therapy → see Alternative column	**po rx:** **Adults** (see Comment for children) **Doxy** 2 mg per kg IV q6h times 20 wks. or (TMP-SMX 5 mg (TMP) per kg + **Doxy** 2 mg per kg) q12h times 20 wks.	**Children <8 yrs old & pregnancy:** For oral regimen, use **AM-CL-ER** 10/20/62.5 mg/kg po bid times 20 wks. Even with compliance, relapse rate is 10%. Max. daily ceftazidime dose: 6 gm.
Haemophilus influenzae	β-lactamase negative β-lactamase positive	**AMP** IV, amox po, TMP-SMX, azithro/clarithro, doxy **AM-CL O Ceph 2/3, P Ceph 3, FQ, azithro/clarithro, telithro³**		
Klebsiella sp.—ESBL pos. & other coliforms⁴	β-lactamase positive	**IMP** or **MER** if resistant, **polymyxin E (colistin)**		25-35% strains β-lactamase positive. ↑ resistance to both TMP-SMX and doxy. See Table 10C, page 67 for dosages. ESBL inactivates all cephalosporins, β-lactam/β-lactamase inhibitor drug activ., co-resistance to all FQs & more predictable: resistance to all FQs & more. Ref.: JAC 51:1119, 2003. Best legionella website: www.legionella.org. Two international observational studies support the superiority of **Levo** over macrolides (CID 40:794 & 800, 2005).
Legionella species	Hospitalized/immunocompromised	**Azithro IV or Levo or Gati or Moxi** See Table 10C, pages 70 & 71 for dosages. Treat for 7-14 days (CID 39:1734, 2004)		

¹ Acinetobacter: susceptibility to IMP & MER may be discordant (CID 41:758, 2005)
² **PIP-TZ** dose: 4.5 gm IV q6h
³ **Telithro** = telithromycin 800 mg po q24h
⁴ **ESBL** = Extended spectrum beta-lactamase

Abbreviations on page 2.

NOTE: All dosage recommendations are for adults (unless otherwise indicated) and assume normal renal function.

TABLE 1 (28)

ANATOMIC SITE/DIAGNOSIS/ MODIFYING CIRCUMSTANCES	ETIOLOGIES (usual)	SUGGESTED REGIMENS¹ PRIMARY	ALTERNATIVE¹	ADJUNCT DIAGNOSTIC OR THERAPEUTIC MEASURES AND COMMENTS
LUNG/Pneumonia/Adults, when culture results available (continued)				
Moraxella catarrhalis	93% β-lactamase positive	O Ceph 2/3, P Ceph 2/3, macrolide,¹ telithro (see footnote 3 page 30), FQ, TMP-SMX. Doxy another option. See Table 10C.		
Pseudomonas aeruginosa	Often ventilator-associated	PIP-TZ 4.5 gm IV q6h + tobra 5 mg per kg IV once q24h (see Table 10D, page 74)	NOTE: High-dose PIP-TZ for P. aeruginosa	
Staphylococcus aureus	Nafcillin/oxacillin susceptible	Nafcillin/oxacillin 2 gm IV q4h.	Vanco 1 gm IV q12h or linezolid 600 mg IV q12h.	Retrospective analysis of 2 prospective randomized double-blind studies of hospital-acquired MRSA showed enhanced survival with linezolid, p 0.03 (Chest 124:1789, 2003); efficacy perhaps related to superior lung concentrations. Concern of possible misinterpretation of post hoc subgroup analysis (Chest 130:314, 2004).
	MRSA	Vanco 1 gm IV q12h.	Linezolid 600 mg IV q12h.	
Stenotrophomonas maltophilia		TMP-SMX	TC-CL,⁵ aztreonam	In vitro synergy refs: AAC 39:2220, 1995; CMR 11:57, 1998
Streptococcus pneumoniae	Penicillin-susceptible	AMP 2 gm IV q6h, amox 1 gm IV q8h, macrolide,¹ pen G IV doxy. O Ceph 2, P Ceph 2/3, telithro 800 mg po q24h. See Table 10C, page 67 for other dosages		
	Penicillin-resistant, high level	FQs with enhanced activity [Gati, Gemi, Levo, Moxi (IV)], linezolid. See Table 5, page 56 for more data if all options not possible (e.g. allergy). linezolid active	high-dose¹⁰ AMP, vanco IV—see Table 5, page 56	
LUNG—Other				
Anthrax, inhalation (applies to oro-pharyngeal & gastrointestinal forms): Treatment (Cutaneous: See page 39)	Bacillus anthracis To report possible bioterrorism event: 770-488-7100	**Adults (including preg-nancy):** CIP 400 mg IV (q12h) or Levo 500 (q24h) IV plus (clindamycin 900 mg IV q8h and/or RIF 300 mg IV q12h) Switch to po when able & lower CIP to 500 mg po bid or doxy 100 mg po bid, & RIF 300 mg po q8h, & RIF 300 mg po bid. Treat times 60 days. Other alternatives: Table 1B, page 48	**Children:** CIP 10 mg per kg IV (q12h) or 15 mg per kg po (q12h) to >8 y/o & <45 kg 100 mg IV q12h; >8 y/o & >45 kg 100 mg IV q12h; >8 y/o & <8 y/o 2.2 mg per kg po bid; <8 y/o 2.2 mg per kg IV q12h plus clindamycin 7.5 mg per kg IV q6h and/or RIF 20 mg per kg (max. 600 mg) IV q24h. Treat times 60 days. See Table 16, page 133 for oral dosage	1. Cidofx may block toxin production 2. Rifampin penetrates CSF & intracellular sites 3. If isolate shown penicillin-susceptible: — Adults: Pen G 4 million units IV q4h — Children: Pen G <12 y/o: 50,000 units per kg IV q6h; >12 y/o: 4 million units IV q4h 4. Constitutive β-lactamases—do not use pen or amp 5. Do not use cephalosporins or TMP-SMX 6. Erythro, azithro activity borderline; clarithro active 7. No person-to-person spread. 8. Antitoxins in development
Refs.: JAMA 287:2236, 2002 & JAMA 286:2549, 2001 Clinical experience: JAMA 286:2549, 2001 CIP rationale: CID 39:303, 2004	Plague, tularemia: see Table 1B, page 48 Chest x-ray: mediastinal widening & pleural effusion (e.g. AnnIM 139:337, 2003; Ln 364:449, 2004)			
Post-exposure prophylaxis	Info: www.bt.cdc.gov	**Adults (including pregnancy): CIP** 500 mg po bid or Levo 500 mg po (q24h) times 60 days **Children:** CIP 20-30 mg per kg per day bid to max. 1 gm per day, or Doxy (as above) times 60 days.	**Adults (including pregnancy): Doxy** 100 mg po bid times 60 d. **Children:** Doxy >8 y/o & >45 kg: 100 mg po bid; >8 y/o & <8 y/o 2.2 mg per kg po bid; <8 y/o 2.2 mg per kg po bid. All for 60 days.	1. Once organism shows suscept. to penicillin, switch to amoxicillin 80 mg per kg per day (div q8h) (max. 500 mg q8h), pregnant pt to amoxicillin 500 mg po tid. 2. Do not use cephalosporins or TMP-SMX. 3. Other FQs (Gati, Moxi) & clarithro should work but no clinical experience.
Aspiration pneumonia + lung abscess Refs.: CID 40:915 & 923, 2005	Transthoracic culture in 90 pts—% of total isolates: anaerobes 34%, Gm-pos. cocci 26%, S. milleri 16%, Klebsiella pneumoniae 25%, Nocardia 66	**Adults (including preg-nancy):** PIP-TZ 3.375 gm IV q6h (For nocardia, see Table 11, page 82)	Ceftriaxone 2 gm IV q24h plus metro 500 mg IV q6h or 1 gm IV q12h	Suggested regimens based on retrospective evaluation of 90 pts with cultures obtained by transthoracic aspirate (CID 40:915 & 923, 2005). Surprising frequency of Klebsiella pneumoniae. Moxi 400 mg IV/po q24h another option (CID 41:764, 2005).
Chronic pneumonia with fever, night sweats and weight loss	M. tuberculosis, coccidiodomycosis, histoplasmosis	See Tables 11, 12, for risk associated with bacteremic S. pneumo see CID 41(Suppl):S187, 2005.		HIV+, foreign-born, alcoholism, contact with TB, travel into developing countries

¹ **Macrolide** = azithromycin, clarithromycin and erythromycin. Dirithromycin serum levels inadequate for bacteremic S. pneumo
² **IV Pen G dosage:** Blood cultures neg., 1 million units IV q4h; blood cultures pos. & no meningitis, 2 million units IV q4h. Another option is continuous infusion (CI) 3 million units loading dose & then CI of 10-12 million units over 12 hrs (Chest 112:1657, 1997).
 Abbreviations on page 2. NOTE: All dosage recommendations are for adults (unless otherwise indicated) and assume normal renal function.

TABLE 1 (29)

ANATOMIC SITE/DIAGNOSIS/ MODIFYING CIRCUMSTANCES	ETIOLOGIES (usual)	SUGGESTED REGIMENS*		ADJUNCT DIAGNOSTIC OR THERAPEUTIC MEASURES AND COMMENTS
		PRIMARY	ALTERNATIVE†	
LUNG/Other (continued) **Cystic fibrosis Acute exacerbation of pulmonary symptoms** Refs.: Ln 361:681, 2003; AJRCCM 168:918, 2003	S. aureus or H. influenzae early in disease, P. aeruginosa later in disease	**For P. aeruginosa: Tobra** 3.3 mg per kg IV q24h. Combine tobra with (**PIP** or **ticarcillin** 100 mg per kg IV q6h) or **ceftaz** 50 mg per kg IV q8h to max. of 6 gm per day. See footnote†	**For S. aureus: (1) MSSA**—**oxacillin/nafcillin** 2 gm IV q4h (Peds dose, Table 16). **(2) MRSA**—**vanco** 1 gm q12h & check serum levels. See footnote†	Other options: **Clarithro** synergistic with tobra vs P. aeruginosa (AAC 46:1105, 2002) + anti-inflammatory properties (Pharmacotherapy 22:227, 2002). **Azithro** modestly improved FEV₁ in pts chronically infected with P. aeruginosa (JAMA 290:1749, 2003). Once daily tobra reported less nephrotoxic (Ln 365:573, 2005). For pharmacokinetics of aminoglycosides in CF, see JAC 50:553, 2002. **NOTE:** Chronic suppression of P. aeruginosa with **inhaled tobra** 300 mg bid times 28 d, then no times 28 d, then repeat cycle (AJRCCM 167:841, 2003)
	Burkholderia (Pseudomonas) cepacia	**TMP-SMX** 5 mg per kg (TMP) IV q6h		B. cepacia has become a major pathogen. Patients develop progressive respiratory failure, 62% mortality at 1 year. **Fail to respond** to APAG, piperacillin, & ceftazidime. Patients with B. cepacia should be isolated from other CF patients. **NOTE:** 3- & 4-drug combinations under study in refractory pts (AAC 43:213, 1999)
Empyema Ref.: CID 22:747, 1996; Pleural effusion review: NEJM 346:1971, 2002				
Neonatal	Staph. aureus	See Pneumonia, neonatal, page 28		Drainage indicated.
Infants/children (1 month–5 yrs)	Staph. aureus, Strep. pneumoniae, H. influenzae	See Pneumonia, age 1 month–5 years, page 28		Drainage indicated.
Child >5 yrs to ADULT—Diagnostic thoracentesis; chest tube for empyema. Acute, usually parapneumonic. For dosage, see Table 10 or footnote page 26	Strep. pneumoniae, Group A strep	**Cefotaxime** or **ceftriaxone** (Dosage, see footnote 1, page 26)	**Vanco**	In large multicenter double-blind trial, intrapleural streptokinase did not improve mortality, reduce the need for surgery or the length of hospitalization (NEJM 352:865, 2005).
	Staph. aureus: Check for MRSA	**Nafcillin** or **oxacillin** (if MSSA) |**Vanco**| if MRSA		Usually complication of S. aureus pneumonia &/or bacteremia.
	H. influenzae	**Ceftriaxone**		Pneumonic Gm-neg. bacilli. ↑ resistance to TMP-SMX.
Subacute/chronic	Anaerobic strep, Strep. milleri, Entero-bacteriaceae, M. tuberculosis	**Clinda** 450–900 mg IV q8h + **ceftriaxone**	**TMP-SMX** |**Vanco**| **PIP-TZ** or **AM-SB** (Dosage, see footnote, page 26)	If organisms not seen, base rx on... R/O tuberculosis or tumor. Pleural biopsy with culture for mycobacteria and histology if TBc suspected (CID 22:747, 1996).
Human immunodeficiency virus infection (HIV+): See SANFORD GUIDE TO HIV/AIDS THERAPY				
CD4 T-lymphocytes <200 per µL or clinical AIDS Acute onset, progressive dyspnea, & diffuse infiltrate **Prednisone first if suspect pneumocystis (see Comment)**	Pneumocystis jiroveci (formerly carinii) most likely, also M. tbc, fungi, Kaposi's sarcoma, & lymphoma. **NOTE:** AIDS pts may develop pneumonia due to DRSP or other pathogens—see next box below	Rx listed here is for **severe** pneumocystis (see Table 13, page 98 for rx regimens for **mild** disease. **Prednisone 1st** (see Comment), then: **TMP-SMX** (IV 15 mg per kg per day div q6h (TMP component) or (**TMP** 5 mg per kg po q8h + **dapsone** 100 mg po q24h) times 21 days, total of 21 days	**TMP-SMX** (1) (**Clinda** (600 mg IV q8h or 300–450 mg po q6h) + **primaquine** 30 mg (base) po q24h) or (**pentamidine isethionate** 4 mg per kg per day IV) times 21 days See Comment	Diagnostic procedure of choice is sputum induction; if negative, bronchoscopy. Pts with PCP or <200 CD4 cells per mm³ should be on anti-PCP prophylaxis for life. **Prednisone 40 mg po times 5 days then 40 mg po q24h po times 5 days then 20 mg q24h po times 11 days is indicated with PCP (pO₂ <70 mmHg), should be given at initiation of anti-PCP rx; don't wait until pt's condition deteriorates** (TMP-SMX or dapsone). In PCP studies negative, consider bacterial pneumonia, TBc, cocci, crypto, Kaposi's sarcoma or lymphoma. **Pentamidine** not active vs bacterial pathogens.
CD4 T-lymphocytes normal Acute onset, purulent sputum &/or pulmonary infiltrates ± pleuritic pain. **Isolate pt until TBc excluded: Adults**	Strep. pneumoniae, H. influenzae, aerobic Gm-neg. bacilli (including P. aeruginosa), Legionella sp.	**P Ceph 3** (Dosages in footnotes on page 26) + **azithro** (**Moxi** IV as alternative (see Comment)		**NOTE:** Strep. pneumoniae resistant to TMP-SMX. If Gm-stain of fresh sputum shows Gm-neg. bacilli, options include **P Ceph 3 AP, TC-CL, PIP-TZ, IMP** or **MER. FQs: Levo** 750 mg po/IV q24h, **Gati** 400 mg IV/po q24h, **Moxi** 400 mg po/IV q24h
As above: Children	Same as adult with HIV + lymphocytic interstitial pneumonia (LIP)	As for HIV+ adults with pneumonia. If diagnosis is LIP rx with steroids.		In children with AIDS, LIP responsible for 1/3 of pulmonary complications, usually >1 yr of age vs PCP, which is seen at <1 yr of age. Clinically: clubbing, hepatosplenomegaly, salivary glands enlarged (like up, gallium), lymphocytosis.

† Other options: (Tobra + aztreonam 50 mg per kg IV q8h) + tobra); (IMP 15-25 mg per kg IV q6h + tobra); **CIP** commonly used **in children**, e.g., CIP IV/po + ceftaz IV (LnID 3:537, 2003).
Abbreviations on page 2.   NOTE: All dosage recommendations are for adults (unless otherwise indicated) and assume normal renal function.

TABLE 1 (30)

ANATOMIC SITE/DIAGNOSIS/ MODIFYING CIRCUMSTANCES	ETIOLOGIES (usual)	SUGGESTED REGIMENS† PRIMARY	ALTERNATIVE†	ADJUNCT DIAGNOSTIC OR THERAPEUTIC MEASURES AND COMMENTS
LUNG/Other (continued) **Viral (interstitial) pneumonia** (See Table 14, page 106)	Consider: Adenovirus, coronavirus (SARS), hantavirus, influenza, metapneumovirus, parainfluenza virus, respiratory syncytial virus	**For Influenza A or B: oseltamivir** 75 mg po bid times 5 d or **zanamivir** 10 mg inhaled bid times 5 d. Start within 48 hrs of symptom onset	**For Influenza A: rimantadine** 100 mg po q12h or **amantadine** 100 mg po q12h	No known efficacious drugs for adenovirus, coronavirus (SARS), hantavirus, influenza, parainfluenza or RSV. Need travel (SARS) & exposure (Hanta) history. RSV as serious as influenza in the elderly (NEJM 352:1749 & 1810, 2005).
LYMPH NODES (approaches below apply to lymphadenitis without an obvious primary source)				
Lymphadenitis, acute **Generalized**	[Etiologies: EBV, early HIV infection, syphilis, toxoplasma, tularemia, Lyme disease, sarcoid, lymphoma, systemic lupus erythematosus, and **Kikuchi-Fujimoto** disease (CID 39:138, 2004). Complete history and physical examination followed by appropriate serological tests. Treat specific agent(s).]			A distinctive form of lymphangitis characterized by subcutaneous swellings along inflamed lymphatic channels. Primary site of skin invasion usually present; regional adenopathy variable.
Regional **Cervical—see cat-scratch disease (CSD), below**	CSD (B. henselae), Grp A strep, Staph. aureus, anaerobes, M. TBc (scrofula), M. avium, M. scrofulaceum, M. malmoense, toxo, tularemia			History & physical exam directs evaluation. If nodes fluctuant, aspirate and base rx on Gram & acid-fast stains. Review of mycobacterial etiology: CID 20:954, 1995. **Kikuchi-Fujimoto** disease causes fever and benign self-limited adenopathy; the etiology is unknown (AJM 171:401, 1996; CID 39:138, 2004).
Inguinal Sexually transmitted	HSV, chancroid, syphilis, LGV			
Not sexually transmitted	GAS, SA, tularemia, LGV			
Axillary	GAS, SA, tularemia, Y. pestis, sporotrichosis, Sporotrichosis, leishmania, Nocardia brasiliensis.	Treatment varies with specific etiology.		
Extremity, with associated nodules (lymphangitis) For full description: AnIM 118:883, 1993	Mycobacterium marinum, M. chelonae, Mycobacterium chelonae.			
Cat-scratch disease— immunocompetent patient Axillary/epitrochlear nodes 46%, neck 26%, inguinal 17%	Bartonella henselae Reviews: AAC 48:1921, 2004; PIDJ 23:1161, 2004.	**Azithro** dosage—**Adults** (>45.5 kg): 500 mg times 1, then 250 mg/day times 4 days. **Peds** (<45.5 kg): liquid azithro 10 mg per kg times 1, then 5 mg per kg per day times 4 days. Rx is controversial—see Comment.	No rx: resolves in 2–6 mos. Needle aspiration of suppurative (not pus) for pain in suppurative nodes. Avoid I&D.	**Clinical:** Approx. 10% nodes suppurate. Atypical presentation in <5% pts, i.e., lung nodules, liver/spleen lesions, Parinaud's oculoglandular syndrome, CNS (encephalitis or aseptic meningitis), peripheral neuropathy, retinitis, FUO. **Dx:** Serology positive. Positive IFA serology. Rarely need biopsy. **Rx:** Only 1 prospective randomized blinded study, used azithro with ↑ rapidity of resolution of enlarged lymph nodes (PIDJ 17:447, 1998).
MOUTH Odontogenic infection, including Ludwig's angina can result in more serious parapharyngeal space infection (see page 36)	Oral microflora: infection polymicrobial	**Clinda** 300–450 mg po q6-8h or 600 mg IV q6-8h	**AM-CL** 875/125 mg po bid or 500/125 mg po tid or 2000/125 mg po bid or **cefotetan** 2 gm IV q12h	Surgical drainage and removal of necrotic tissue essential. β-lactamase producing organisms are ↑ in frequency. Ref.: Carnad Dental Assn J 64:508, 1998. Other parenteral alternatives: AM-SB, PIP-TZ, or TC-CL
Buccal cellulitis Children <5 yrs	H. influenzae	**Cefuroxime** or **ceftriaxone**	**AM-CL** or **TMP-SMX**. Dosage: see Table 16, page 133	With Hib immunization, invasive H. influenzae infections have ↓ by 95%. Now occurring in infants prior to immunization.
Herpetic stomatitis	Herpes simplex virus 1 & 2	See Table 14		
Aphthous stomatitis, recurrent, HIV+neg	[Etiology: unknown]	Topical steroids (Kenalog in Orabase) may ↓ pain and swelling; if AIDS see SANFORD GUIDE TO HIV/AIDS THERAPY.		
MUSCLE **"Gas gangrene"** Contaminated traumatic wound Can be spontaneous without trauma (CID 28:159, 1999)	Cl. perfringens, other histotoxic Clostridium sp.	(**Clinda** 900 mg IV q8h) + (**pen G** 24 million units per day div q4-6h) [**Vanco** not for this]	**Ceftriaxone** 2 gm IV q12h or **erythro** 1 gm q6h IV (not by bolus)	Surgical debridement primary rx. Hyperbaric oxygen therapy. Consider if debridement not complete or possible (NEJM 334:1642, 1996). Clinda decreases toxin production.
Pyomyositis Review: AJM 117:420, 2004	Staph. aureus, Group A strep, (rarely Gm-neg. bacilli), variety of anaerobic organisms	(**Nafcillin** or **oxacillin** 2 gm IV q4h) or (**P Ceph 1** (**cefazolin** 2 gm IV q8h)) if **MSSA**	**Vanco** 1 gm q12h if **MRSA**	Common in tropics: rare, but occurs, in temperate zones (IDCP 7:265, 1998). Now seen in HIV/AIDS. Follows exercise or muscle injury, see Necrotizing fasciitis. Add **metro** if anaerobes suspected/proven (IDCP 8:260, 1999).

Abbreviations on page 2. NOTE: All dosage recommendations are for adults (unless otherwise indicated) and assume normal renal function.

TABLE 1 (31)

ANATOMIC SITE/DIAGNOSIS/ MODIFYING CIRCUMSTANCES	ETIOLOGIES (usual)	SUGGESTED REGIMENS*		ADJUNCT DIAGNOSTIC OR THERAPEUTIC MEASURES AND COMMENTS
		PRIMARY	ALTERNATIVE†	
PANCREAS: Reviews—*Ln 361:1447, 2003; JAMA 291:2865, 2004*				
Acute alcoholic (without necrosis) (idiopathic) pancreatitis	Not bacterial	None CT-diagnosed		1–9% become infected but prospective studies show no advantage of prophylactic antimicrobials (*Ln 346:652, 1995*). Observe for pancreatic abscesses or necrosis which require rx.
Pancreatic abscess, infected pseudocyst, post-necrotizing pancreatitis	Enterobacteriaceae, enterococci, S. aureus, S. epidermidis, anaerobes, candida	Need culture of abscess/infected pseudocyst to direct therapy		Can often get specimen by fine-needle aspiration.
Antimicrobial prophylaxis, necrotizing pancreatitis	As above			Infection of necrotic pancreas occurs in 30–50% of pts leading to multiple clinical trials. An International Consensus Panel reviewed all available data & concluded that prophylactic antibacterial &/or antifungal agents should not be used (*CCM 92:2524, 2004*).
PAROTID GLAND "Hot" tender parotid swelling	S. aureus, oral flora, & aerobic Gm-neg. bacilli (rare), mumps, rarely enteroviruses/influenza	Nafcillin or oxacillin 2 gm IV q4h		Predisposing factors: stone(s) in Stensen's duct, dehydration. Rx depends on ID of specific etiologic organism.
"Cold" tender parotid swelling	Granulomatous disease (e.g., mycobacteria, fungi, sarcoidosis, Sjögren's syndrome), drugs (iodides, et al.), diabetes, cirrhosis, tumors			History/lab results may need biopsy for dx
PERITONEUM/PERITONITIS: *Reference: CID 37:997, 2003*				
Primary (spontaneous) bacterial peritonitis, SBP) Rev. *CID 27:669, 1998* ESBL ref. *CID 28:683, 1999* Microbiology *CID 33:1513, 2007*	Enterobacteriaceae 63%, S. pneumo 15%, enterococci 6–10%, anaerobes <1%. Extended β-lactamase positive Klebsiella species	**Cefotaxime 2 gm IV q8h (if life-threatening 2 gm q4h) OR TC-CL or PIP-TZ or AM-SB OR ceftriaxone 2 gm IV q24h OR [ERTA 1 gm IV q24h]** **If resistant E. coli/Klebsiella species (ESBL+), then: IMP or MER or FQ: CIP, Levo, Gati, Moxi (Dosage in footnote)⁹**	(**CIP 400 mg IV q12h or Levo 750 mg IV q24h) +**	One-year **risk of SBP** in pts with ascites and cirrhosis as high as 29% (*Gastro 104:1133, 1993*) 30–40% of pts have bacteremia. Diagnosis: paracentesis with ascitic fluid & blood culture bottles. **Duration of rx unclear.** Suggest 2 wks if blood culture pos. One report suggests repeat paracentesis after 48 hrs of cefotaxime. If PMNs <250 per mm³ and ascitic fluid sterile, success with 5 days rx (*AJM 97:169, 1994*) IV albumin (1.5 gm per kg at dk 1 & 3 gm per kg day 3) may ↓ frequency of renal impairment (p 0.002) & ↓ hospital mortality (p 0.01) (*NEJM 341:403, 1999*).
Prevention of SBP⁶ Cirrhosis & ascites		TMP-SMX-DS 1 tab po 5 days per wk or CIP 750 mg po qd	TMP-SMX [22:1171, 1995	
Secondary (bowel perforation, ruptured appendix, ruptured diverticula) Refs.: *NEJM 338:1521, 1998 & CID 37:997, 2003*	Enterobacteriaceae, Bacteroides sp., enterococci, P. aeruginosa (3+–15%)	**Mild-moderate disease—Inpatient rx:** (e.g. focal periappendiceal peritonitis, periappendiceal abscess, endomyometritis) **PIP-TZ 3.375 gm IV q6h or 4.5 gm q8h OR AM-SB 3 gm IV q6h OR ERTA 1 gm IV q24h** **Severe life-threatening disease—ICU patient:** **IMP 500 mg IV q6h OR MER 1 gm IV q8h**	(**CIP 400 mg IV q12h or Levo 750 mg IV q24h) + metro 1 gm IV q12h) or FQ: CFP 2 gm IV q12h + metro) or tigecycline 100 mg IV times 1 dose, then 50 mg q12h** [(**AMP** 2 gm IV q4h + **metro** 500 mg q6h) + **CIP** 400 mg q12h)] OR [**AMP** 2 gm IV q4h + **APAG** + **metro** 500 mg q6h]¹⁰ (Dosage in Table 10D, page 74)	Must "cover" both Gm-neg. aerobic & Gm-neg. anaerobic bacteria. **Drugs active only vs aerobic Gm-neg. bacilli:** clinda, metro. **Drugs active vs both aerobic/anaerobic Gm-neg. bacteria:** cefoxitin, cefotetan, TC-CL, PIP-TZ, AM-SB, IMP, MER, Gati, Moxi. Increasing resistance:

	Cefoxitin	Cefotetan	Clindamycin
% R	17–87	5–13	16–44

Essentially no resistance to **metro**, **PIP-TZ** (*CID 39:Suppl 1:S126, 2000*). Case reports of resistance to **CIP/Levo,** but insufficient clinical data to alter recommendations. *CID 40:e67, 2005; JCM 42:4127, 2004.* Mechanisms of resistance *CID 39:92, 2004.* **Ertapenem** not active vs P. aeruginosa/Acinetobacter species. Based on in vitro activity, could sub **Gati/Moxi** for **CIP/Levo.** **With severe pen allergy,** can "cover" Gm-neg. aerobes with CIP or aztreonam (Table 10D, page 74). Less need for aminoglycosides. **metro** 1 gm loading then 0.5 gm q6h or 1 gm q12h. **AP Pen** (ticarcillin 4 gm q6h). **Remember IMP/MER are β-lactams.** |
| | | **Concomitant surgical management important.** | | |

¹ Parenteral IV therapy for peritonitis: **TC-CL** 3.1 gm q6h, **AM-SB** 3 gm q6h, **IMP** 0.5 gm q6h, **MER** 1 gm q8h, **FQ** (**CIP** 400 mg q12h, **Oflox** 400 mg q12h, **Levo** 750 mg q24h, **Gati** 400 mg q24h, **Moxi** 400 mg q4-8h), **AMP** 1 gm q4-6h, **P Ceph 3** (cefotaxime 2 gm q8h, ceftazidime 2 gm q8h, cefepime 2 gm q12h, cefotetan 2 gm q12h, cefoxitin 2 gm q6h, ceftriaxone 1 gm q24h), **APAG** (see Table 10D, page 74), **P Ceph 2** (**CFP** 2 gm q12h) cefoperazone...
PIP 4 gm q6h, **aztreonam** 2 gm q8h).   NOTE: All dosage recommendations are for adults (unless otherwise indicated) and assume normal renal function.

Abbreviations on page 2.

TABLE 1 (32)

ANATOMIC SITE/DIAGNOSIS/ MODIFYING CIRCUMSTANCES	ETIOLOGIES (usual)	SUGGESTED REGIMENS*		ADJUNCT DIAGNOSTIC OR THERAPEUTIC MEASURES AND COMMENTS
		PRIMARY	ALTERNATIVE†	
PERITONEUM/PERITONITIS (continued) **Associated with chronic ambulatory dialysis** (defined as > 100 WBC per mcL, > 50% PMNs)	Staph. aureus (most common), Staph. epidermidis, Gm-neg. bacilli, aeruginosa 7%, Gm-neg. bacilli 11%, sterile 20%, M. fortuitum (rare)	If of moderate severity, can rx by adding drug to dialysis fluid—see Table 17 for dosage. Reasonable empiric combinations: (**vanco** + **ceftazidime**) or (**vanco** + **APAG**). If renal failure, Table 17 & via addition to dialysis fluid. Excellent ref. Perit Dialysis Int 13:14, 1993		For diagnosis: concentrate several hundred mL of removed dialysis fluid by centrifugation. Gram stain and culture. A positive Gram stain will guide initial therapy. If culture blood culture bottles. A positive Gram stain will guide initial therapy. If culture neg. Staph. epidermidis, consider "saving" dialysis catheter. If multiple Gm-neg. bacilli cultured, consider bowel perforation and catheter removal.
PHARYNX **Pharyngitis/Tonsillitis**—Reviews: NEJM 344:205, 2001; AnIM 139:113, 2003. Guideline for Group A strep: CID 35:113, 2002 **Exudative or diffuse erythema** Rheumatic fever ref.: Ln 366:155, 2005	Group A,C,G strep, "viral", infectious mononucleosis (NEJM 329:156, 1993), C. diphtheriae, A. haemolyticum, Mycoplasma pneumoniae In adults, only 10% pharyngitis due to Group A strep	**Pen V** IM [NEJM 344:205, 2001; AnIM 139:113, 2003. Guideline for Group A strep: CID 35:113, 2002 (Group A,C,G strep, "viral",] **O Ceph 2** times 4–6 days (CID 38:1526 & 1535, 2004) or **clinda** or **azithro** times 5 days, or **clarithro** times 10 days or **clarithro** times 10 days or **erythro** times 10 days (adjust clarithro, clinda (AAC 48:473, 2004)	**Pen V** IM 1 dose See footnote** for adult and pediatric dosages Acetaminophen effective for pain relief (BrJ Gen Prac 50:817, 2000). Children—Linezolid should work.	Rapid strep test or culture. (Some debate: JAMA 291:1587, 2004; & 292:167, 2004) **In children & adults—**No penicillin or cephalosporin-resistant **S. pyogenes**, but now **macrolide-resist. S. pyogenes** (7% 2000–2003). Culture & susceptibility testing if clinical failure with azithro/clarithro (CID 41:599, 2005). **S. pyogenes Groups C & G cause pharyngitis but not a risk for post-strep rheumatic fever.** To prevent rheumatic fever, eradicate Group A strep. Requires 10 days of pen V po. 4–6 day rx of po O Ceph 2, 5 days of po azithro, 10 days of clarithro. In controlled trial, better eradication rate with 10 days clarithro (91%) than 5 days azithro (82%)(CID 32: 1798,2001)
Asymptomatic post-rx carrier Multiple repeated culture-positive episodes (CID 25:574, 1997)	Group A strep	No rx required	**Because of risk of concomitant genital C. trachomatis, add either (azithro 1 gm po times 1) or (azithro 100 mg po q12h times 7 days). See page 17 for more options.**
Whitish plaques, HIV+ (thrush) **Vesicular, ulcerative** **Membranous**—Diphtheria or C. diphtheriae **Vincent's angina**	Candida albicans (see Table 11, page 78) Coxsackie A9, B1-5, ECHO (multiple types) Enterovirus 71, Herpes simplex 1,2 C. diphtheriae Vincent's angina (anaerobes/spirochetes)	**Antibiotics not indicated, but for HSV: acyclovir** 400 mg tid po times 10 days **Antitoxin + erythro** 7–14 days (CID 35:717, 1995) or **penicillin** G **VK** 500 mg po q6h times 5 days **Pen G** 4 million units IV q4h	[Antibacterial agents not indicated.] **Clinda** or **AM-CL** po Parenteral **benzathine pen** **G** + **RIF** (see Comment) Dosages in footnote⁶	Routine post-rx throat culture not advised. Small % of pts have recurrent culture-pos. Group A strep with symptomatic gonococcal, anal epithelium harbors Group A strep. Infection w/ active viral infection in carrier of Group A strep. Addition of **RIF** may ↓ the carrier rate: max of 300 mg (p.o.) times 10 days. Diphtheria occurs in immunized individuals. Antibiotics may ↓ toxin production; ↓ spread of organisms. Penicillin superior to erythro in randomized trial (CID 27:845, 1998). May be complicated by F. necrophorum bacteremia, see jugular vein phlebitis (Lemierre's), page 36

¹ Primary rationale for rx is eradication of Group A (GAS) and prevention of acute rheumatic fever (ARF). PEDIATRIC DOSAGE: Benzathine penicillin 25,000 units per kg IM up to 1.2 million units. **Pen V** 25–50 mg per kg per day div. q6h was associated with clearance of GAS on pharyngeal cultures (CID 19:1110, 1994). Treatment studies have been based on cultures, not actual prevention of ARF. Treatment decreases duration of symptoms.

² Treatment of Group A strep: **All po unless otherwise indicated. PEDIATRIC DOSAGE: Benzathine penicillin** 25,000 units per kg per day div q6h times 10 days; **erythro estolate** 20 mg per kg per day times 10 days; **cefuroxime axetil** 20 mg per kg per day div. bid for 4–10 days (PIDJ 14:295, 1995); **cefpodoxime proxetil** 10 mg per kg per day div bid times10 days; **cefdinir** 7 mg per kg q12h times 5–10 days or 14 mg per kg q24h times 10 days; **cefprozil** 15 mg per kg per day div. bid times 10 days; **clarithro** 15 mg per kg per day div. bid times 10 days; **clinda** 20–30 mg per kg per day div. q8h times 10 days ADULT DOSAGE: **Benzathine penicillin** 1.2 million units IM times 1; **Pen V** 500 mg po bid or 250 mg qid times 10 days; **erythro** (all formulations) 500 mg po bid or 250 mg qid times 10 days; **cefuroxime axetil** 250 mg q12h times 10 days; **cefpodoxime proxetil** 100 mg po q12h times 10 days; **cefdinir** 300 mg po bid or 600 mg q24h times 10 days; **cefprozil** 500 mg q24h times 10 days; **clarithro** 250 mg po bid or clarithro-ER 500 mg po q24h times 10 days; **azithro** 500 mg times 1 and then 250 mg q24h times 4 days; **dirithromycin** 500 mg q24h times 5 days.

³ **clarithro** 250 mg bid times 10 days, **azithro** 500 mg times 1 and then 250 mg q24h times 4 days; pharyngitis, increasing number of studies show efficacy of 4–6 days.

NOTE: All dosage recommendations are for adults (unless otherwise indicated) and assume normal renal function.

Abbreviations on page 2.

TABLE 1 (33)

ANATOMIC SITE/DIAGNOSIS/ MODIFYING CIRCUMSTANCES	ETIOLOGIES (usual)	SUGGESTED REGIMENS* PRIMARY	ALTERNATIVE†	ADJUNCT DIAGNOSTIC OR THERAPEUTIC MEASURES AND COMMENTS
PHARYNX *(continued)* **Epiglottitis** Children	H. influenzae (rare), S. pyogenes, S. pneumoniae, S. aureus	**Peds dosage:** Cefo-taxime 50 mg per kg IV q8h or ceftriaxone 50 mg per kg IV q24h	**Peds dosage: AM-SB** 100-200 mg per kg per day div q6h or **TMP-SMX** 8-12 mg TMP component per kg per day div q12h. See footnote[1]	Have tracheostomy set "at bedside." Chloro is effective, but potentially less toxic alternative agents available. Review (adults): JAMA 272:1358, 1994)
Adults	(Group A strep), H. influenzae (rare)	**ceftriaxone** **Adult dosage:** See footnote[1]	**TC-CL** or **clinda** or **PIP-TZ** or **AM-SB** (Dosage, see footnote 1)	
Parapharyngeal space infection Poor dental hygiene, dental extractions, foreign bodies (e.g. toothpicks, fish bones)	Spaces include: sublingual, submaxillary (Ludwig's angina, used loosely for these), lateral pharyngeal, retropharyngeal, pretracheal] Polymicrobic: Strep sp., anaerobes, Eikenella corrodens	(**Clinda** 600-900 mg IV q8h) or (**pen G** 24 million units by cont. infusion or div q4-6h (4h) + **metro** 1 gm IV load and then 0.5 gm IV q8h))	**Cefoxitin** 2 gm IV q8h or **clinda** or **TC-CL** or **PIP-TZ** or **AM-SB**, see footnote 1	Close observation of airway; 1/3 require intubation. MRI or CT to identify abscess; if present, surgical drainage. **Metro** may be given 1 gm IV q12h.
Jugular vein septic phlebitis (Lemierre's disease) (PIDJ 22:921, 2003; CID 31:524, 2000)	Fusobacterium necro-phorum in vast majority	**Pen G** 24 million units q24h by cont. infusion or div q4-6h	**Clinda** 600-900 mg IV q8h	Usual rx includes external drainage of lateral pharyngeal space. Emboli, pulmonary and systemic common. Erosion into carotid artery can occur.
Laryngitis (hoarseness)/tracheitis	Viral (90%)	Not indicated		
SINUSES, PARANASAL Sinusitis, acute: current terminology: acute rhinosinusitis Obstruction of sinus ostia, usually by virus (colds) for 7 days or less. Refs.: Otolaryn-Head & Neck Surgery 130:1, 2004; AnIM 134:495 & 498, 2001. For rhinovirus infections (common cold), see Table 14, page 17. Pediatric Guidelines: Peds 108:798, 2001	Strep. pneumoniae 31%, H. influenzae 21%, M. catarrhalis 2%, Group A strep 2%, anaerobes 6%, viruses 15%, Staph aureus 4%. By CT scans, sinus mucosa inflamed in 87% of young adults with common cold; develop bacterial rhinosinusitis	Reserve antibiotic rx for pts given decongestants/ analgesics for 7 days who don't improve or worsen. If severe (facial pain, fever), treat sooner—usually requires hospitalization. For mild/mod. disease: Ask if antibiotics in prior month **NO:** Amox-HD or AM-CL-ER or cefdinir or cefpodox-ime or cefprozil or telithro	**YES:** AM-CL-ER (adults) or resp. FQ (adults). For pen allergy see Comments Use AM-CL susp. in peds (Otitis) In general, treat times 10 days, exceptions in adult and pediatric doses, footnote[2] and footnote 3 page 9	**Rx goals:** (1) Resolve infection, (2) prevent complications, e.g., meningitis, brain abscess, (3) avoid chronic sinus disease, (4) avoid unnecessary antibiotic rx. High rate of spontaneous resolution. For pts with pen/cephalosporin allergy, e.g., hives, anaphylaxis, treatment options: telithro, clarithro, azithro, TMP-SMX, doxy or FQs. Telithro listed 1st because of activity vs S. pneumo, resistant to clarithro/azithro. Avoid FQs if under age 18. Dosages in footnote[2] page 35. If allergy just skin rash, po cephalosporin OK. Usual rx 10 days. In 1 study, results of 3 & 10 d. of TMP-SMX the same (JAMA 273:1015, 1995). telithro approved for 5 days. Watch for pts with fever & fascial erythema; ↑ risk of S. aureus infection, requires IV **nafcillin/oxacillin (antistaphylococcal penicillin, penicillinase-resistant for MSSA or vanco for MRSA).** Pts age 1-18 yrs with clinical diagnosis of sinusitis randomized to placebo, amox, or AM-CL for 14 d. **No difference** in multiple measures of efficacy (Peds 107:619, 2001). Similar study in adults: AnIM 163:1793, 2003. Hence, without bacteriologic endpoints, data are hard to interpret. AM-CL-ER ref: AJM 117(Suppl 3A):23S, 2004.
Clinical failure after 3 days	As above, consider diagnostic: tap/aspirate	**Mild/Mod. Disease:** AM-CL-ER or cefpodoxime, cefprozil, cefdinir, or telithro	**Severe Disease:** (cefdinir, cefpodoxime, cefprozil or Gati, Gemi, Levo, Moxi Treat 10 days. & Comment	

---

[1] **Ceftriaxone** 2 gm IV q24h; **cefotaxime** 2 gm IV q4-8t; **AM-SB** 2 gm IV q4-8t; **PIP-TZ** 3.375 gm IV q6h; **TC-CL** 3.1 gm IV q4-6h; **TMP-SMX** 8-10 mg per kg per day (based on TMP component) div q6h, q8h, or q12h.

[2] **Adult doses for sinusitis (all oral):** Amoxicillin high dose (all oral): Amoxicillin high dose 1 gm po tid; 5 mg per kg times 1 then 5 mg per kg per day times 4 days, **clarithro** 500 mg po bid or **clarithro** XR 1 gm po q24h; **doxy** 100 mg bid; **TMP-SMX** 1 DS po bid. **Adult doses for sinusitis (all oral): AM-CL-ER** (Augmentin XR) 2000/125 mg bid; **amox high dose** (should work) 1 gm po tid or 875 mg po q12h (not FDA indication but should work); **respiratory FQs** (**Gati** 400 mg q24h; **Gemi** 320 mg q24h (not FDA indication but should work); **Levo** 750 mg q24h; **Moxi** 400 mg q24h); **O Ceph** (**cefdinir** 300 mg q12h or 600 mg q24h; **cefpodoxime** 200 mg bid, **cefprozil** 250-500 mg bid; **cefuroxime axetil** 250-500 mg bid (results after 3- and 10-day rx similar), **telithro** 800 mg q24h). **TMP-SMX** "double-strength" (TMP 160 mg) bid (results after 3- and 10-day rx similar). *NOTE: All dosage recommendations are for adults (unless otherwise indicated) and assume normal renal function.*

Abbreviations on page 2.

TABLE 1 (34)

ANATOMIC SITE/DIAGNOSIS/ MODIFYING CIRCUMSTANCES	ETIOLOGIES (usual)	SUGGESTED REGIMENS* PRIMARY	ALTERNATIVE†	ADJUNCT DIAGNOSTIC OR THERAPEUTIC MEASURES AND COMMENTS
SINUSES, PARANASAL/Sinusitis, Diabetes mellitus with acute ketoacidosis; neutropenia; deferoxamine rx	**Acute** (continued) Rhizopus sp. (mucor), aspergillus	See Table 11, pages 75 & 82. Ref.: *NEJM 337:254, 1997*		
Hospitalized or nasotracheal or nasogastric intubation	Gm-neg, bacilli 47% (pseudomonas, acinetobacter, E. coli common), Gm + (S. aureus) 35%, yeasts 18%. Polymicrobial in 80%	Remove nasotracheal tube and if fever persists, recommend nasal sinus aspiration for C/S prior to empiric rx. **IMP** 0.5 gm IV q6h or **MER** 1 gm IV q8h. Add vanco for MRSA if Gram stain suggestive.	**Ceftaz** 2 gm IV q8h + **vanco** or **CFP** 2 gm IV q12h + **vanco**. Vanco if MRSA	After 7 d. of nasotracheal or gastric tubes, 95% have x-ray "sinusitis" (fluid in sinuses), but on transnasal puncture only 38% culture + [AJRCCM 150:776, 1994]. For pts requiring mechanical ventilation for ≥1 wk. bacterial sinusitis occurs in <10% [CID 27:851, 1998]. May need fluconazole if yeast on Gram stain of aspirate. Review: *CID 25:1441, 1997* Epidemiology study: *CID 27:463, 1998.*
Sinusitis, chronic **Adults**	Prevotella, anaerobic strep, & fusobacterium—common anaerobes. Strep sp. haemophilus, P. aeruginosa, S. aureus, & moraxella- anaerobes. [CID 35:428, 2002]	Antibiotics usually not effective	Otolaryngology consultation. If acute exacerbation, rx as acute	Pathogenesis unclear and may be polybacterial: damage to ostiomeatal complex during acute bacterial disease, allergy ± polyps, occult immunodeficiency, and/or odontogenic disease (periodontitis in maxillary teeth).
SKIN				
Acne vulgaris [*JAMA 292:726, 2004; NEJM 352:1463, 2005; Ln 352:2188, 2004; Cochrane Database Syst Rev 2000, 2:CD002086*]				
Comedonal acne, "blackheads," "whiteheads," earliest form, no inflammation	Excessive sebum production & ductal obstruction. No Propionibacterium acnes	Topical **tretinoin** (cream 0.025 or 0.05%) or (gel 0.01 or 0.025%).	All once-q24h: Topical **adapalene** 0.1% gel or topical **azelaic acid** 20% cream or topical **tazarotene** 0.1% cream	Goal is prevention, ↓ number of new comedones and create an environment unfavorable to P. acnes. Adapalene causes less irritation than tretinoin. Azelaic acid less potent but less irritating than retinoids. Expect 40–70% ↓ in comedones in 8-12 weeks.
Mild inflammatory acne: small papules or pustules	Proliferation of P. acnes + abnormal desquamation of follicular cells	Topical **erytho** 3% + **benzoyl peroxide** 5%, bid	Can substitute **clinda** 1% gel for erytho	In random, controlled trial, topical benzoyl peroxide + erythro of equal efficacy to oral minocycline & tetracycline and not affected by antibiotic resistance of propionibacteria [*Ln 364:2188, 2004*].
Inflammatory acne: comedones, papules & pustules. Less common: deep nodules (cysts)	Progression of above events	Oral alts.: (**doxy** 100 mg bid) or (**minocycline** 50 mg bid). Others: **tetracycline**, **erytho**, TMP-SMX, **clinda** (Topical **erytho** 3% + **benzoyl peroxide** 5% bid) + oral antibiotic. See **Comment** for mild acne	**Metro** topical cream bid	Systemic **isotretinoin** reserved for pts with severe widespread nodular cystic lesions that fail oral antibiotic rx. 4–5 mo. course of 0.1–1 mg per kg per day. Aggressive/violent behavior reported. Tetracyclines stain developing teeth. Doxy can cause photosensitivity. Minocycline side-effects: urticaria, vertigo, pigment deposition in skin or oral mucosa.
Acne rosacea *NEJM 352:793, 2005*	? skin mite: Demadex folliculorum	Azelaic acid gel bid, topical		More if satisfaction with azelaic acid [*J Am Acad Derm 40(6, Pt.1):961, 1999*]. More options listed in *NEJM 352:793, 2005*
Anthrax, cutaneous, inhalation (pulmonary, mediastinal) **To report bioterrorism event:** 770-488-7100; **for info:** www.bt.cdc.gov Refs.: *JAMA 281:1735, 1999, & MMWR 50:909, 2001*	B. anthracis See *Lung, page 31, and Table 1B, page 48*	**Adults (including pregnancy):** CIP 500 mg IV bid or **Levo** 500 mg IV q24h times 60 days. **Children: CIP** 20-30 mg per kg day IV div q12h or per kg day IV div q12h (to max. 1 gm per day) times 60 days	**Adults (including pregnancy): Doxy** 100 mg po bid times 60 days. **Children: Doxy** >8 y & >45 kg: 100 mg po bid; >8 y & ≤45 kg & <8 y, 2.2 mg per kg po bid. All for 60 days.	If penicillin susceptible, then: 1 **Adults: Amox** 500 mg po q8h times 60 days **Children: Amox** 80 mg per kg day div tid (max. 500 mg q8h) 2 Usual treatment of cutaneous anthrax is 7-10 days, 60 days in setting of bioterrorism with presumed aerosol exposure 3 Other **FQs** (Gati, Levo, Moxi) should work based on in vitro susceptibility data
Bacillary angiomatosis: For other immunocompromised (HIV-), bone marrow transplant) Also see *SANFORD GUIDE TO HIV/AIDS*	Bartonella henselae and quintana	**Clarithro** 500 mg po bid or ext release 1 gm po q24h or (**CIP** 500-750 mg po q24h or CIP 500-750 mg po bid (see **Comment**)	**Erythro** 500 mg po qid or **doxy** 100 mg po bid	In immunocompromised pts with severe disease, doxy 100 mg po/V bid + RIF 300 mg po bid reported effective [*IDC No. Amer 12:37, 1998; Ada Pit 11:1, 1996*]

Bacillary angiomatosis: For other immunocompromised (HIV-), see Cat-scratch disease lymphadenitis, page 33, and Bartonella, page 41

Abbreviations on page 2. NOTE: All dosage recommendations are for adults (unless otherwise indicated) and assume normal renal function.

TABLE 1 (35)

ANATOMIC SITE/DIAGNOSIS/ MODIFYING CIRCUMSTANCES	ETIOLOGIES (usual)	SUGGESTED REGIMENS* PRIMARY	ALTERNATIVE†	ADJUNCT DIAGNOSTIC OR THERAPEUTIC MEASURES AND COMMENTS
SKIN (continued)				
Bite: Remember tetanus prophylaxis—see Table 20. See **Table 20C for rabies prophylaxis**				
Bat, raccoon, skunk	Strep. & staph from skin; rabies	See **Table 20C for rabies prophylaxis**		In Americas, **antirabies rx indicated**: rabies immune globulin + vaccine. *(See Table 20D, pages 144–145)*
Cat (Ref.: *NEJM* 340:85 & 138, 1999)	**Pasteurella multocida**, Staph. aureus	**AM-CL** 875/125 mg po bid or 500/125 mg po tid	**Cefuroxime axetil** 0.5 gm po q12h or **doxy** 100 mg po bid. **Do not use cephalexin.** Sens. to FQs in vitro.	80% cat bites become infected. **P. multocida resistant to dicloxacillin, cephalexin, clinda; many strains resistant to erythro** (most sensitive to azithro but no clinical data). P. multocida infection develops within 24 hrs. Observe for osteomyelitis. If culture + for only P. multocida, can switch to pen G IV or pen VK po.
Cat-scratch disease: see page 33				
Catfish sting	Toxins	See Comments		Presents as immediate pain, erythema and edema. Resembles strep cellulitis. May become secondarily infected; AM-CL may be reasonable choice for prophylaxis.
Dog (Ref.: *NEJM* 340:85 & 138, 1999)	**P. multocida**, S. aureus, Bacteroides sp, Fusobacterium sp, EF-4, Capnocytophaga	**AM-CL** 875/125 mg po bid or 500/125 mg po tid	**Clinda** 300 mg po qid + FQ (adults) or **clinda + TMP-SMX** (children)	Only 5% dog bites become infected. Prophylaxis may be worthwhile *(AnEM 23:535, 1994)*. Consider antirabies rx: rabies immune globulin + vaccine *(Table 20C)*. Capnocytophaga in splenectomized pts may cause local eschar, sepsis with DIC. **P. multocida resistant to diclox, cephalexin, clinda and erythro.**
Human (Ref. for bacteriology, see *CID* 37:1481, 2003)	Viridans strep (100%), Staph epidermidis 53%, corynebacterium 41%, **Staph. aureus 29%, eikenella 15%**, bacteroides 82%, peptostrep 26%	**Early** (not yet infected): **AM-CL** 875/125 mg po bid times 5 days. **Later:** Signs of infection (usually in 3–24 hrs): **(AM-SB** 1.5 gm IV q6h or **cefoxitin** 2 gm IV q8h) or **TC-CL** 3.1 gm IV q6h or **(PIP-TZ** 3.375 gm IV q6h or 4.5 gm q8h)) Pen allergy: **Clinda + (either CIP or TMP-SMX)**	**AM-CL** 875/125 mg po bid **P Ceph 3 or TC-CL or AM-SB or IMP**	**Eikenella resistant to clinda, nafcillin/oxacillin, metro, P Ceph 1, and erythro; susceptible to FQs and TMP-SMX.**
Pig (swine)	Polymicrobic: Gm+ cocci, Gm– bacilli, anaerobes, Pasteurella sp.	**AM-CL** 875/125 mg po bid	Pen allergy: see Table 14A, page 112	Information limited but infection is common and serious *(Ln 348:888, 1996)*
Prairie dog	Monkeypox	No rx recommended		
Primate, non-human	Herpesvirus simiae	**Acyclovir** times 14 days	See Table 14B, page 114	*CID* 20:421, 1995
Rat	Spirillum minus & Streptobacillus moniliformis	**AM-CL** 875/125 mg po bid	**Doxy**	Antirabies rx is not indicated
Seal	Mycoplasma	Tetracycline times 4 wks		Can take weeks to appear after bite *(Ln 364:448, 2004)*.
Snake: pit viper (Ref. *NEJM* 347:347, 2002)	Pseudomonas sp, Enterobacteriaceae, Staph. epidermidis, Clostridium sp.			Primary therapy is antivenom. Penicillin generally used but would not be effective vs organisms isolated. Ceftriaxone should be more effective vs organisms isolated
Spider bite: Most necrotic ulcers attributed to spiders are probably due to another cause, e.g., cutaneous anthrax *(Ln 364:549, 2004)* or MRSA infection				
Widow (Latrodectus)	Not infectious	None		May be confused with "acute abdomen." Diazepam or calcium gluconate helpful to control pain, muscle spasm; tetanus prophylaxis.
Brown recluse (Loxosceles) *NEJM* 352:700, 2005	Not infectious. Overdiagnosed! Spider distribution limited to South Central & desert SW of USA	Bite usually self-limited &, self-healing. No therapy of proven efficacy	**Dapsone** 50 mg po q24h often used despite marginal supportive data	Dapsone causes hemolysis (check for G6PD deficiency). Can cause hepatitis; baseline & weekly liver panels suggested.
Boils—Furunculosis—Subcutaneous abscesses in drug addicts ("skin poppers").				
Active lesions See Table 6, page 57	Staph. aureus, both MSSA & MRSA—concern for community-acquired MRSA	**If afebrile & abscess <5 cm in diameter:** I&D, apply hot packs. No drug. **If ≥5 cm in diameter: TMP-SMX-DS** 2 tabs po bid times 5-10 days.	**Febrile, large &/or multiple abscesses:** I&D, culture abscess, & maybe blood; hot packs. **(TMP-SMX-DS** 2 tabs po bid **+ RIF** 300 mg bid) times 10 days	Carbuncles = multiple connecting furuncles. Epidemic of **community-acquired MRSA**, currently susceptible to TMP-SMX, clinda, minocycline, & linezolid. If erythro-resistant, probably clinda-resistant. **Alternatives for febrile pt, multiple abscesses: Linezolid** 600 mg po bid times 10 days or **dalbavancin** 1000 mg IV times 1 dose.

Abbreviations on page 2   NOTE: All dosage recommendations are for adults (unless otherwise indicated) and assume normal renal function.

39

TABLE 1 (36)

ANATOMIC SITE/DIAGNOSIS/MODIFYING CIRCUMSTANCES	ETIOLOGIES (usual)	SUGGESTED REGIMENS* PRIMARY	ALTERNATIVE†	ADJUNCT DIAGNOSTIC OR THERAPEUTIC MEASURES AND COMMENTS
SKIN/Boils—Furunculosis—Subcutaneous abscesses in drug addicts *(continued)*				
To lessen number of recurrences	MSSA & MRSA	Guided by in vitro susceptibilities: (**Diclox** or **TMP-SMX-DS** 2 tabs po bid) + **RIF** 300 mg po qd24h, all times 10 days	Nasal & under fingernail treatment with **mupirocin ointment** bid	Plus: Shower with Hibiclens q24h times 3 days & then 3 times per week. Others have tried 5% povidone-iodine cream intranasal qid times 5 days. Reports of S. aureus resistant to mupirocin. Not sure about bacitracin ointment, no controlled/comparative studies vs MRSA. Role of topical prophylaxis of bacterial skin colonization in prevention of S. aureus infection in placebo-controlled study *(AnIM 143:419 & 484, 2004)*
Hidradenitis suppurativa	Lesions secondarily infected: S. aureus, Enterobacteriaceae, pseudomonas, anaerobes	Aspirate, base rx on culture		Caused by keratinous plugging of apocrine glands of axillary and/or inguinal areas.
Burns. For overall management: *NEJM 350:810, 2004—step-by-step case outlined & explained*				
Initial burn wound care *(CID 37:543, 2003)*	Not infected	Early excision & wound closure; shower hydrotherapy. Role of topical antimicrobics unclear	**Silver sulfadiazine** cream, 1%, apply 1–2 times per day or 0.5% **silver nitrate** solution or **mafenide acetate** cream. Apply bid.	Many pts ultimately require surgical excision.
Burn wound sepsis	Strep. pyogenes, Enterobacter sp., S. aureus, S. epidermidis, S. aureus, often P. aeruginosa, Fungi rare, Herpesvirus rare	(**Vanco** 1 gm IV q12h) + (**amikacin** 10 mg per kg loading dose then 7.5 mg per kg IV q12h) + (**PIP** 4 gm IV q4h (give ½ q24h dose in subeschar tissues with lymphedema & recurrent erysipelas, often q24h) alternative for vanco		Marrow-induced neutropenia can occur during 1st wk of sulfadiazine but resolves even if use is continued. Silver nitrate leaches electrolytes from wounds & stains everything. Mafenide inhibits carbonic anhydrase and can cause metabolic acidosis.
				Monitor serum levels, 1/2 of most antibiotics ↓. Staph. aureus (and/or MRSA) localizes to burn wound, if toxic, consider toxic shock syndrome. Candida sp. colonizes but seldom invade. Pneumonia is the major infectious complication, often staph. Complications include septic thrombophlebitis. Dapto (4 mg per kg IV q24h) alternative for vanco.
		Variety of skin grafts and skin substitutes, see *JAMA 283:717, 2000*		
Cellulitis, erysipelas: Be wary of MRSA (erythro)-resistant (Group A strep, occ. Group B C, G. Staph. aureus (uncommon but difficult to exclude)	Strep. pyogenes. *NEJM 350:904, 2004.* **NOTE:** Consider diseases that masquerade as cellulitis *(AnIM 142:47, 2005)*			
Extremities, not associated with venous catheter *(see diabetes melitus below)*		**Pen G** 1–2 million units IV q6h OR **P Ceph 1** or **cefazolin** 1 gm IV q8h If not severe, **dicloxacillin** 500 mg po q6h or **cefazolin** 1 gm IV q8h. See Comment	**Erythro** or **P Ceph 1** or **clarithro** or **dirithro** or **tigecycline** *(Dosage, see footnote page 12 or Table 10C)*	**"Spontaneous" erysipelas** of leg in non-diabetic is usually due to strep. Erysipelas of face can mimic S. pyogenes erysipelas of an extremity. Forced to treat empirically for MRSA until in vitro susceptibilities available.
Facial, adult (erysipelas)	Group A strep, Staph. aureus (to include MRSA), S. pneumo	**Vanco** 1 gm IV q12h	**Dapto** 4 mg per kg per day	**Choice of empiric therapy must have activity vs S. aureus.** S. aureus erysipelas of face can mimic S. pyogenes erysipelas of an extremity.
Diabetes melitus and erysipelas *(See Foot, "Diabetic", page 12)*	Group A strep, Staph. aureus, Enterobacteriaceae, clostridia (rare)			Prompt surgical debridement indicated to rule out necrotizing fasciitis and to obtain cultures. If septic, consider x-ray of extremity to demonstrate gas. **Prognosis is dependent on blood supply: assess arteries.** See diabetic foot, page 12.
Erysipelas 2° to lymphedema (congenital = Milroy's disease); post-breast surgery with lymph node dissection	S. pyogenes, Groups A, C, G	**Early mild: TMP-SMX-DS** 2 tabs po bid + **RIF** 300 mg po bid. **For severe disease: IMP** or **MER** or **ERTA** IV + **(linezolid** 600 mg IV/po bid or **vanco** IV) *Dosages, see footnote. Diabetic foot.*		
		Benzathine pen G 1.2 million units IM q4 wks⁻ (of minimal benefit in reducing recurrences in pts with underlying predisposing conditions *CID 25:685, 1997*)		Indicated only if pt is having frequent episodes of cellulitis. Pen V 250 mg po bid should be effective but not aware of clinical trials. In pen-allergic pts: erythro 500 mg po q24h, azithro 250 mg po q24h, or clarithro 500 mg po q24h
Dandruff (seborrheic dermatitis)	Malassezia species	**Ketoconazole shampoo** 2% or **selenium sulfide** 2.5% *(see page 8, chronic external otitis)*		
Decubitus or venous stasis or arterial insufficiency ulcers; with sepsis	Polymicrobic: S. pyogenes (Gps A,C,G), enterococcus + aerobic strep, Enterobacteriaceae, Pseudomonas sp., Bacteroides sp., Staph. aureus	**IMP** or **MER** or **ERTA** or **PIP-TZ** or **TC-CL** or **ERTA**	**(CIP, Gati, Levo,** or **Moxi)** *Dosages, see footnotes pages 12, 19, 24, 45*	Without sepsis & extensive cellulitis local care may be adequate. Debride as needed. Topical mafenide or silver sulfadiazine adjunctive. RYO underlying osteomyelitis. May need wound coverage with skin graft or skin substitute *(JAMA 283:716, 2000)*
Erythema multiforme	H. simplex type 1, mycoplasma, Strep. pyogenes, drugs (sulfonamides, phenytoin, penicillins)			**Rx:** Acyclovir if due to H. simplex

Abbreviations on page 2.   NOTE: All dosage recommendations are for adults (unless otherwise indicated) and assume normal renal function.

TABLE 1 (37)

ANATOMIC SITE/DIAGNOSIS/ MODIFYING CIRCUMSTANCES	ETIOLOGIES (usual)	SUGGESTED REGIMENS*		ADJUNCT DIAGNOSTIC OR THERAPEUTIC MEASURES AND COMMENTS
		PRIMARY	**ALTERNATIVE†**	
SKIN (continued)				
Erythema nodosum	Sarcoidosis, inflammatory bowel disease, M. tbc, coccidioidomycosis, yersinia, sulfonamides			Rx: **NSAIDs**; **glucocorticoids** if refractory
Erythrasma	Corynebacterium minutissimum	**Erythro** 250 mg po q6h times 14 days		Coral red fluorescence with Wood's lamp. Alt: 2% aqueous clinda topically
Folliculitis	Many etiologies: S. aureus, candida, P. aeruginosa, malassezia, demodex	See individual entities. See Whirlpool folliculitis, page 41.		
Furunculosis	Staph. aureus	See Boils, pages 38–39		
Hemorrhagic bullous lesions Hx of sea water-contaminated abrasion or eating raw seafood, shock	Vibrio vulnificus, V. damsela	**Ceftazidime** 2 gm IV q8h + **doxy** 100 mg IV bid	Either **cefotaxime** 2 gm IV q8h or **Ceftaz** 750 mg po bid or 400 mg IV bid	~½ pts have chronic liver disease with mortality in 50% (NEJM 312:343, 1985). In Taiwan, where a number of cases are seen, the impression exists that ceftazidime is superior to tetracyclines (CID 15:271, 1992), hence both.
Herpes zoster (shingles) See Table 14				
Impetigo, ecthyma—usually children **Group A strep impetigo** "Honey-crust" lesions (non-bullous)	Staph. aureus + streptococci	**Mupirocin** ointment 2% tid or **fusidic acid cream†** 2% times 3–5 days	**Azithro** or **clarithro** or **erythro** or **Ceph 2**	In meta-analysis that combined strep & staph impetigo, mupirocin had higher cure rates than placebo. Mupirocin superior to oral erythro. Penicillin inferior to erythro. Few placebo-controlled trials. Ref.: Cochrane Database Systemic Reviews, 2004 (2): CD003261.
Staph. aureus impetigo Bullous (if ruptured, thin "varnish-like" crust)	MSSA & MRSA	**For MSSA:** po therapy with **dicloxacillin, oxacillin, cephalexin, AM-CL, azithro, clarithro,** or **mupirocin** ointment	**For MRSA: Mupirocin** ointment, **TMP-SMX-DS, minocycline**	
		For dosages, see Table 10C		
Infected wound, extremity—Post-trauma (for bites, see page 38; for post-operative, see below)	Polymicrobic: Staph. aureus (MSSA & MRSA), Group A strep, Enterobacteriaceae, anaerobic organisms, Cl. tetani, (if water exposure, Aeromonas sp.)			**Culture & sensitivity, check Gram stain. Tetanus toxoid if indicated.**
Mild to moderate; uncomplicated		**TMP-SMX-DS** 2 tabs po bid or **clinda** 300–450 mg po bid (see Comment)	**Minocycline** 100 mg po bid or **linezolid** 600 mg po bid (see Comment)	**Mild infection:** Suggested drugs focus on S. aureus & Strep species. If suspect Gm-neg. bacilli, **add AM-CL-ER** 1000/62.5 two tabs po bid. If MRSA suspected, may have inducible resistance to clinda.
Febrile with sepsis—hospitalized		**IMP-SB** or **TC-CL** or **PIP-TZ** or **IMP** or **MER** + **vanco** 1 gm IV q12h	**Vanco** 1 gm IV q12h (see Comment) + **CIP** (V—dose in Comment)	**Fever—sepsis:** Alternative to vanco is **linezolid** 600 mg IV/po q12h. If Gm-neg. bacilli & severe pen allergy, CIP 400 mg IV q12h or Levo 750 mg IV q24h.
Infected wound, post-operative—Gram stain negative Surgery not involving GI or female genital tract	Staph. aureus, Group A, B, or G strep			Check Gram stain of exudate. If Gm-neg, bacilli, **add** β-lactam/β-lactamase inhibitor: AM-CL-ER po or (ERTA or PIP-TZ or TC-CL) IV. Dosage on page 19.
Without sepsis (mild)		**TMP-SMX-DS** 2 tabs po bid	**Clinda** 300–450 mg po bid	
With sepsis (severe)	MSSA/MRSA	**Vanco** 1 gm IV q12h	**Dapto** 6 mg per kg IV q24h	
Surgery involving GI tract (includes oropharynx, esophagus) or female genital tract—fever, neutrophilia	coliforms, bacteroides & other anaerobes	**[(PIP-TZ or Ceph 3 + metro) or ERTA or IMP or MER] if seriously ill. Mild infection:** AM-CL-ER po q12h (see page 41) Add **TMP-SMX-DS** 2 tabs po bid if MRSA (see page 41)		For all treatment options, see Peritonitis, page 34. Most important: Drain wound & get cultures. Can sub linezolid for vanco. Can sub CIP or Levo for β-lactams.
Meleney's synergistic gangrene: See Necrotizing fasciitis				
Infected patient, febrile—Gram stain: Gram-positive cocci in clusters	S. aureus, possibly MRSA	**Oral: TMP-SMX-DS** 2 tabs po bid or **clinda** 300–450 mg po bid (see page 41) **IV: Vanco** 1 gm IV q12h	Do culture & sensitivity **IV: Vanco** 1 gm IV q12h or **daptomycin** 4 mg per kg IV q24h or 6 mg per kg q24h if septic	↑ in community-acquired MRSA (CA-MRSA). Need culture & sensitivity to verify. Other po options for CA-MRSA include minocycline 100 mg po q12h (inexpensive) & linezolid 600 mg po q12h (expensive). If MRSA clinda-sensitive but erythro-resistant, watch out for inducible resistance. If resistance, IV alternatives are **tigecycline** 100 mg times 1 dose, then 50 mg per day.

Abbreviations on page 2.   NOTE: All dosage recommendations are for adults (unless otherwise indicated) and assume normal renal function.

TABLE 1 (38)

ANATOMIC SITE/DIAGNOSIS/ MODIFYING CIRCUMSTANCES	ETIOLOGIES (usual)	SUGGESTED REGIMENS* PRIMARY	ALTERNATIVE†	ADJUNCT DIAGNOSTIC OR THERAPEUTIC MEASURES AND COMMENTS
SKIN (continued)				
Necrotizing fasciitis ("flesh-eating bacteria") Post-surgery, trauma, strepto- coccal skin infections

See Gas gangrene, page 33, and S. aureus, page 46 | **4 types:** (1) Streptococci, Grp A, C, G. (2) Clostridia sp.. (3) polymicrobic: aerob- ic + anaerobic strep + Ente- robacteriaceae (fascial plane). (4) Community-acquired MRSA | For treatment of clostridia, see Muscle, gas gangrene, page 33. The terminology of **polymicrobic** wound infections is not precise: necrotizing fasciitis, Meleney's synergistic gangrene, Fournier's gangrene, necrotizing fasciitis have a common pathophysiology. **All require prompt surgical debridement** as well as antibiotics. Dx of necrotizing fasciitis requires incision and probing; if no resistance to probing, subcutaneously (fascial plane). dx = necrotizing fasciitis. **Need Gram stain/culture** to determine if etiology is strep, clostridia, polymicrobial, or S. aureus. **Treatment: Pen G** if strep or clostridia. **IMP** or **MER** if polymicrobial, add **vanco** if MRSA suspected. **NOTE:** If strep necrotizing fasciitis, reasonable to treat with penicillin & clinda (*SMJ 96:968, 2003*); if clostridia ± gas gangrene, add clinda to penicillin ref: *NEJM 352:1445, 2005* | | |
Puncture wound—nail Through tennis shoe: P. aeruginosa		Local debridement to remove foreign body & tetanus prophylaxis		Osteomyelitis evolves in only 1-2% of plantar puncture wounds.
Staphylococcal scalded skin syndrome Ref.: *PIDJ 19:819, 2000*	Toxin-producing S. aureus	**Nafcillin** or **oxacillin** 2 gm IV q4h (children 150 mg per kg per day div. q6h) times 5–7 days for MSSA. **vanco** 1 gm IV bid for MRSA (children 40–60 mg per kg per day div. q6h).		Toxin causes **intraepidermal split** and positive Nikolsky sign. Drugs cause epidermal/dermal split, **called toxic epidermal necrolysis**—more serious (*Ln 351:1417, 1998*). Biopsy differentiates.
Ulcerated skin lesions	Consider anthrax, tularemia, plague, and others			**P. aeruginosa** (ecthyma gangrenosum), plague, blastomycosis, spider (rarely), mycobacteria, leishmania, arterial insuffi- ciency, venous stasis, and others
Whirlpool (Hot Tub) folliculitis See Folliculitis, page 40	Pseudomonas aeruginosa	Usually self-limited, treatment not indicated		Decontaminate hot tub: drain and chlorinate. Also associated with exfoliative beauty aids (loofah sponges) (*J Clin Microbiol 31:480, 1993*).
SPLEEN. For post-splenectomy prophylaxis, see Table 15B, page 125				
Acute	Staph. aureus, streptococci			
Endocarditis, bacteremia	Polymicrobic			
Contiguous from intra-abdominal site	Candida sp.			
Immunocompromised				
SYSTEMIC FEBRILE SYNDROMES				
Spread by infected TICK, FLEA, or LICE: *CID 35:684, 2002* **Babesiosis:** *CID 29:888, 1999)*. Epidemiologic history crucial **Babesiosis:** See *NEJM 343:1454, 2000* & *CID 31:1117* B. microti et al. Etiol.: B. microti et al. Vector: Usually Ixodes ticks Host: White-footed mouse & others	Babesiosis, Lyme disease, & granulocytic Ehrlichiosis have same reservoir & tick vector. Exposure endemic areas May to Sept. Can result from blood transfusion (*JAMA 281:927, 1999*). Lyme, subclinical illness likely in asplenic pts, pts with HIV Dx: Giemsa-stained blood smear; antibody test available. PCR under study **Rx: Exchange transfusions successful adjunct, used early, in severe disease.**		
Babesiosis, if asymptomatic, young, has spleen, and immunocompetent		(**Atovaquone** 750 mg po q12h) + **azithro** 500 mg po day 1, then 250 mg/day times 7 days **OR** [**Clinda** 1.2 gm IV bid or 600 mg po tid times 7 days + **quinine** 650 mg po tid times 7 days. **Ped. dos- age: Clinda** 20–40 mg per kg per day and **quinine** 25 mg per kg per day] plus **exchange transfusion**		
Bartonella Infections: *CID 35:684, 2002*				
Asymptomatic bacteremia	B. quintana	**Doxy** 100 mg po/IV times 15 days		Can lead to endocarditis &/or trench fever, found in homeless, esp. if lice/leg pain.
Acute bacteremia	B. quintana			
Cat-scratch disease	B. henselae	**Azithro** 500 mg po day 1, then 250 mg po q24h times 4 days		Usually self-limited, can involve CNS, liver in immunocompetent pts
B. angiomatosis-bacteremia	B. henselae, B. quintana	(**Clarithro** 500 mg po bid or **doxy** 100 mg po bid) or **clarithro** ER 1 gm po q24h or **azithro** 250 mg po q24h or CIP 500–750 mg po bid times 8 wks		Manifestations of Bartonella infections: **Immunocompetent Patient:** Bacteremia/endocarditis/FUO encephalitis Cat scratch disease Vertebral osteo Trench fever
Peliosis hepatis—pts with AIDS	B. henselae, B. quintana	**Gentamicin** 3 mg per kg IV once q24h times minimum 14 days + **doxy** 500 mg po bid q24h times 4–6 wks		**HIV/AIDS Patient:** Bacillary angiomatosis Bacillary peliosis Bacteremia/endocarditis/FUO
Endocarditis (see page 23) (*AAC 47:2204, 2003*)	B. henselae, B. quintana	**Doxy** 100 mg po (doxy alone if **no** endocarditis)		Hard to detect with automated blood culture systems. Need lysis-centrifugation and/or direct subculture onto chocolate agar at 7 & 14 days. Diagnosis often by antibody titer ≥1:800.
Trench fever (FUO)	B. quintana	**Doxy** 100 mg po bid (doxy alone)		Same as Urban Trench Fever (page 43)

Abbreviations on page 2. NOTE: All dosage recommendations are for adults (unless otherwise indicated) and assume normal renal function.

TABLE 1 (39)

ANATOMIC SITE/DIAGNOSIS/ MODIFYING CIRCUMSTANCES	ETIOLOGIES (usual)	SUGGESTED REGIMENS* PRIMARY	ALTERNATIVE†	ADJUNCT DIAGNOSTIC OR THERAPEUTIC MEASURES AND COMMENTS
SYSTEMIC FEBRILE SYNDROMES				
Ehrlichiosis: CDC def. is one of: (1) 4x↑ IFA antibody, (2) detection of Ehrlichia DNA in blood or CSF by PCR, (3) visible morulae in WBC, and IFA ≥1:64 *[MMWR 46/RR-10):1-55, 1997]*	Spread by infected: **TICK, FLEA or LICE** *(continued)*			
Human monocytic ehrlichiosis (HEM) *[JAMA 292:2263, 2004]*	*Ehrlichia chaffeensis* (Lone Star tick is vector)	**Doxy** 100 mg po/IV bid times 7-14 days	**Tetracycline** 500 mg po qid times 7-14 days. No current recommendation for children or pregnancy. See Comment	30 states: mostly SE of line from NJ to Ill. to Missouri to Oklahoma to Texas. History of outdoor activity and tick exposure. April-Sept. Fever, rash (36%), leukopenia and thrombocytopenia. Blood smears no help. PCR for early dx.
Human granulocytic ehrlichiosis (HGE) *[JAMA 292:2263, 2004]*	*Anaplasma (Ehrlichia) phagocytophilum* (Ixodes sp. ticks are vector). Dog variant is Ehrlichia ewingii *[NEJM 341:148 & 195, 1999]*	**Doxy** 100 mg bid po or IV times 7-14 days	**Tetracycline** 500 mg po times 7-14 days. Not in children or pregnancy. See Comment	Upper Midwest, NE, West Coast & Europe. H/O tick exposure. April-Sept. Febrile flu-like illness after outdoor activity. No rash. Leukopenia/thrombocytopenia common. **Dx:** Up to 80% have positive blood smear. Antibody test for confirmation. **Rx:** RIF successful in pregnancy *[CID 27:213, 1998]* but worry about resistance developing. Based on in vitro studies, no clear alternative rx—Levo activity questionable *[AAC 47:413, 2003]*
Lyme Disease NOTE: Think about concomitant tick-borne disease—babesiosis *[JAMA 275:1657, 1996]* or ehrlichiosis *[JAMA 275:199, 1996]*. Tick bite, possible bodies acquired in endemic area	*Borrelia burgdorferi*	**If endemic area,** if nymphal tick partially engorged & deer tick present: **doxy** 200 mg po times 1 dose with food	**If not endemic area,** not engorged, not deer tick: No treatment	Prophylaxis study in endemic area: erythema migrans developed in 3% of the control group and 0.4% doxy group *[NEJM 345:79 & 133, 2001]*. Reviews: *LnID 3:489 & 761, 2003; Ln 362:1639, 2003. www.cdc.gov*
Early (erythema migrans) *See Comment*		**Doxy** 100 mg po bid, or **amoxicillin** 500 mg po tid or **cefuroxime axetil** 500 mg po bid times 14-21 days. All regimens for 14-21 days. (10 days as good as 20. *AnIM 138:697, 2003)*	**Doxy** 100 mg po bid or **erythro** 250 mg po qid. See Comment for peds doses	High rate of clinical failure with azithro & erythro *[Drugs 57:157, 1999]*. **Peds** (all po for 14-21 days): **Amox** 50 mg per kg per day in 3 div. doses or **cefuroxime axetil** 30 mg per kg per day in 2 div. doses or **erythro** 30 mg per kg per day in 3 div. doses.
Carditis *See Comment*		**Ceftriaxone** 2 gm IV (q24h) or **(cefotaxime** 2 gm IV q4h) or **(pen G** 24 million units IV q24h) times 14-21 days	**Doxy** (see Comments) or **amoxicillin** 500 mg po tid times 14-21 days or **cefuroxime axetil** 250-500 mg po tid times 14-21 days	Lesions usually hemogenous—not target-like *[AnIM 136:423, 2002]*. First degree AV block: Oral regimen. High degree AV block (PR >0.3 sec.): IV therapy—permanent pacemaker not necessary
Facial nerve paralysis (isolated finding, early)		**(Doxy** 100 mg po bid) or **(amoxicillin** 500 mg po tid) times 14-21 days	**Ceftriaxone** 2 gm IV q24h times 14-21 days	LP suggested to exclude neurologic disease. If LP neg., oral regimen OK. If abnormal or not done, suggest parenteral regimen.
Meningitis, encephalitis For encephalopathy, see Comment		**Ceftriaxone** 2 gm IV q24h times 14-28 days	**(Pen G** 20 million units IV q24h) or **(cefotaxime** 2 gm IV q8h) times 14-28 days	Encephalopathy: memory difficulty, depression, somnolence or headache; CSF abnormalities. 89% had objective CSF abnormalities. 18/18 pts improved with ceftriaxone 2 gm per day times 30 days *[JID 180:377, 1999]*
Arthritis		**(Doxy** 100 mg po bid) or **(amoxicillin** 500 mg po qid), both times 30-60 days or **ceftriaxone** 2 gm IV q24h times 14-28 days	**Ceftriaxone** 2 gm IV q24h times 7-10 days or **(pen G** 20-24 million units per day IV) times 14-28 days	Choice should not include doxy. amoxicillin 500 mg po qid times 21 days
Pregnant women		None indicated.		
Asymptomatic seropositivity post-rx				No benefit from rx *[NEJM 345:85, 2001]*
Plague **As biological weapon:** *[JAMA 283:2281, 2000, and Table 1B, page 48]*	*Yersinia pestis* Reservoir: rat Vector: rat flea	**Gentamicin** 2 mg per kg IV loading dose then 1.7 mg per kg IV q8h or **strepto-mycin** 1 gm IM/IV q12h	**Doxy** 100 mg IV/po bid or **(chloro** 500 mg IV/po qid)	Reference IV streptomycin *[CID 19:1150, 1994]*. Septicemic form can occur without buboes. **CIP** effective in vitro + in animal models *[JAC 41:301, 1998]*. CIP success in 1 pt *[CID 30:132, 2003]*
Relapsing fever Can be tick-borne or louse-borne *[MMWR 39:649, 2003]*	*Borrelia recurrentis, B. hermsii,* & other borrelia sp.	**Doxy** 100 mg po bid	**Erythro** 500 mg po qid	Jarisch-Herxheimer (fever, ↑ pulse, ↑ resp., ↓ blood pressure) in most patients (occurs in ~2 hrs). Not prevented by prior steroids. **Dx:** Examine peripheral blood smear during fever for spirochetes. Can relapse up to 10 times.

† In endemic area (New York), high % of both adult ticks and nymphs were jointly infected with both HGE and *B. burgdorferi* and *B. burgdorferi* *[NEJM 337:49, 1997]*.

NOTE: All dosage recommendations are for adults (unless otherwise indicated) and assume normal renal function.

TABLE 1 (40)

ANATOMIC SITE/DIAGNOSIS/ MODIFYING CIRCUMSTANCES	ETIOLOGIES (usual)	SUGGESTED REGIMENS*		ADJUNCT DIAGNOSTIC OR THERAPEUTIC MEASURES AND COMMENTS
		PRIMARY	ALTERNATIVE†	
SYSTEMIC FEBRILE SYNDROMES:				
Rickettsial diseases. Review—Disease in travelers (*CID 39:1493, 2004*)				
Spotted fevers (NOTE: Rickettsial pox not included)				
Rocky Mountain spotted fever (RMSF) (*AJTMH 63:21, 2000; AIM 163:769, 2003*) NOTE: Can mimic ehrlichiosis.	R. rickettsii (*Dermacentor* ticks)	**Doxy** 100 mg po/IV times 1 for 2 days after temp. normal	**Chloro** use found as risk factor for fatal RMSF (*IJID 184:1437, 2001*)	Fever, rash (95%), petechiae 40–50%. **Rash spreads from distal extremities to trunk.** Dx: immunohistology on skin biopsy; confirmation with antibody titers. Highest incidence in Mid-Atlantic states; also seen in Oklahoma, S. Dakota, Montana. NOTE: Only 3–18% of pts present with fever, rash, and hx of tick exposure; **esp. in children many early deaths & empiric doxy reasonable** (*MMWR 49: 888, 2000*).
Other spotted fevers, e.g. Boutonneuse fever. In sub-Saharan Africa, R. africae R. africae review: *LnID 3:557, 2003*	6 species; e.g. R. conorii et al (multiple ticks). In sub-Saharan Africa, R. africae	**Doxy** 100 mg po bid times 7 days	Clarithro 7.5 mg per kg q12h & azithro 10 mg per kg per day times 1 for 3 days equally effective in children with Mediterranean spotted fever (*CID 34:154, 2002*) R. africae review *CID 36:1411, 2003* R. parkeri in U.S. *CID 38:805, 2004*	
Typhus group—Consider in returning travelers with fever				
Louse-borne	R. prowazekii (body louse)	**Doxy** 100 mg IV/po bid times 7 days	**Chloro** 500 mg IV/po qid times 7 days	**Brill-Zinsser disease** (*Ln 357:1198, 2001*) is a relapse of remote past infection, e.g. WW II. Trunk rash spreads centrifugally—opposite of RMSF. A winter disease.
Murine typhus (cat flea typhus similar)	R. typhi (rat reservoir and flea vector)	**Doxy** 100 mg IV/po bid times 7 days	**Chloro** 500 mg IV/po qid times 7 days	Most U.S. cases south Texas and southern Calif. Flu-like illness. Rash in < 50%. Dx based on suspicion; confirmed serologically.
Scrub typhus	O. tsutsugamushi (rodent reservoir; vector is larval stage of mites (chiggers))	**Doxy** 100 mg IV/po bid times 7 days. NOTE: Reports of doxy and chloro resistance from northern Thailand (*Ln 348:86, 1996*). In prospective random trial single 500 mg dose of **azithro** as effective as doxy (*CID 39:1329, 2004*).		Limited to Far East (Asia, India). Cases imported into U.S. Evidence of chigger bite, flu-like illness. Rash like louse-borne. **RIF** alone 450 mg bid po times 7 days reported effective (*Ln 356:1057, 2000*). Worry about RIF resistance.
Tularemia, typhoidal type Ref. bioterrorism: see *Table 1B, page 48, & JAMA 285:2763, 2001*	Francisella tularensis (Vector depends on geography; ticks, biting flies, mosquitoes (identified)	**Gentamicin** or **tobra** 5 mg per kg per day div. q8h IV times 7–14 days	Add **chloro** IV times 14 days or **CIP** reported effective in 12 children (*PIDJ 19:449, 2000*)	Typhoidal form in 5–30% pts. No lymphadenopathy. Diarrhea, pneumonia common. Dx: blood cultures. Antibody confirmation. Rx. Jarisch-Herxheimer reaction may occur. Clinical failures with rx with P Ceph 3 (*CID 17:976, 1993*).
Urban trench fever (endocarditis) (*AAC 47:2204, 2003*)	Bartonella quintana Vector: Body louse	**Gentamicin** 3 mg per kg IV once q24h times min of 14 days **+ doxy** 200 mg po single q24h dose times 28 days		One of many Bartonella syndromes; see pages 23 & 41
Other Zoonotic Systemic Bacterial Febrile Illnesses: Obtain careful epidemiologic history				
Brucellosis Review: *NEJM 352:2325, 2005*				
Adult or child > 8 years	Brucella sp. B. abortus—cattle B. suis—pigs B. melitensis—goats B. canis—dogs	[**Doxy** 100 mg po bid times 6 wks + **gentamicin** times 2–3 wks (see *Table 10D, page 74*)] or [doxy times 6 wks + **streptomycin** 1 gm IM q24h times 2–3 wks] See Comment	[**Doxy + RIF** 600–900 mg po q24h, both times 6 wks] or [**TMP-SMX** 1 DS tab (160 mg) po q12h times 6 wks + **gentamicin** times 2 wks]	**Clinical disease:** Protean. Fever in 91%. **Malodorous perspiration almost pathognomonic.** Osteoarticular disease in approx. 20%; epididymitis/orchitis 6%. **Lab:** Mild hepatitis. Leukopenia & relative lymphocytosis. **Diagnosis:** Serology; bone marrow culture; real-time PCR if available. **Treatment:** Drugs must penetrate macrophages & act in acidic milieu. **Pregnancy:** TMP-SMX-DS + RIF reasonable
Child < 8 years		TMP-SMX 5 mg per kg TMP po q12h times 6 wks + **gentamicin** 2 mg per kg IV/IM q8h times 2 wks	[**Doxy** + **ceftriaxone** 1 gm q6h or **ceftriaxone** 1 gm q24h times 6 wks] or [**AMP** 0.5–1 gm IV q6h + gentamicin]	
Leptospirosis (*CID 36:1507 & 1514, 2003; LnID 3:757, 2003*)	Leptospira—in urine of domestic livestock, dogs, small rodents	**Pen G** 1.5 million units IV q6h or **ceftriaxone** 1 gm q24h. Duration: 7 days	**Doxy** 100 mg po or IV/IM q12h or **AMP** 0.5–1 g/m IV q6h	**Severity varies.** Two-stage mild anicteric illness to severe icteric disease (Weil's disease) with renal failure and myocarditis. **Rx:** Penicillin, doxy, & cefotaxime of equal efficacy in severe lepto (*CID 39:1417, 2004*).

Abbreviations on page 2.   NOTE: All dosage recommendations are for adults (unless otherwise indicated) and assume normal renal function.

TABLE 1 (41)

ANATOMIC SITE/DIAGNOSIS/ MODIFYING CIRCUMSTANCES	ETIOLOGIES (usual)	SUGGESTED REGIMENS*		ADJUNCT DIAGNOSTIC OR THERAPEUTIC MEASURES AND COMMENTS
		PRIMARY	ALTERNATIVE†	
SYSTEMIC FEBRILE SYNDROMES: Other Zoonotic Systemic Bacterial Febrile Illnesses *(continued)*				
Salmonella bacteremia (enteric fever most often caused by S. typhi)	Salmonella enteritidis—a variety of serotypes	CIP 400 mg IV q12h times 14 days (switch to po to 750 mg bid when clinically possible)	Ceftriaxone 2 gm IV q24h times 14 days (switch to po CIP when possible)	Usual exposure is contaminated poultry and eggs. Many others. Myriad of complications to consider, e.g. mycotic aneurysm (10% of adults over age 50. AJM 110:60, 2001), septic arthritis, osteomyelitis, septic shock. Sporadic reports of resistance to CIP. Ref: CID 37:1141, 2005
Miscellaneous Systemic Febrile Syndromes				
Kawasaki syndrome 6 weeks to 12 yrs of age, peak at 1 yr of age; 85% below age 5. (Ln 364:533, 2004)	Acute self-limited vasculitis with ↑ temp, rash, conjunctivitis, stomatitis, cervical adenitis, red hands/feet & coronary artery aneurysms (25% if untreated)	IVIG 2 gm per kg over 12 hrs + ASA 20-25 mg per kg qid THEN ASA 3-5 mg per kg per day po q24h times 6-8 wks	If still febrile after 1st dose of IVIG, give a 2nd dose (PIDJ 17:1144, 1998)	IV gamma globulin (2 gm per kg over 10 hrs) in pts rx before 10th day of illness ↓ coronary artery lesions (Ln 347:1128, 1996) See Table 14B, page 115 for IVIG adverse effects and expense.
Rheumatic Fever, acute Ref: Ln 366:155, 2005	Post-Group A strep, pharyngitis (not Group B, C, or G) (See Pharyngitis, page 35)	(1) ↓ symptom relief: ASA 80-100 mg per kg per day in children; 4-8 gm per day in adults. (2) Eradicate Group A strep: Pen times 10 days (3) Start prophylaxis: see below.		Prevents rheumatic fever even when started 7-9 days after onset of illness.
Prophylaxis Primary prophylaxis (previous documented rheumatic fever)		Benzathine pen G 1.2 million units IM (see Pharyngitis, p. 32)	Penicillin V 250 mg po bid times 10 days, prevents rheumatic fever.	
Secondary prophylaxis		Benzathine pen G 1.2 million units IM	Alternative: Penicillin V 250 mg po bid. Duration of 2° prophylaxis varies: with carditis continue 10 yrs or until age 18 (or longer); without carditis continue 5 yrs or until age 21. (JAMA 268:2069-2073, 1992)	
Typhoid Fever (typhoid fever, enteric fever) (Ln 366:749, 2005; LnID 5:623, 2005)	Salmonella typhi, S. paratyphi NOTE: In vitro resistance to nalidixic acid predicts clinical failure of CIP (FQs) (Ln 366:749, 2005)	CIP 500 mg IV times 10 days or (ceftriaxone 2 gm IV q24h times 14 days). If associated abscess, add dexamethasone a few minutes before antibiotic. (See Comment)	dexamethasone dose: 3 mg per kg then 1 mg per kg q6h times 8 doses ↓ mortality (NEJM 310:82, 1984). Complications: perforation of terminal ileum &/or cecum, osteo, septic arthritis, mycotic aneurysm (approx. 10% over age 50. AJM 110:62, 2001), meningitis. Other rx options: Controlled trial of CIP vs chloro. Efficacy equivalent. After 5 days, blood culture positive: CIP 18%, chloro 38% (AAC 47:1727, 2003). Children & adolescents: Ceftriaxone (75 mg per kg per day) and azithro (20 mg per kg per day to 1 gm max.) equal efficacy. More relapses with ceftriaxone (CID 38:951, 2004).
Sepsis: Following suggested empiric therapy pt is bacteremic; mimicked by fungal, rickettsial infections and pancreatitis				
Neonatal—early onset <1 week old	Group B strep, E. coli, klebsiella, enterobacter, Staph. aureus (uncommon), listeria (rare in U.S.)	AMP 25 mg per kg IV q8h + cefotaxime 50 mg per kg IV q12h	(AMP + APAG 2.5 mg per kg IV/IM q12h) or (AMP + cefotaxime 50 mg per kg IV/IM q12h)	Blood cultures are key but only 5–10% +. Discontinue antibiotics after 72 hrs if cultures and course do not support diagnosis. In Spain, listeria predominates; in S. America, salmonella.
Neonatal—late onset 1-4 weeks old	As above + H. influenzae & S. epidermidis	AMP 25 mg per kg IV q8h + cefotaxime 50 mg per kg IV q8h or (AMP 25 mg per kg IV q6h or cefotaxime 75 mg per kg IV q24h)	AMP + APAG 2.5 mg per kg IV or IM	If MSSA/MRSA a concern, add vanco.
Child; not neutropenic	Strep, pneumoniae, meningococci, Staph. aureus (MSSA & MRSA), H. influenzae now rare	Cefotaxime 50 mg per kg IV q8h or ceftriaxone 100 mg per kg IV q24h + vanco 15 mg per kg IV q6h	Aztreonam 7.5 mg per kg q6h + linezolid (see Table 16, page 133 for dose)	Major concerns as S. pneumoniae & community-acquired MRSA. Coverage for Gm-neg. bacilli included but H. influenzae infection now rare. Meningococcemia mortality remains high (Ln 356:961, 2000).

Abbreviations on page 2.   NOTE: All dosage recommendations are for adults (unless otherwise indicated) and assume normal renal function.

TABLE 1 (42)

ANATOMIC SITE/DIAGNOSIS/ MODIFYING CIRCUMSTANCES	ETIOLOGIES (usual)	SUGGESTED REGIMENS*		ADJUNCT DIAGNOSTIC OR THERAPEUTIC MEASURES AND COMMENTS
		PRIMARY	ALTERNATIVE†	
SYSTEMIC FEBRILE SYNDROMES/Sepsis *(continued)*				
Adult: not neutropenic; NO HYPOTENSION but LIFE-THREATENING!—For Septic Shock, see page 46				Systemic inflammatory response syndrome (SIRS): 2 or more of the following:
Source unclear—consider intra-abdominal or skin source. **Life-threatening!**	Aerobic Gm-neg. bacilli, S. aureus, streptococci, others	(IMP or MER or ERTA) + vanco	**Dapto** 6 mg per kg IV q24h (or TC-CL). PIP-TZ or TC-CL	1. temperature above 38° or <36°C 2. Heart rate >90 beats per min. 3. Respiratory rate >20 breaths per min. 4. WBC >12,000 per mcL or >10% bands
			Could substitute linezolid for vanco or dapto; however, linezolid bacteriostatic vs S. aureus. *Dosages in footnote*[1]	**Sepsis:** SIRS + a documented infection (+ culture) **Severe sepsis:** Sepsis + organ dysfunction or hypoperfusion abnormalities (lactic acidosis, oliguria, ↓mental status) **Septic shock:** Sepsis-induced hypotension (systolic BP <90 mm/Hg) not responsive to 500 mL IV fluid challenge + peripheral hypoperfusion.
If suspect biliary source *(see p. 10)*	Enterococci + aerobic Gm-neg. bacilli	**AM-SB, PIP-TZ**, or **TC-CL**	**[CIP 3 : metro: (CIP or Levo) : metro.** Dosages–footnote[1]	
If illicit use IV drugs	S. aureus	**Vanco** (if high prevalence of MRSA). Some empirically use vanco + oxacillin pending susceptibility results. Dosages–footnote[1]		
If suspect intra-abdominal source	Mixture aerobic & anaerobic Gm-neg. bacilli		[See secondary peritonitis, page 34	
If petechial rash	Meningococcemia			Need TMP-SMX to prevent PCP. Hard to predict which leukemia/lymphoma/solid tumor at ↑ risk of PCP.
If suspect urinary source	Aerobic Gm-neg. bacilli & enterococci	[See pyelonephritis, page 26		
Neutropenia: Child or Adult (absolute PMN count <500 per mm³).				
Prophylaxis—afebrile				
Post-chemotherapy, impending neutropenia	Aerobic Gm-neg. bacilli, Pneumocystis (PCP)	**Ceftriaxone** 2 gm IV q12h (until sure no meningitis); consider Rocky Mountain spotted fever—*see page 43*		Meta-analysis demonstrates substantive reduction in mortality with **CIP** 500 mg po bid or q24h (*AnIM 142:979, 2005*). Similar results in observational study using **Levo** 500 mg po q24h (*CID 40:1087 & 1094, 2005*). Also *NEJM 353:977, 988 & 1052, 2005.*
Pneumocystis therapy in AIDS patient.	↑ risk pneumocystis	**TMP-SMX-DS** po bid—adults; 10 mg per kg per day div bid po—children		Combined regimen justified by combined effect of neutropenia and immuno-suppression.
Allogeneic hematopoietic stem-cell transplant	↑ risk pneumocystis, herpes viruses, candida	**TMP-SMX** as above + (either **acyclovir** or **ganci-clovir**) + **fluconazole**		Need TMP-SMX to prevent PCP. Hard to predict which leukemia/lymphoma/solid tumor at ↑ risk of PCP.
Empiric therapy—febrile neutropenia (≥38.3°C x1 or ≥38°C for ≥1 hr)				
Low-risk adults	As above	**CIP** 750 mg po bid + **AM-CL 875** mg po bid		**Treat as outpatients with 24/7 access to inpatient care if: no focal findings, no hypotension, no COPD, no fungal infection, age <60 & >16.** Neutropenic children with neg. blood cultures safely switched to po cefixime 4 mg per kg q12h (*CID 32:36, 2001*).
(Def. low risk in Comment)				
High-risk adults and children	Aerobic Gm-neg. bacilli; ceph-resistant viridans strep, MRSA	**Monotherapy: CFP** or **ceftaz** or **IMP** or **MER**	**Combination therapy:** **(Gent** or **tobra** + **(TC-CL** or **PIP-TZ))**	Increasing resistance of viridans streptococci to penicillins, cephalosporins & FQs (*CID 34:1469 & 1524, 2002; CID 31:1126, 2000; JAC 47: 47, 2001*). No formal trials, but [APAG
			Dosages: Footnote[1] and Table 10	
		Include empiric vanco if suspect IV access infected; colonized with drug-resistant S. pneumo or MRSA; blood culture pos. for Gm.-pos. cocci; pt hypotensive		
Persistent fever and neutropenia after 5 days of empiric antibacterial therapy—see CID 34:730, 2002—General guidelines				
	Candida species, aspergillus	**Add** either **caspofungin** 70 mg IV day 1, then 50 mg IV q24h **OR voriconazole** 6 mg per kg IV q12h times 2 doses, then 3 mg per kg IV q12h		**V**Conventional ampho B more fever & nephrotoxicity & lower efficacy than liposomal ampho B (*NEJM 340:764, 1999*); both caspofungin & voriconazole better tolerated & perhaps more efficacious than liposomal ampho B (*NEJM 346:225, 2002 & 351:1391 & 1445, 2005*).

[1] **P Ceph 3 (cefotaxime** 2 gm IV q8h; use q4h if life-threatening; **ceftizoxime** 2 gm IV q4h; **ceftriaxone** 2 gm IV q24h). **ceftazidime** 3 gm IV q4h). **ticarcillin** 3 gm IV q4h. **TC-CL** 3.1 gm IV q4h. **PIP-TZ** 3.375 gm IV q4h or **AM-SB** 3 gm IV q8h. **PAG** (see Table 10). **gentamicin** 5 mg per kg q24h. **MER** 1 gm IV q8h. **CIP** 400 mg IV q12h. **oxacillin** 2 gm IV q4h, **aztreonam** 2 gm IV q6h, **IMP** 0.5 gm IV q6h or 1 gm IV q8h, **clinda** 450-900 mg IV q8h, **P Ceph 4 (cefepime** 2 gm IV q12h) or **(ceftazidime** 2 gm IV q8h). **P Ceph 4 [CFP** 2 gm IV q12h (q8h if neutropenic)], **levo** 750 mg IV q24h, **linezolid** 600 mg IV q12h. **Ceph 3 (cefotaxime** 2 gm IV q4h) **P Ceph 3** 2 gm IV q12h (q8h if neutropenic)] & assume normal renal function.
NOTE: All dosage recommendations are for adults (unless otherwise indicated) and assume normal renal function.

Abbreviations on page 2.

TABLE 1 (43)

ANATOMIC SITE/DIAGNOSIS/ MODIFYING CIRCUMSTANCES	ETIOLOGIES (usual)	SUGGESTED REGIMENS		ADJUNCT DIAGNOSTIC OR THERAPEUTIC MEASURES AND COMMENTS
		PRIMARY	ALTERNATIVE†	
SYSTEMIC FEBRILE SYNDROMES (continued)				
Shock syndromes				
Septic shock: Fever & hypotension Bacteremic shock, endotoxin shock Overall review (CID 365:63, 2005) Antimicrobial therapy: CCM 32(Suppl):S495, 2004 Management comments: CCM 32:858, 2004	Bacteria with aerobic Gm-neg. bacteria or Gm+ cocci	**Proven therapy: (1)** Replete intravascular volume, **(2)** correct, if possible, disease that allowed bloodstream invasion, **(3) appropriate empiric antimicrobial rx.** see suggestions under life-threatening sepsis, page 45. **(4)** Decreased indication for recombinant **activated Protein C** (drotrecogin alfa), see Comment. **(5) Low-dose steroids** if document relative adrenal insufficiency (see Comment for criteria). [Hydrocortisone 50 mg IV q6h + fludrocortisone (Florinef) 50 mcg via NG tube per day x 7 days. (6) Add vasopressin in pts with low dose pressin reported effective for catecholamine-resistant septic shock (Sem Resp Crit Care Med 25:705, 2004). (6) Low glucose control: 80–110 mg per dL		**Activ. Protein C: Drotrecogin (Xigris):** In a prospective randomized double-blind study (NEJM 344:699, 2001, 28-d mortality ↓ from 31 to 25% in sickest pts. Now in less ill pts (APACHE II score <25) showed no benefit. Xigris not indicated in pts with single organ dysfunction & surgery within last 30 days due to evidence of increased mortality (NEJM 353:1332, & 1398, 2005). **Hemorrhage** major adverse **cost** of drug: 2% (drotrecogin, 2% placebo) in initial NEJM trial. If major bleeding present, discontinue drotrecogin IV infusion. Can restart 2 hrs before & restart 12 hrs after surgery. **Average cost** of therapy: ~ $6800. **Low-dose steroids** in controlled random double-blind trial, rx if low baseline cortisol & s9 mcg per dL response to 250 mg IV cosyntropin 28-day mortality 63% placebo & steroid group (JAMA 288:862 & 886, 2002). Results in question because "total" & not "free" cortisol was measured (NEJM 350:1629, 2004). Confirm. trial in process. **Targeted glucose levels:** Tight plasma glucose control appears to reduce mortality (AJM 164:2005, 2004).
Septic shock: postsplenectomy (asplenia)	S. pneumoniae, N. meningitidis, H. influenzae, Capnocytophaga (DF-2)	**Ceftriaxone** 2 gm IV q24h† (1 to 2 gm q12h if meningitis)	**Levo** 500 mg or **Moxi** 400 mg, then 750 mg or 400 mg q24h	Howell–Jolly bodies in peripheral blood smear confirm absence of functional spleen. DIC often results in symmetrical **peripheral gangrene of digits** due to severe DIC. For prophylaxis, see Table 15A, page 124.
Toxic shock syndrome, Clostridium sordellii (CID 35:1441, 2002) Post-partum, post-abortion, post-mifepristone MMWR 54:724, 2005	Clostridium sordellii	Other management as above. Fluids, aq. **penicillin G** 18–20 million units per day div. q4–6h + **clindamycin** 900 mg IV q8h.	—	[Several deaths reported after use of mifepristone (RU486) & misoprostol (Cytotec: ref. fda.gov/cder/drug/advisory/mifeprex.htm). Clinically: often edema, rapid progression, hypotension, hemoconcentration, neutrophilia.
Toxic shock syndrome, staphylococcal: "Superantigen" mediated Staph. aureus of vagina (tampon-assoc.), surgical/traumatic wounds, endometrium, burns	Staph. aureus (tampon-shock toxin-mediated)	**Nafcillin or oxacillin** 2 gm IV q4h (or if MRSA, **vanco** 1 gm IV q12h) + **IVIG**	**Cefazolin** 1–2 gm IV q8h (or if MRSA, **vanco** 1 gm IV q12h) + **IVIG**	Nafcillin/oxacillin/cefazolin have no effect on initial syndrome, but ↓ recurrences. Seek occult abscess. TSS may occur with "clean" colonized post-op wounds. Case fatality 5%. **IVIG reasonable rx** (see Strep/occcus TSS)—dose 1 gm per kg day 1, then 0.5 gm per kg days 2 & 3.
Toxic shock syndrome, streptococcal [Ref: JID 179(Suppl.2):S366–374, 1999] Associated with invasive disease, i.e., myositis, nec-rotizing fasciitis; secondary strep infection of varicella. Secondary causes TSS reported [JID 179:255, NEJM 335:547 & 334:240, 1996; CID 27:150, 1988]	Group A, B, C, & G Strep. pyogenes	For necrotizing fasciitis without toxic shock: see page 41 **Pen G** 24 million units per day div. q4–6h IV + **clinda** 900 mg IV q8h IVIG associated with a ↓ in sepsis-related organ failure (CID 37:333 & 341, 2003)	**Ceftriaxone** 2 gm IV q24h† or **clinda** 900 mg IV q8h + **IVIG**	**Definition:** Isolation of Group A strep, hypotension and ≥2 of: renal impairment, coagulopathy, liver involvement, ARDS, generalized rash, soft tissue necrosis (JAMA 269:390, 1993). Associated with invasive disease. Mortality 30–50%. Clinda ↓ toxin production. Use of NSAID may predispose to/& mask severity of necrotizing fasciitis. **Surgery usually required.** Mortality 80% even with early rx (CID 14:2, 1992). Clinda ↓ toxin production. Use of NSAID many predispose toxic TSS & may fall in fulminant S. pyogenes infections. Discussion of possible reasons pen G may fall in fulminant S. pyogenes infections. see JID 167:1401, 1993).
Other Toxin-Mediated Syndromes—no fever unless complicated				
Botulism (CID 41:1167, 2005) Bad sign (CID 366:374, 1999)	IVIG associated with a ↓ in sepsis-related organ failure 1 gm per kg day 1, then 0.5 gm per kg days 2 & 3.			
Food-borne JAMA 285:1059, 2001; Table 1B, page 48; www.bt.cdc.gov Time of presentation bad sign (CID 39:357 & 363, 2004)	C. botulinum	For all types: Follow vital capacity, other support. If no ileus, purge GI tract	Trivalent (types A, B, E) antitoxin from State Health Dept. or CDC (see Comment)	**Equine antitoxin:** Obtain from State Health Depts. or CDC (404-639-2206 M-F OR 404-639-2888 evenings/weekends). Skin test first & desensitize if necessary. **Antimicrobials** may make infant botulism worse. Untested in wound botulism. When used, pen G 10–20 million units per day usual dose. If complications (pneumonia, UTI) occur, avoid antimicrobials with assoc. neuromuscular blockade, i.e., aminoglycosides, tetracycline.
Infant	Human botulinum immunoglobulin (BIG) IV, single dose. Call 510-540-2646 Do not use equine antitoxin		No antibiotics; may lyse C. botulinum in gut and ↑ toxin load	**Differential dx:** Guillain-Barré, myasthenia gravis, tick paralysis, organophosphate toxicity, West Nile virus.

NOTE: All dosage recommendations are for adults (unless otherwise indicated) and assume normal renal function.

TABLE 1 (44)

ANATOMIC SITE/DIAGNOSIS/ MODIFYING CIRCUMSTANCES	ETIOLOGIES (usual)	SUGGESTED REGIMENS*		ADJUNCT DIAGNOSTIC OR THERAPEUTIC MEASURES AND COMMENTS
		PRIMARY	ALTERNATIVE†	
SYSTEMIC FEBRILE SYNDROMES/Other Toxin-Mediated Syndromes/Botulism (continued)				
Wound		Debridement & anaerobic cultures. Trivalent equine antitoxin (see Appendix). Proven value of antibiotics untested. Role of antibiotics untested.		Can result from spore contamination of tar heroin.
Tetanus	C. tetani	Pen G 24 million units per day in div. dose or **doxy** 100 mg IV q12h times 7–10 days	**Metro** 500 mg po q6h or IV 1 gm IV q12h times 7–10 days (See Comment)	Multifaceted treatment: Wound debridement, tetanus immunoglobulin (250–500 units IM), antimicrobials, & tetanus toxoid (tetanus does not confer immunity). Options for control of muscle spasms: continuous infusion of midazolam, IV propofol, and/or intrathecal baclofen. CID 38:321, 2004.
VASCULAR				
Cavernous sinus thrombosis	Staph. aureus, Group A strep, H. influenzae, aspergillus/mucor/rhizopus	Vanco 1 gm IV q12h + **ceftriaxone** 2 gm IV q24h	(**Dapto** 6 mg per kg IV q24h^NFDA or **linezolid** 600 mg IV q12h) + **ceftriaxone** 2 gm IV q24h	CT or MRI scan for diagnosis. Heparin indicated (Ln 338:597, 1991). If patient diabetic with ketoacidosis or post-desferoxamine rx or neutropenic, consider fungal etiology: aspergillus, mucor, rhizopus, see Table 11A, pages 75 & 82.
IV line infection (see IDSA Guidelines: CID 32:1249, 2001): Heparin lock, midline catheter, non-tunneled central venous catheter (subclavian, internal jugular), peripherally inserted central catheter (PICC) Avoid femoral vein if possible. ↑ risk of infection and/or thrombosis (JAMA 286:700, 2001)	Staph. epidermidis, Staph. aureus (MSSA/MRSA)	**Treatment:** (For Prevention, see below) Vanco 1 gm IV q12h See Comment. Other rx and duration: (1) If S. aureus, remove catheter. Can use TEE result to determine if 2 or 4 wks of rx. (2) If S. epidermidis, can try to "save" catheter 80% cure after 7–10 days of rx.	**Linezolid alternative—see Comment.**	If no response to, or intolerant of, **vanco** switch to **daptomycin** 6 mg per kg IV q24h. If no response to, or intolerant of, **vanco** switch to daptomycin 6 mg per kg IV q24h. If definitely no endocarditis or osteomyelitis, could use **linezolid** 600 mg IV po bid. **Quinupristin-dalfopristin** an option if vanco cross-allergenic is not an issue): 1000 mg IV, **Dalbavancin** an option if vanco cross-allergenic is not an issue): 1000 mg IV q24h. Culture removed catheter. With "roll" method, >15 colonies (NEJM 312:1142, 1985) suggests infection. Lines do not require "routine" changing when not infected. When infected, do if (See Comment). For multimicrobial-impregnated catheters may ↓ infection risk, the debate is likely (CID 37:65, 2003 & 38:1287, 2004 & 39:1829, 2004).
Tunnel infection indwelling venous catheters and ports (Broviac, Hickman, Groshong, Quinton), dual lumen hemodialysis catheters (Perma-cath)	Staph. epidermidis, Staph. aureus, (Candida sp.). Rarely, leuconostoc or lactobacillus—both resistant to vanco (see Table 2)	"antibiotic lock" rx infections may respond to "antibiotic lock" rx & allow salvage of catheter. Drug (vanco, gent, CIP) at 1–5 mg per mL mixed with 50–100 units heparin (or saline) in 2–5 mL volume: fill catheter when not in use. Continue 2 wks. **For S. aureus, need full course of parenteral therapy** (AAC 44:1818, 2000 & 55:90, 2005)		If S. aureus & catheter left in, vanco cure 80% of infections limited to exit site but only 25% cure of infection in subcutaneous tunnel between skin and subclavian vein. If S. aureus & catheter left in, vanco cure rate 10% at exit site & 0% with tunnel infection (AJM 88:137, 1990). Similar statistics for infected "ports" (CID 29:102, 1999). Infected hemodialysis access catheters should be removed (AJKD 127: 275, 1997).
Impaired host (burn, neutropenic)	As above + Pseudomonas sp. Enterobacteriaceae, Corynebacterium jeikeium, Candida sp.	(Vanco + P Ceph 3 AP) or (P Ceph 3 + **APAG**)	(vanco + AP Pen) or IMP or **AP Pen** (Dosage, see page 45)	Usually have associated septic thrombophlebitis. Biopsy of vein to rule out fungi. If fungal, surgical excision + amphotericin B. Surgical drainage, ligation or removal often indicated.
Hyperalimentation	As with tunnel infection plus, Candida sp. (non-albicans & azole-resistant Candida species)	If candida: **voriconazole** 3 mg per kg bid IV or **caspofungin** 70 mg IV day 1, then 50 mg IV q24h		Remove venous catheter and discontinue antimicrobial agents if possible. Ophthalmologic consultation recommended. **Rx all patients with blood cultures.** See Table 11A, Candidiasis.
Intravenous lipid emulsion	Staph. epidermidis Malassezia furfur	Vanco 1 gm IV q12h Amphotericin B		Discontinue intralipid. AJM 90:129, 1991
IV line infection: **Prevention** (CID 35:1281, 2002; NEJM 348:1123, 2003). 1. Maximal sterile barrier precautions during catheter insertion 2. Use 2% chlorhexidine for skin antisepsis 3. If infection rate high despite # 1 & 2, use either chlorhexidine/silver sulfadiazine or minocycline/rifampin-impregnated catheters.				Tunneled catheters: Small study, ↓ infection rate when catheter locked with gentamicin (5 mg per mL) + heparin 5000 units per mL), p < 0.02 (Kidney Int 66:801, 2004). 4. If possible, use subclavian vein
Septic pelvic vein thrombophlebitis (puerperal sepsis): Postpartum or postabortion or postpelvic surgery	Streptococci, bacteroides, Enterobacteriaceae	(P Ceph 3, cefoxitin TC-CL, PIP-TZ, or AM-SB)	IMP or MER or ERTA or (clinda + aztreonam or APAG) Dosages: Table 10B	↓ use of anticoagulation or recommended. Need not add antifungal unless Candida grows from blood. Add heparin if no response. Cefotetan has methyltetrazole side-chain which is associated with hypoprothrombinemia (prevent with vitamin K).

Abbreviations on page 2.

NOTE: All dosage recommendations are for adults (unless otherwise indicated) and assume normal renal function.

TABLE 1B: PROPHYLAXIS AND TREATMENT OF ORGANISMS OF POTENTIAL USE AS BIOLOGICAL WEAPONS *(See page 2 for abbreviations)*

DISEASE	ETIOLOGY	SUGGESTED EMPIRIC TREATMENT REGIMENS		SPECIFIC THERAPY AND COMMENTS
		PRIMARY	**ALTERNATIVE**	

Anthrax
Cutaneous, Inhalational, gastrointestinal
Refs.: *LN* 364:393 & 449, 2001; *NEJM* 345:1607 & 1621, 2001; *CID* 35:851, 2002
 	
or
www.bt.cdc.gov
 	
Also see *Table 1, pages 31 & 37*
 	
To report bioterrorism event:
770-488-7100
 	
Rationale for CIP: *CID* 39:303, 2004
	Bacillus anthracis
	Post-exposure prophylaxis
	Ref.: *Med Lett* 43:91, 2001
	
	------------ 	
	Treatment—
	Cutaneous anthrax
	NEJM 345:1611, 2001
	
	------------ 	
	Treatment—**Inhalational, gastrointestinal, or oropharyngeal**
	
	Characteristic signs & symptoms—**Present**: Dyspnea, N/V;
	Absent: Rhinorrhea, sore throat.
	(*AnIM* 139:337, 2003)
		Adults (including pregnancy): Doxy 100 mg po bid or **Levo** 500 mg po q24h) times 60 days
		Children: CIP 20-30 mg/kg per day div q12h times 60 days
		
		Adults (including pregnancy):
		(**CIP** 500 mg po bid or **Levo** 500 mg po q24h) times 60 days
		Children: CIP 20-30 mg per day div q12h times 60 days
		
		Adults (including pregnancy):
		(**CIP** 400 mg IV q12h) or (**Levo** 500 mg IV q24h) or (**doxy** 100 mg IV q12h) + **clinda** 900 mg IV q8h + **RIF** 300 mg IV q12h
		(switch to po when able) & **doxy** to 500 mg po bid; **clinda** to 450 mg po q8h, & **RIF** 300 mg po bid
		Treat times 60 days. *See Table 16, page 133 for oral dosage*
			Adults (including pregnancy): Doxy 100 mg po bid times 60 days
			Children (see *Comment*): **Doxy** >8 y/o & >45 kg: 100 mg po bid; >8 y/o & ≤45 kg: 2.2 mg per kg po bid; ≤8 y/o: 2.2 mg per kg po bid. All for 60 days
			
			Adults (including pregnancy): Doxy 100 mg po bid times 60 days
			Children: Doxy >8 y/o & > 45 kg: 100 mg po bid; >8 y/o & ≤45 kg: 2.2 mg per kg po bid; ≤8 y/o: 2.2 mg per kg po bid. All for 60 days
			
			Children: (**CIP** 10 mg per kg IV q12h or 15 mg per kg po q12h) or (**Doxy** >8 y/o & >45 kg: 100 mg IV q12h; >8 y/o & ≤45 kg: 2.2 mg per kg IV q12h; ≤8 y/o: 2.2 mg per kg IV q12h) + (**clinda** 7.5 mg per kg IV q6h) & (**RIF** 20 mg per kg IV q12h)
			Treat times 60 days. *See Table 16, page 133*
				1. Once organism shows susceptibility to penicillin, switch children to **amoxicillin** 80 mg per kg per day div q8h (max. 500 mg q8h); switch pregnant pt to **amoxicillin** 500 mg po tid.
				2. Other **FQs** (Gati, Moxi) & clarithro should work but no clinical experience.
				
				1. If penicillin susceptible, then: **Adults: Amox** 500 mg po q8h times 60 days
				Children: Amox 80 mg per kg per day div q8h (max. 500 mg q8h) times 60 days
				2. Other **FQs** (Gati, Levo, Moxi) should work based on in vitro susceptibility data.
				
				1. Clinda may block toxin production.
				2. Rifampin penetrates CSF & intracellular sites.
				3. If isolate shown penicillin-susceptible:
				  a. **Adult: Pen G** 4 million units IV q4h
				  Child: Pen G 1 y/o: 50,000 units per kg IV q6h; >12 y/o: 4 million units IV q4h.
				  c. Constitutive & inducible β-lactamases—do not use pen or AMP alone.
				4. Do not use cephalosporins or TMP-SMX.
				5. Erythro, azithro activity borderline, clarithro active.
				6. FQs active against vegetative forms.

Botulism: *CID* 41:1167, 2005; *JAMA* 285:1059, 2001 **Food-borne** *See Table 1, page 46*	*Clostridium botulinum*	Supportive care for all types. Follow vital capacity. Submit suspect food for toxin testing. Ref.: *CID* 39:357 & 363, 2004 Fluid/electrolyte balance. Optimize circulatory volume.	Antibiotics have no effect on toxin	
Hemorrhagic fever viruses Ref.: *JAMA* 287:2391, 2002 *See Table 14, page 106*	Ebola, Lassa, Hanta, yellow fever, & others	For Lassa & Hanta: **Ribavirin** LD 30 mg per kg IV (max. 2 gm) IV times 1, then 16 mg per kg IV (max. 1 gm per dose) q6h times 4 days, then 8 mg per kg IV (max. 500 mg) q8h times 6 days	Ribavirin active in vitro, not FDA-approved for this indication. Pregnancy: Children: LD 30 mg per kg IV times 1. Howev- NOTE: Ribavirin contraindicated in pregnancy, er, in this setting, the benefits outweigh the risks.	
Botulinum toxin *See Table 1, page 46*		**Trivalent antitoxin** (types A, B, E): single 10 ml vial per pt. diluted in saline IV (slowly)		
Plague Ref.: *JAMA* 283:2281, 2000 **Inhalation pneumonic plague** *See Table 1, page 42*	*Yersinia pestis* **Treatment** ------------ **Post-exposure prophylaxis**	**Gentamicin** 5 mg per kg IV q24h or **streptomycin** 15 mg per kg IV bid Tobramycin should work. **Doxy** 100 mg po bid times 7 days	(**Doxy** 200 mg IV times 1, then 100 mg po or IV bid) or (**CIP** 500 mg po bid or 400 mg IV q12h) or **gentamicin** plus **doxy** Ref.: *CID* 38:663, 2004 **CIP** 500 mg po bid times 7 days	1. **Chloro** also active: 25 mg per kg IV q6h 2. In a mass casualty situation, may have to treat po. 3. Pediatric doses: *see Table 16, page 133* 4. Isolate during first 48 hrs of therapy. 5. For community with pneumonic plague epidemic. Pediatric doses: *see Table 16, page 133*. Pregnancy: *As for non-pregnant adults*
Smallpox Ref.: *NEJM* 346:1300, 2002 *See Table 14, page 113*	Variola virus	Smallpox vaccine up to 4 days after exposure: isolation; gloves, gown, & NAS respirator	**Cidofovir** protected mice against aerosol cowpox (*JID* 181:10, 2000)	***Immediately notify State Health Dept.*** & State notifies CDC (770-488-7100). Vaccinia immune globulin of no benefit. For vaccination complications, see *JAMA* 288:1901, 2002.
Tularemia **Inhalational tularemia** Ref.: *JAMA* 285:2763, 2001 *See Table 1, page 43*	*Francisella tularensis* **Treatment** ------------ **Post-exposure prophylaxis**	**Streptomycin** 15 mg per kg IV bid or **gentamicin** 5 mg per kg IV q24h times 10 days **Doxy** 100 mg po bid times 14 days	**Doxy** 100 mg IV or po bid times 14-21 days or **CIP** 400 mg IV (or 750 mg po) bid times 14-21 days **CIP** 500 mg po bid times 14 days	For pediatric doses, see *Table 16, page 133*. Pregnancy: *As for non-pregnant adults* **Tobramycin** should work. For pediatric doses, see *Table 16, page 133* Pregnancy: *As for non-pregnant adults*

TABLE 2: RECOMMENDED ANTIMICROBIAL AGENTS AGAINST SELECTED BACTERIA

BACTERIAL SPECIES	ANTIMICROBIAL AGENT (See page 2 for abbreviations)		
	RECOMMENDED	ALTERNATIVE	ALSO EFFECTIVE[1] (COMMENTS)
Alcaligenes xylosoxidans (Achromobacter xylosoxidans)	IMP, MER, AP Pen	TMP-SMX. Some strains susc. to ceftaz (AAC 32: 276, 1988)	Resistant to APAG; P Ceph 1, 2, 3, 4; aztreonam; FQ (AAC 40:772, 1996)
Acinetobacter calcoaceticus–baumannii complex	IMP or MER or [FQ + (amikacin or ceftaz)]	AM-SB (CID 24:932, 1997; CID 34:1425, 2002). Sulbactam^A,B also effective (AAC 42:793, 1998); colistin (CID 36:1111, 2003)	Up to 10% isolates resistant to IMP; resistance to FQs, amikacin increasing. Doxy + amikacin effective in animal model (JAC 45: 493, 2000). (See Table 5, page 56)
Actinomyces israelii	AMP or Pen G	Doxy, ceftriaxone	Clindamycin, erythro
Aeromonas hydrophila	FQ	TMP-SMX or (P Ceph 3, 4)	APAG; ERTA; IMP; MER; tetracycline (some resistant to carbapenems)
Arcanobacterium (C.) haemolyticum	Erythro	Benzathine Pen G	Sensitive to most drugs, resistant to TMP-SMX (AAC 38:142, 1994)
Bacillus anthracis (anthrax): inhalation [See Table 1B, page 48]			
Bacillus cereus, B. subtilis	Vancomycin, clindamycin	FQ, IMP	
Bacteroides fragilis (ssp. fragilis) "DOT" group of bacteroides	Metronidazole	Clindamycin	Cefoxitin, ERTA, IMP, MER, TC-CL, PIP-TZ, AM-SB, cefotetan, AM-CL (not cefotetan)
Bartonella (Rochalimaea) henselae, quintana See Table 1, pages 33, 37, 41	Azithro or clarithro or CIP (bacillary angiomatosis) or azithro (cat-scratch) (PIDJ 17:447, 1998; AAC 48:1921, 2004)	Erythro or doxy	Other drugs: TMP-SMX (IDC No. Amer 12:137, 1998). Consider doxy + RIF for severe bacillary angiomatosis (IDC No. Amer 12:137, 1998); doxy + gentamicin optimal for endocarditis (AAC 47:2204, 2003)
Bordetella pertussis	Erythro	TMP-SMX	An erythro-resistant strain reported in Arizona (MMWR 43:807, 1994)
Borrelia burgdorferi, B. afzelii, B. garinii	Ceftriaxone, cefuroxime axetil, doxy, amox (See Comments)	Penicillin G (HD), cefotaxime	Clarithro. Choice depends on stage of disease, Table 1, page 42
Borrelia sp.	Doxy	Erythro	Penicillin G
Brucella sp.	Doxy + either gentamicin or streptomycin (IDCP 7, 2004)	(Doxy + RIF) or (TMP-SMX + gentamicin)	FQ + RIF (AAC 41:80, 1997; EID 3:213, 1997; CID 21:283, 1995). Minocycline + RIF (J Chemother 15:248, 2003).
Burkholderia (Pseudomonas) cepacia	TMP-SMX or MER or CIP	Minocycline or chloramphenicol	(Usually resistant to APAG, AG, polymyxins) (AAC 37: 123, 1993 & 43:213, 1999; Inf Medicine 18:49, 2001) (Some resistant to carbapenems). Combination rx may be necessary (AJRCCM 161:1206, 2000).
Burkholderia (Pseudomonas) pseudomallei See Table 1, page 30, & Ln 361:1715, 2003	Initially, IV ceftaz or IMP (CID 29:381, 1999)	Then, combination po chloro, doxy, & TMP-SMX	(In Thailand, 12–80% strains resistant to TMP-SMX. FQ active in vitro. Combination of chloro, TMP-SMX, doxy more effective than doxy alone for maintenance rx (CID 29:375, 1999). MER also effective (AAC 48: 1763,2004)
Campylobacter jejuni	Erythro	FQ (↑ resistance, NEJM 340: 1525,1999)	Clindamycin, doxy, azithro, clarithro (see Table 5, page 57)
Campylobacter fetus	IMP	Gentamicin	AMP, chloramphenicol, erythro
Capnocytophaga ochracea (DF-1) and canimorsus (DF-2)	Clindamycin or AM-CL AM-CL	CIP, Pen G	P Ceph 3, IMP, cefoxitin, FQ, (resistant to APAG, TMP-SMX). C. haemolytica & C. granulosa are often resistant to β-lactams & aminoglycosides [CID 35 (Suppl.1):S17, 2002].
Chlamydophila pneumoniae	Doxy	Erythro, FQ	Azithro, clarithro, telithro
Chlamydia trachomatis	Doxy or azithro	Erythro or oflox	Levofloxacin
Chryseomonas (Flavobacterium) meningosepticum	Vancomycin ± RIF (CID 26:1169, 1998)	CIP, levofloxacin	In vitro susceptibilities may not correlate with clinical efficacy (AAC 41:1301, 1997; CID 26:1169, 1998)
Citrobacter diversus (koseri), C. freundii	CARB	FQ	APAG
Clostridium difficile	Metronidazole (po)	Vancomycin (po)	Bacitracin (po)
Clostridium perfringens	Pen G ± clindamycin	Doxy	Erythro, chloramphenicol, cefazolin, cefoxitin, AP Pen, CARB
Clostridium tetani	Metronidazole or Pen G	Doxy	CARB
Corynebacterium jeikeium	Vancomycin	Pen G + APAG	
C. diphtheriae	Erythro	Clindamycin	RIF. Penicillin reported effective (CID 27:845, 1998)
Coxiella burnetii (Q fever) acute disease	Doxy (see Table 1, page 23)	Erythro	In meningitis consider FQ (CID 20:489, 1995). Endocarditis: doxy + (hydroxy-chloroquine) (JID 188:1322, 2003; LnID 3:709, 2003).
chronic disease	(CIP or doxy) + RIF	FQ + doxy x3 yrs (CID 20:489, 1995)]	Chloroquine + doxy (AAC 37:1773, 1993). γ gamma interferon (Ln 20:546, 2001)
Ehrlichia chaffeensis, Ehrlichia ewubguum Anaplasma (Ehrlichia) phagocytophilium	Doxy	Tetracycline, RIF (CID 27:213, 1998)	CIP, oflox, chloramphenicol also active in vitro. Resistant to clinda, TMP-SMX, IMP, AMP, erythro, & azithro (AAC 41:76, 1997).

TABLE 2 (2)

BACTERIAL SPECIES	ANTIMICROBIAL AGENT (See page 2 for abbreviations)		
	RECOMMENDED	**ALTERNATIVE**	**ALSO EFFECTIVE† (COMMENTS)**
Eikenella corrodens	Penicillin G or AMP or AM-CL	TMP-SMX, FQ	Doxy, cefoxitin, cefotaxime, IMP (Resistant to clindamycin, cephalexin, erythromycin, and metronidazole)
Enterobacter species	Recommended agents vary with clinical setting. *See Tables 1 & 4*		
Enterococcus faecalis *See Table 5, page 56*			
Enterococcus faecium, β-lactamase +, high-level aminoglycoside resist., vancomycin resist.: *See Table 5, page 56*			
Erysipelothrix rhusiopathiae	Penicillin G or AMP	P Ceph 3, FQ	IMP, AP Pen (vancomycin), APAG, TMP-SMX resistant
Escherichia coli	Recommended agents vary with clinical setting *See Tables 1 & 4*		
Francisella tularensis (tularemia) *See Table 1B, page 48*	Gentamicin, tobramycin, or streptomycin	Doxy or CIP	Chloramphenicol, RIF. Doxy/chloro bacteriostatic → relapses
Gardnerella vaginalis (bacterial vaginosis)	Metronidazole	Clindamycin	See Table 1, page 20 for dosage
Hafnia alvei	*Same as Enterobacter spp.*		
Helicobacter pylori *See Table 1, page 19*			Drugs effective in vitro often fail in vivo.
Hemophilus aphrophilus	[(Penicillin or AMP) ± gentamicin] or [AM-SB ± gentamicin]	P Ceph 3 ± gentamicin	(Resistant to vancomycin, clindamycin, methicillin)
Hemophilus ducreyi (chancroid)	Azithro or ceftriaxone	Erythro, CIP	Most strains resistant to tetracycline, amox, TMP-SMX
Hemophilus influenzae Meningitis, epiglottitis & other life-threatening illness	Cefotaxime, ceftriaxone	TMP-SMX, CARB, AMP (AMP if β-lactamase negative) (U.S. 25–30% AMP resistance, Japan 35%)	Chloramphenicol (downgraded from 1st choice because of hematotoxicity). 9% of U.S. strains resistant to TMP-SMX (*AAC 41:292, 1997*)
non-life threatening illness	AM-CL, O Ceph 2/3, TMP-SMX, AM-SB	FQ	Azithro, clarithro, telithro
Klebsiella ozaenae/rhinoscleromatis	FQ	RIF + TMP-SMX	(*Ln 342:122, 1993*)
Klebsiella species	Recommended agents vary with clinical setting *See Tables 1 & 4*		
Lactobacillus species	(Pen G or AMP) ± gentamicin	Clindamycin, erythro	**May be resistant to vancomycin**
Legionella sp. *(42 species & 60 serotypes recognized) (Sem Resp Inf 13:90, 1998)*	FQ, or azithro, or (erythro ± RIF)	Clarithro	TMP-SMX, doxy. Most active FQs in vitro: Gemi, Gati, Levo, Moxi. *See AnIM 129: 328, 1998*. Telithro active in vitro.
Leptospira interrogans	Penicillin G	Doxy	Ceftriaxone (*CID 36:1507, 2003*), cefotaxime (*CID 39:1417, 2004*)
Leuconostoc	Pen G or AMP	Clindamycin, erythro, minocycline	APAG **NOTE: Resistant to vancomycin**
Listeria monocytogenes	AMP	TMP-SMX	Erythro, penicillin G (high dose), APAG may be synergistic with β-lactams. **Cephalosporin-resistant!**
Moraxella (Branhamella) catarrhalis	AM-CL or O Ceph 2/3, TMP-SMX	Azithro, clarithro, dirithromycin, telithro	Erythro, doxy, FQs
Morganella species	Recommended agents vary with clinical setting *See Tables 1 & 4*		
Mycoplasma pneumoniae	Erythro, azithro, clarithro, dirithro, telithro,or FQ	Doxy	(Clindamycin and β lactams NOT effective)
Neisseria gonorrhoeae (gonococcus)	Ceftriaxone, cefixime, cefpodoxime	Ofloxacin & other FQs *(Table 1, pages 17–18)*, spectinomycin	Kanamycin (used in Asia). FQ resistance in Asia: rare in U.S., but ↑ (*MMWR 47:405, 1998*)
Neisseria meningitidis (meningococcus)	Penicillin G	Ceftriaxone, cefuroxime, cefotaxime	Sulfonamide (some strains), chloramphenicol. Chloro-resistant strains found in SE Asia (*NEJM 339:868, 1998*) (Prophylaxis: page 8)
Nocardia asteroides	TMP-SMX, sulfonamides (high dose)	Minocycline	Amikacin + (IMP or ceftriaxone or cefuroxime) for brain abscess
Nocardia brasiliensis	TMP-SMX, sulfonamides (high dose)	AM-CL	Amikacin + ceftriaxone
Pasteurella multocida	Pen G, AMP, amox	Doxy, AM-CL, P Ceph 2, TMP-SMX	Ceftriaxone, cefpodoxime, FQ (active in vitro), azithro (active in vitro) (*DMID 30:99, 1998; AAC 43:1475, 1999*)
Plesiomonas shigelloides	CIP	TMP-SMX	AM-CL, P Ceph 1,2,3,4, IMP, MER, tetracycline, aztreonam
Proteus mirabilis (indole–)	AMP	TMP-SMX	Ceftriaxone, cefpodoxime, FQ (active in vitro). β-lactamase (including ESBL) production now being described in P. mirabilis (*J Clin Micro 40:1549, 2002*)
vulgaris (indole +)	P Ceph 3 or FQ	APAG	CARB, aztreonam, BL/BLI
Providencia sp.	Amikacin or P Ceph 3 or FQ	TMP-SMX	AP Pen + amikacin, IMP
Pseudomonas aeruginosa	AP Pen, AP Ceph 3, IMP, MER, tobramycin, CIP, aztreonam. For serious inf., use AP β-lactam + tobramycin or CIP (*LnID 4:519, 2004*)	For UTI, single drugs usually effective: AP Pen, AP Ceph 3, cefepime, IMP, MER, APAG, CIP, aztreonam	Resistance to β-lactams (IMP, ceftaz) may emerge during rx. β-lactam addition adds nothing to activity of TC or PIP against P. aeruginosa. Clavulanic acid has been shown to antagonize TC in vitro (*AAC 43:882, 1999*). *See also Table 5A*). Editors recommend combination therapy for serious infections, but value of combinations remains controversial (*LnID 5:192, 2005*).

TABLE 2 (3)

BACTERIAL SPECIES	ANTIMICROBIAL AGENT (See page 2 for abbreviations)		
	RECOMMENDED	ALTERNATIVE	ALSO EFFECTIVE[1] (COMMENTS)
Rhodococcus (C. equi)	IMP, APAG, erythro, vancomycin, or RIF (consider 2 agents)	CIP (variable) [resistant strains SE Asia (CID 27: 370, 1998)], TMP-SMX, te-tracycline, or clindamycin	Vancomycin active in vitro but intra-cellular location of R. equi may impair efficacy (Sem Resp Inf 12:57, 1997; CID 34:1379, 2002)
Rickettsiae species	Doxy	Chloramphenicol	FQ, clari, azithro effective for Mediter-ranean spotted fever in children (CID 34:154, 2002).
Salmonella typhi	FQ, ceftriaxone	Chloramphenicol, amox, TMP-SMX, azithro (for uncomplicated disease: AAC 43:1441, 1999)	Multi drug resistant strains (chloram-phenicol, AMP, TMP-SMX) common in many developing countries, seen in immigrants. FQ resistance now being reported (AJTMH 61:163, 1999).
Serratia marcescens	P Ceph 3, ERTA, IMP, MER, FQ	Aztreonam, gentamicin	TC-CL, PIP-TZ
Shigella sp.	FQ or azithro	TMP-SMX and AMP (resistance common in Middle East, Latin America). Azithro ref.: AnIM 126:697, 1997	
Staph. aureus, methicillin-susceptible	Oxacillin/nafcillin	P Ceph 1, vancomycin, teicoplanin[NUS], clinda-mycin, dalbavancin	ERTA, IMP, MER, BL/BLI, FQ, erythro, clarithro, dirithromycin, azithro, telithro, quinu-dalfo, linezolid, dapto
Staph. aureus, methicillin-resistant (health-care associated)	Vancomycin	Teicoplanin[NUS] TMP-SMX (some strains resistant), quinu-dalfo, linezolid, daptomycin, dalbavancin	Fusidic acid[NUS], >60% CIP-resistant in U.S. (Fosfomycin + RIF), novobiocin. Partially vancomycin-resistant strains (GISA, VISA) & highly resistant strains now described—see Table 6, page 57.
Staph. aureus, methicillin-resistant [community-acquired (CA-MRSA)]			CA-MRSA usually not multiply-resistant (Ln 359: 1819, 2002; JAMA 286: 1201, 2001). Obtain ref. to erythro & variably to FQ. Vanco, teico[NUS], daptomycin or dalbavancin can be used for pts requiring hospitalization (see Table 6, page 57).
Mild-moderate infection	(TMP-SMX or doxy or mino) ± RIF (CID 40: 1429, 2005).	Clinda (if susceptible to erythro & clinda)	
Severe infection	Vanco or teico[NUS]	Linezolid or daptomy-cin or dalbavancin	
Staph. epidermidis	Vancomycin ± RIF	RIF + (TMP-SMX or FQ), dalbavancin, daptomycin	Cephalothin or nafcillin/oxacillin if sensitive to nafcillin/oxacillin but 75% are resistant. FQs. (See Table 5)
Staph. haemolyticus	TMP-SMX, FQ, nitro-furantoin	Oral cephalosporin	Recommendations apply to UTI only.
Staph. lugdunensis	Oxacillin/nafcillin or penicillin G (if β-lactamase neg.) (Inf Dis Alert 22:193, 2003)	P Ceph 1 or vancomycin or teico[NUS]	Approx. 75% are penicillin-susceptible. Usually susceptible to gentamicin, RIF (AAC 32:2434, 1990).
Staph. saprophyticus (UTI)	Oral cephalosporin or AM-CL	FQ	Susceptible to most agents used for UTI; occ. failure of sulfonamides, nitro-furantoin reported (JID 155:170, 1987). Resistant to fosfomycin.
Stenotrophomonas (Xanthomonas, Pseudo-monas) maltophilia	TMP-SMX	TC-CL or (aztreonam + TC-CL) (AAC 41:2612, 1997)	In vitro synergy (TC-CL + TMP-SMX) and (TC-CL + CIP), AAC 39:2220, 1995; CMR 11:57, 1998]
Streptobacillus moniliformis	Penicillin G or doxy	Erythro, clindamycin	
Streptococcus, anaerobic (Peptostreptococcus)	Penicillin G	Clindamycin	Erythro, doxy, vancomycin
Streptococcus pneumoniae penicillin-susceptible	Penicillin G	Multiple agents effect-ive, e.g., amox	See footnote 2 page 9
penicillin-resistant (MIC ≥2.0)	(Vancomycin ± RIF) or (Gati, Levo, or Moxi) See footnote 1 page 6 and Table 5, page 56)		For non-meningitis infections: P Ceph 3/4, CARB, quinu-dalfo, linezolid, telithro
Streptococcus pyogenes, Groups A, B, C, G, F, Strep. milleri (constellatus, intermedius, anginosus)	Penicillin G or V (some add gentamicin for serious Group B strep infections & some add clinda for serious invasive Group A strep infections) (SMJ 96:968, 2003)	All β lactams, erythro, azithro, dirithromycin, clarithro, telithro	Macrolide resistance increasing.
Vibrio cholerae	Doxy, FQ	TMP-SMX	Strain 0139 is resistant to TMP-SMX
Vibrio parahemolyticus	Antibiotic rx does not ↓ course		Sensitive in vitro to FQ, doxy
Vibrio vulnificus, alginolyticus, damsela	Doxy + ceftaz	Cefotaxime, FQ (e.g., levo, AAC 46:3580, 2002)	APAG often used in combination with ceftaz
Yersinia enterocolitica	TMP-SMX or FQ	P Ceph 3 or APAG	CID 19:655, 1994
Yersinia pestis (plague)	See Table 1B, page 48		

[1] These agents are more variable in effectiveness than the "Recommended" or "Alternative". Selection of "Alternative" or "Also Effective" agents is based on in vitro susceptibility testing, pharmacokinetics, host factors such as auditory, renal, hepatic function, and cost.

TABLE 3: SUGGESTED DURATION OF ANTIBIOTIC THERAPY IN IMMUNOCOMPETENT PATIENTS[1,2]

CLINICAL SITUATION		DURATION OF THERAPY (Days)
SITE	**CLINICAL DIAGNOSIS**	
Bacteremia	Bacteremia with removable focus (no endocarditis)	10–14 (CID 14:75, 1992) (See Table 1)
Bone	Osteomyelitis, adult; acute	42
	adult; chronic	Until ESR normal (often > 3 months)
	child; acute; staph. and enterobacteriaceae[3]	21
	child; acute; strep., meningococci, hemophilus[3]	14
Ear	Otitis media with effusion	<2 yrs: 10 (or 1 dose ceftriaxone); ≥2 yrs: 5–7
	Recent meta-analysis suggests 3 days of azithro (JAC 52:469, 2003) or 5 days of "short-acting" antibiotics effective for uncomplicated otitis media (JAMA 279:1736, 1998), but may be inadequate for severe disease (NEJM 347:1169, 2002).	
Endocardium	Infective endocarditis, native valve	
	Viridans strep	14 or 28 (See Table 1, pages 21–22)
	Enterococci	28 or 42 (See Table 1, page 22)
	Staph. aureus	14 (R-sided only) or 28 (See Table 1, pages 22–23)
Gastrointestinal Also see Table 1	Bacillary dysentery (shigellosis)/traveler's diarrhea	3
	Typhoid fever (S. typhi): Azithro	5 (children/adolescents)
	Ceftriaxone	14*
	FQ	5–7
	Chloramphenicol	14
		*[Short courses less effective (AAC 44:450, 2000)]
	Helicobacter pylori	10–14
	Pseudomembranous enterocolitis (C. difficile)	10
Genital	Non-gonococcal urethritis or mucopurulent cervicitis	7 days doxy or single dose azithro
	Pelvic inflammatory disease	14
Heart	Pericarditis (purulent)	28
Joint	Septic arthritis (non-gonococcal) Adult	14–28 (Ln 351:197, 1998)
	Infant/child	Rx as osteomyelitis above
	Gonococcal arthritis/disseminated GC infection	7 (See Table 1, page 17)
Kidney	Cystitis (bladder bacteriuria)	3
	Pyelonephritis	14 (7 days if CIP used)
	Recurrent (failure after 14 days rx)	42
Lung	Pneumonia, pneumococcal	Until afebrile 3–5 days (minimum 5 days)
	Pneumonia, enterobacteriaceae or pseudomonal	21, often up to 42
	Pneumonia, staphylococcal	21–28
	Pneumocystis carinii, in AIDS;	21
	other immunocompromised	14
	Legionella, mycoplasma, chlamydia	7–14
	Lung abscess	Usually 28–42[4]
Meninges[5] (CID 39:1267, 2004)	N. meningitidis	7
	H. influenzae	7
	S. pneumoniae	10–14
	Listeria meningoencephalitis, gp B strep, coliforms	21 (longer in immunocompromised)
Multiple systems	Brucellosis (See Table 1, page 43)	42 (add SM or gent for 1st 7–14 days)
	Tularemia (See Table 1, pages 33, 43)	7–14
Muscle	Gas gangrene (clostridial)	10
Pharynx Also see Pharyngitis, Table 1, page 35	Group A strep pharyngitis	10 O Ceph 2/3, azithromycin effective at 5 days (JAC 45, Topic TI 23, 2000). 3 days less effective (Inf Med 18:515, 2001)
	Diphtheria (membranous)	7–14
	Carrier	7
Prostate	Chronic prostatitis (TMP/SMX)	30–90
	(FQ)	28–42
Sinuses	Acute sinusitis	10–14[6]
Skin	Cellulitis	Until 3 days after acute inflammation disappears
Systemic	Lyme disease	See Table 1, page 42
	Rocky Mountain spotted fever (See Table 1, page 43)	Until afebrile 2 days

[1] It has been shown that early change from parenteral to oral regimens (about 72 hours) is cost-effective with many infections, i.e., intra-abdominal (AJM 91:462, 1991)

[2] The recommended duration is a minimum or average time and should not be construed as absolute

[3] These times are with proviso: sx & signs resolve within 7 days and ESR is normalized (J.D. Nelson, APID 6:59, 1991)

[4] After patient afebrile 4-5 days, change to oral therapy

[5] In children relapses seldom occur until 3 days or more after termination of rx. Practice of observing in hospital for 1 or 2 days after rx is expensive and non-productive. For meningitis in children, see Table 1, page 6.

[6] If pt not sx-free at 10 days, sinus puncture and/or rx for 7 more days (NEJM 326:319, 1992). One study reports 3 days of TMP-SMX effective (JAMA 273:1015, 1995). Therapy with azithro for 3 & 6 days as effective as 10 days of AM/CL (AAC 47:2770, 2003).

TABLE 4
COMPARISON OF ANTIMICROBIAL SPECTRA*
(These are generalizations; there are major differences between countries, areas and hospitals depending upon antibiotic usage patterns—verify for individual location. See Table 5 for resistant bacteria)

PENICILLINS, CARBAPENEMS, AZTREONAM, FLUOROQUINOLONES

Column groups: Anti-staphylococcal Penicillins (Methicillin, Nafcillin/Oxacillin, Cloxacillin^NUS/Diclox.); Amino-Penicillins (AMP/Amox, Amox/Clav, AMP-Sulb); Anti-Pseudomonal Penicillins (Ticarcillin, Ticar-Clav, Pip-Tazo, Piperacillin); Carbapenems (Ertapenem, Imipenem, Meropenem); Aztreonam; Fluoroquinolones (Ciprofloxacin, Ofloxacin, Lomefloxacin, Pefloxacin^NUS, Levofloxacin, Moxifloxacin, Gemifloxacin, Gatifloxacin)

Organisms	Penicillin G	Penicillin V	Methicillin	Nafcillin/Oxacillin	Cloxacillin^NUS/Diclox.	AMP/Amox	Amox/Clav	AMP-Sulb	Ticarcillin	Ticar-Clav	Pip-Tazo	Piperacillin	Ertapenem	Imipenem	Meropenem	Aztreonam	Ciprofloxacin	Ofloxacin	Lomefloxacin	Pefloxacin^NUS	Levofloxacin	Moxifloxacin	Gemifloxacin	Gatifloxacin
GRAM-POSITIVE:																								
Strep, Group A,B,C,G	+	+	+	+	+	+	+	+	+	+	+	+	+	+	+	0	±	±	0	0	+	+	+	+
Strep. pneumoniae	+	+	+	+	+	+	+	+	+	+	+	+	+	+	+	0	±	±	0	0	+	+	+	+
Viridans strep	±	±	±	±	±	±	±	±	±	±	±	±	±	±	±	0	0	0	0		+	+	+	+
Strep. milleri	+	+	+	+	+	+	+	+	+	+	+	+	+	+	+	0	0	0			+	+	+	+
Enterococcus faecalis	+	+	0	0	0	+	+	+	±	±	+	±	+	±	0	0	**	**			0	+	+	+
Enterococcus faecium	±	±	0	0	0	±	±	±	±	±	±	±	0	0	0	0	0	0	0		0	±	±	±
Staph. aureus (MSSA)	0	0	+	+	+	0	+	+	0	+	+	0	+	+	+	0	+	+	+	+	+	+	±	±
Staph. aureus (MRSA)	0	0	0	0	0	0	0	0	0	0	0	0	0	0	0	0	0	0	0	0	0	±	±	±
Staph. epidermidis	0	0	+	+	+	0	+	+	±	±	+	±	+	+	+	0	+	+						
C. jeikeium	0	0	0	0	0	0	0	0	0	0	0	0	0	0	0	0	0	0						
L. monocytogenes	+	0	0	0	0	+		+				+	±	±	+	0	+	0	0	0	+	+	+	+
GRAM-NEGATIVE:																								
N. gonorrhoeae	0	0	0	0	0	0	+	+	+	+	+	+	+	+	+	+	+	+	+	+	+	+	+	+
N. meningitidis	+	0	0	0	0	+	+	+	+	+	+	+	+	+	+	+	+	+			+	+	+	+
M. catarrhalis	0	0	0	0	0	0	+	+	0	+	+	±	+	+	+	+	+	+	+	+	+	+	+	+
H. influenzae	0	0	0	0	0	±	+	+	±	+	+	±	+	+	+	+	+	+	+	+	+	+	+	+
E. coli	0	0	0	0	0	±	+	+	+	+	+	+	+	+	+	+	+	+	+	+	+	+	+	+
Klebsiella sp.	0	0	0	0	0	0	+	+	0	+	+	±	+	+	+	+	+	+	+	+	+	+	+	+
Enterobacter sp.	0	0	0	0	0	0	0	0	±	+	+	+	0	+	+	+	+	+	+	+	+	+	+	+
Serratia sp.	0	0	0	0	0	0	0	0	±	+	+	+	+	+	+	+	+	+	+	+	+	+	+	+
Salmonella sp.	0	0	0	0	0	±	+	+	±	+	+	+	+	+	+	+	+	+	+	+	+	+	+	+
Shigella sp.	0	0	0	0	0	±	+	+	±	+	+	+	+	+	+	+	+	+	+	+	+	+	+	+
Proteus mirabilis	0	0	0	0	0	+	+	+	+	+	+	+	+	+	+	+	+	+	+	+	+	+	+	+
Proteus vulgaris	0	0	0	0	0	0	+	+	+	+	+	+	+	+	+	+	+	+	+	+	+	+	+	+
Providencia sp.	0	0	0	0	0	0	+	+	+	+	+	+	+	+	+	+	+	+	+	+	+	+	+	+
Morganella sp.	0	0	0	0	0	0	±	+	+	+	+	+	+	+	+	+	+	+	+	+	+	+	+	+
Citrobacter sp.	0	0	0	0	0	0	0	0	+	+	+	+	+	+	+	+	+	+	+	+	+	+	+	+
Aeromonas sp.	0	0	0	0	0	0	±	+	+	+	+	+	+	+	+	+	+	+	+	+	+	+	+	+
Acinetobacter sp.	0	0	0	0	0	0	0	+	+	+	+	+	0	+	+	±	±	±		±	±	±	±	±
Ps. aeruginosa	0	0	0	0	0	0	0	0	+	+	+	+	0	+	+	+	+	±	+		±	±		±
B. (Ps.) cepacia§	0	0	0	0	0	0	0	0	0	0	0	0	0	0	0	0	0	0	0	0	0	±		0
S. (X.) maltophilia§	0	0	0	0	0	0	0	0	0	±	±	0	0	0	0	0	0	0	0	0	±	+		
Y. enterocolitica	0	0	0	0	0	0	±	±	±	+	+	+	+	+	+	+	+	+	+	+	+	+	+	+
Legionella sp.	0	0	0	0	0	0	0	0	0	0	0	0	0	0	0	0	+	+			+	+	+	+
P. multocida	+	+	+	0	0	+	+	+	+	+	+	+	+	+	+	+	+	+			+	+	+	+
H. ducreyi	+					0	+										+	+	+		+	+	+	+
MISC.:																								
Chlamydia sp.	0	0	0	0	0	0	0	0	0	0	0	0	0	0	0	0	+	+	+	+	+	+	+	+
M. pneumoniae	0	0	0	0	0	0	0	0	0	0	0	0	0	0	0	0	+	+	+	+	+	+	+	+
ANAEROBES:																								
Actinomyces	+	±	0	0	0	+	+	+	+	+	+	+	+	+	+	0								
Bacteroides fragilis§	0	±	0	0	0	0	+	+	0	+	+	0	+	+	+	0	0	0	0		0	±	±	±
P. melaninogenica§	+	0	0	0	0	+	+	+	+	+	+	+	+	+	+	0	0	0	0	0	0	+	+	+
Clostridium difficile	+[1]							+[1]			+[1]		+[1]	+[1]	+[1]	0	0				0	0	0	0
Clostridium (not difficile)	+	+				+	+	+	+	+	+	+	+	+	+	0	±	±	0		+	+	+	+
Peptostreptococcus sp.	+	+	+	+	+	+	+	+	+	+	+	+	+	+	+	0	±	±	0		+	+		+

+ = usually effective clinically or >60% susceptible; ± = clinical trials lacking or 30–60% susceptible; 0 = not effective clinically or <30% susceptible; blank = data not available

§ B. melaninogenicus → Prevotella melaninogenica, Pseudomonas cepacia → Burkholderia cepacia, Xanthomonas → Stenotrophomonas

** Most strains ±, can be used in UTI, not in systemic infection

[1] No clinical evidence that penicillins or fluoroquinolones are effective for C. difficile enterocolitis (but they may cover this organism in mixed intra-abdominal and pelvic infections)

TABLE 4 (2)

Organisms	1st Generation Cefazolin	2nd Generation Cefotetan	2nd Generation Cefoxitin	2nd Generation Cefuroxime	3rd/4th Generation Cefotaxime	3rd/4th Ceftizoxime	3rd/4th Ceftriaxone	3rd/4th Ceftazidime	3rd/4th Cefepime	1st Gen Cefadroxil	1st Gen Cephalexin	Oral 2nd Cefaclor/Loracarbef*	Oral 2nd Cefprozil	Oral 2nd Cefuroxime axetil	Oral 3rd Cefixime	Oral 3rd Ceftibuten	Oral 3rd Cefpodox/Cefdinir/Cefditoren
GRAM-POSITIVE:																	
Strep, Group A,B,C,G	+	+	+	+	+	+	+	+	+	+	+	+	+	+	+	+	+
Strep. pneumoniae[1]	+	+	+	+	+	+	+	+[1]	+	+	+	+	+	+	+	±	+
Viridans strep	+	+	+	+	+	+	+	±[1]	+	+	+	+	0	+	+	0	+
Enterococcus faecalis	0	0	0	0	0	0	0	0	0	0	0	0	0	0	0	0	0
Staph. aureus (MSSA)	+	+	+	+	+	+	+	±	+	+	+	+	+	+	0	0	+
Staph. aureus (MRSA)	0	0	0	0	0	0	0	0	0	0	0	0	0	0	0	0	0
Staph. epidermidis	±	±	±	±	±	±	±	±	±	±	±	±	±	±	0	0	±
C. jeikeium	0	0	0	0	0	0	0	0	0	0	0	0	0	0	0	0	0
L. monocytogenes	0	0	0	0	0	0	0	0	0	0	0	0	0	0	0	0	0
GRAM-NEGATIVE																	
N. gonorrhoeae	+	±	±	+	+	+	+	±	+	0	0	±	±	+	+	+	+
N. meningitidis	0	±	±	+	+	±	+	±	+	0	0	±	±	±	±	±	+
M. catarrhalis	±	+	+	+	+	+	+	+	+	0	0	±	+	+	+	+	+
H. influenzae	+	+	+	+	+	+	+	+	+		0	±	+	+	+	+	+
E. coli	+	+	+	+	+	+	+	+	+	+	+	+	+	+	+	+	+
Klebsiella sp.	+	+	+	+	+	+	+	+	+	+	+	+	+	+	+	+	+
Enterobacter sp.	0	±	0	±	+	+	+	+	+	0	0	0	0	0	0	±	+
Serratia sp.	0	+	0	0	+	+	+	+	+	0	0	0	0	0	±	±	0
Salmonella sp.					+	+	+	+	+		0				+	+	+
Shigella sp.					+	+	+	+	+		0				+	+	+
Proteus mirabilis	+	+	+	+	+	+	+	+	+	+	+	+	+	+	+	+	+
Proteus vulgaris	0	+	+	+	+	+	+	+	+	0	0	0	0	0	+	+	±
Providencia sp.	0	±	+	0	+	+	+	+	+	0	0	0	0	0	+	+	
Morganella sp.	0	+	±	±	+	+	+	+	+	0	0	0	0	±	0	0	0
C. freundii	0	0	0	0	0	0	0	0	0	0	0	0	0	0	0	0	0
C. diversus	0	±	±	±	+	+	+	+	+	0	0	0	0		+		
Citrobacter sp.	0	±	±	±	+	+	+	+	+		0	±	0	±	+	+	+
Aeromonas sp.	0	+	±	+	+	+	+	+	+						+	+	
Acinetobacter sp.	0	0	0	0	+	+	+	+	±	0	0	0	0	0	0	0	0
Ps. aeruginosa	0	0	0	0	±	±	±	+	+	0	0	0	0	0	0	0	0
B. (Ps.) cepacia[§]	0	0	0	0	±	±	±	+	±	0	0	0	0	0	0	0	0
S. (X.) maltophilia[§]	0	0	0	0	0	0	0	±	0	0	0	0	0	0	0	0	
Y. enterocolitica	0	±	±	+	+	+	+	+	+	0	0				+	+	
Legionella sp.	0	0	0	0	0	0	0	0	0	0	0	0	0	0	0	0	0
P. multocida					+	+					0				+		+
H. ducreyi			+			+	+								+		
ANAEROBES:																	
Actinomyces					+	+											
Bacteroides fragilis	0	±[2]	+	0	0	±	0	0	0		0		0	0	0		0
P. melaninogenica[§]		+	+	+	+	+	±	+	0				+	+	+		
Clostridium difficile			0			0	0		0								
Clostridium (not difficile)		+	+	+	+	+	+	+					+	+	+		
Peptostreptococcus sp.		+	+	+	+	+	+	+	+			+	+	+			

+ = usually effective clinically or >60% susceptible; ± = clinical trials lacking or 30–60% susceptible; 0 = not effective clinically or <30% susceptible; blank = data not available.

§ B. melaninogenicus → Prevotella melaninogenica, P. cepacia → Burkholderia cepacia, Xanthomonas → Stenotrophomonas

* A 1-carbacephem best classified as a cephalosporin

[1] Ceftaz 8–16 times less active than cefotax/ceftriax, effective only vs Pen-sens. strains (AAC 39:2193, 1995). Oral cefuroxime, cefprozil, cefpodoxime most active in vitro vs resistant S. pneumo (PIDJ 14:1037, 1995).

[2] Cefotetan is less active against B. ovatus, B. distasonis, B. thetaiotamicron

TABLE 4 (3)

Column groups: **AMINOGLYCOSIDES** (Gentamicin, Tobramycin, Amikacin, Netilmicin[AUS]) · Chloramphenicol · **MACROLIDES** (Clindamycin, Erythro/Dirithro, Azithromycin, Clarithromycin) · **KETOLIDE** (Telithromycin) · **TETRACYCLINES** (Doxycycline, Minocycline) · **GLYCYLCYCLINE** (Tigecycline) · **GLYCOPEPTIDES** (Vancomycin, Teicoplanin, Dalbavancin) · Fusidic Acid[AUS] · Trimethoprim · TMP-SMX · **URINARY TRACT AGENTS** (Nitrofurantoin, Fosfomycin) · **MISCELLANEOUS** (Rifampin, Metronidazole, Linezolid, Quinupristin-dalfopristin, Daptomycin, Colistimethate (Colistin))

Organisms	Gen	Tob	Amk	Net[AUS]	Chloram	Clinda	Eryth/Dir	Azithro	Clarithro	Telithro	Doxy	Mino	Tige	Vanco	Teico	Dalba	Fusidic[AUS]	Trimeth	TMP-SMX	Nitrofur	Fosfo	Rifampin	Metro	Linez	Q-D	Dapto	Colistin
GRAM-POSITIVE:																											
Strep Group A,B,C,G	0	0	0	0	+	+	+	+	+	+	+	±	+	+	+	+	±	±	+[1]	+		+	0	+	+	+	0
Strep. pneumoniae	0	0	0	0	+	+	+	+	+	+	±	+	+	+	+	+	±	±	±	+		+	0	+	+	+	0
Enterococcus faecalis	S	S	S	S	±	0	0	0	0	0	0	±	0	+	+	+	0	±	±[1]	+	+	+	0	+	±	+	0
Enterococcus faecium	S	0	0	0	±	0	0	0	0	0	0	0	±	+	+	+	0	±	±	+	+	+	0	+	+	+	0
Staph.aureus(MSSA)	+	+	+	+	±	+	±	+	+	+	±	+	+	+	+	+	+	±	+	+	+	+	0	+	+	+	0
Staph.aureus(MRSA)	0	0	0	0	0	0	0	0	0	0	±	±	+	+	+	+	±	±	+	+		+	0	+	+	+	0
Staph. epidermidis	±	±	±	±	0	0	0	0	0	0	0	0	±	+	+	+	±	±	±	+		+	0	+	+	+	0
C. jeikeium	0	0	0	0	0	0	0	0	0	0	0	0	±	+	+	+	0					+	0	+	+	+	0
L. monocytogenes	S	S	S	S	+		+	+	+	+	0	0	±	+	+		0		+			+	0	+	0	+	0
GRAM-NEGATIVE:																											
N. gonorrhoeae	0	0	0	0		+	0	±	±	±		±	±				0	0		+		0		0	+		0
N. meningitidis	0	0	0	0		0	+	0	+		+	+	+				0	0	0			+	0	0		0	0
M. catarrhalis[§]	+	+	+	+			+	+	+	+	+	+	+						+			+	0	0		0	
H. influenzae	+	+	+	+		0	±	±	±	±	+	+	+					±	+			+	0	+	±	0	+
Aeromonas	0										+	+	+	0					+			0	0		±	±	
E. coli	+	+	+	+		+	0	0	0	0	0	±	±	0	0	0	0	0	0[1]	+	+	0	0	0	0	0	+
Klebsiella sp.	+	+	+	+		±	0	0	0	0	0	±	±	0	0	0	0	±	±	+		0	0	0	0	0	+
Enterobacter sp.	+	+	+	+		±	0	0	0	0	0	±	±	0	0	0	0	±	±	0	0	0	0	0	0	0	+
Salmonella sp.	+	+	+	+		0	0	0	±	0	0	±	±	0	0	0	0	±	±			0	0	0	0	0	
Shigella sp.	+	+	+	+		0	0	0	±	0	0	±	±	0	0	0	0	±	±		0	0	0	0	0	0	
Serratia marcescens	+	+	+	+		0	0	0	0	0	0	±	±	0	0	0	0	0	±		0	0	0	0	0	0	
Proteus vulgaris	+	+	+	+		0	0	0	0	0	0	±	±	0	0	0	0	±	±	0		0	0	0	0	0	0
Acinetobacter sp.	0	+	0									+	+					0	±			0	0	0	0	0	+
Ps. aeruginosa	+	+	+	+		0	0	0	0	0	0	0	0	0	0	0	0	0	0	0	±	0	0	0	0	0	+
B. (Ps.) cepacia[§]	0	0	0	0		0	0	0	0	0	0	0	±	0	0	0	0	0	+	0		0	0	0	0	0	0
S. (X.) maltophilia[§]	0	0	0	0		0	0	0	0	0	0	0	+	0	0	0	0	0	+	0		0	0	0	0	0	0
Y. enterocolitica	+					0	0	0	0	0	0	0	±						+			0	0	0	0	0	0
F. tularensis	+										+											0	0	0	0	0	0
Brucella sp.	+					0	+	0	0	0	+	+			0	0	0		+			+	0	0	0	0	0
Legionella sp.	+					+	+	+	+		+	+	+					±	+	+		+	0	0	0	0	
H. ducreyi						+	+	+	+										+			0	0	0	0	0	
V. vulnificus	±	±	±			+					+	+						0				0	0	0	0	0	
MISC.:																											
Chlamydophila sp.	0	0	0	0			+	+	+	+	+	+	+					0	0			+	0	+	+		
M. pneumoniae	0	0	0	0		0	+	+	+	+	+	+						0	0			+	0	0			
Rickettsia sp.	0	0	0	0			±				+	+	+	0	0	0			0	0		+	0	0			
Mycobacterium avium							+	+	+					0	0	0						0	0	0			
ANAEROBES:																											
Actinomyces	0	0	0	0	+	+	+	+	+		+	+		+	+	+						0					
Bacteroides fragilis	0	0	0	0	+	±	0	0	0	0		±	±	0	0		0	0	0			0	+	0		±	
P. melaninogenica[§]	0	0	0	0	+	+	+	+	+		±	+	±	0	0		0	0	0			0	+			±	
Clostridium difficile	0	0	0	0	±									+	+	+							+	+	+		
Clostridium (not difficile) **					+		±	±			+	+	+	+	+	+	+						+	+	+		
Peptostreptococcus sp.	0	0	0	0	+	+	+	+	+		+	+	+	+	+	+	+						+	+	+		

+ = usually effective clinically or >60% susceptible; ± = clinical trials lacking or 30–60% susceptible; 0 = not effective clinically or <30% susceptible; S = synergistic with penicillins (ampicillin); blank = data not available. Antimicrobials such as azithromycin have high tissue penetration and some such as clarithromycin are metabolized to more active compounds, hence in vivo activity may exceed in vitro activity.

[1] Although active in vitro, TMP-SMX is not clinically effective for Group A strep pharyngitis or for infections due to E. faecalis.

[§] B. melaninogenicus → Prevotella melaninogenica, P. cepacia → Burkholderia cepacia, Xanthomonas → Stenotrophomonas

** Vancomycin, metronidazole given po active vs C. difficile; IV vancomycin not effective

TABLE 5: TREATMENT OPTIONS FOR SELECTED HIGHLY RESISTANT BACTERIA (See page 2 for abbreviations)

ORGANISM/RESISTANCE	THERAPEUTIC OPTIONS	COMMENT
E. faecalis. Resistant to:		
Penicillin G or AMP (MIC >500 mcg per mL); β-lactamase neg. (JAC 40:161, 1997).	Penicillin G or AMP (systemic infections). Nitrofurantoin, fosfomycin (UTI only). Usually resistant to Synercid.	Non BL + strains of E. faecalis resistant to penicillin and AMP described in Spain, but unknown in U.S. and elsewhere (AAC 40:2420, 1996). Linezolid effective in 60–70% of cases (AnIM 138:135, 2003). Daptomycin, tigecycline active in vitro (JAC 52:123, 2003).
Penicillin (β-lactamase producers)		Appear susceptible to AMP and penicillin by standard in vitro methods. Must use direct test for β-lactamase with chromogenic cephalosporin (nitrocefin) to identify. Rare since early 1990s.
E. faecium. Resistant to:		
Vanco and high levels (MIC >500 mcg per mL) of streptomycin and gentamicin	Penicillin G or AMP (systemic infections). Nitrofurantoin (UTI only)	For strains with pen/AMP MICs of >8 ≤64 mcg per mL, anecdotal evidence that high-dose (300 mg per kg per day) AMP may be effective. Daptomycin, tigecycline active in vitro (JAC 52:123, 2003).
Penicillin, AMP, vanco, & high-level resist. to streptomycin and gentamicin (NEJM 342:710, 2000)	Linezolid 600 mg per kg IV q12h and quinu-dalfo 7.5 mg per kg IV q8h are bacteriostatic against most strains of E. faecium. Use combinations of cell wall-active antibiotics with other agents (including FQ, chloramphenicol, RIF, or doxy). Chloramphenicol alone effective in some cases of quinu-dalfo bacteremia (Clin Micro Inf 7:17, 2001). Nitrofurantoin or fosfomycin may work for UTI	For strains with Van B phenotype (vanco R, teico S), teicoplanin[NUS], preferably in combination with streptomycin or gentamicin (if not highly AG resistant), may be effective. Synercid roughly 70% effective in clinical trials (CID 30:790, 2000 & 33:1816, 2001). Linezolid shows similar efficacy. Comparable but somewhat lower rates (58% linezolid, 43% Q/D) response rates in cancer pts (JAC 53:646, 2004). Emergence of resistance with therapeutic failure has occurred during monotherapy with either quinu-dalfo or linezolid (NEJM 346:867, 2002). Daptomycin active in vitro against most strains (JAC 52:123, 2003). Infectious disease consultation imperative!
S. aureus. Resistant to:		
Methicillin (health-care associated) (CID 32:108, 2001) For community-acquired MRSA infections, see Table 6	Vanco (+ RIF for persistent bacteremia ≥7 days) on vanco or teico-planin[NUS] (see Table 6)	Alternatives: teicoplanin[NUS], daptomycin (AAC 49:770, 2003), linezolid (Chest 124:1789, 2003), dalbavancin (EMID 48:137, 2004). TMP-SMX (test susceptibility first), minocycline & doxy (some strains). Vanco (JID 41(Suppl 5):S303, 2005), or quinu-dalfo (CID 34:1481, 2002). Fusidic acid[NUS], fosfomycin, RIF may be active, use only in combination to prevent in vivo emergence of resistance. Staphy-lococci (MIC ≤2 mcg per mL) may appear susceptible to clindamycin in vitro. Clinda therapy may result in therapeutic failure (CID 37:1257, 2003). Test for inducible resistance (double-disk) (JCM 42:2777, 2004). If resistance found, and Macro test (+), Clinda should not be used. (LY333328) (MMWR 51:902, 2002; NEJM 348:1342, 2003).
Vanco, methicillin (VRMRSA) (NEJM 339:520, 1998; CID 32:108, 2001; MMWR 51:902, 2002; NEJM 348:1342, 2003)	Unknown, but even then. Linezolid, quinu-dalfo, daptomycin active in vitro	Most clinical isolates of VRMRSA have had only low levels (MIC ≤16 mcg per mL) of vanco resistance (AAC 40:135, 1997). Some call these strains VISA or GISA. Only anecdotal data on therapeutic regimens. Most susceptible to TMP-SMX, minocycline, doxycycline. RIF and AGs (CID 32:108, 2001). RIF should always be combined with a 2nd therapeutic agent to prevent emergence of RIF resistance during therapy, 4 clinical isolates of MRSA (MIC >64) MRSA described. Organisms still susceptible to RIF, TMP-SMX (MMWR 51:902, 2004; JAC 48:1342, 2003).
S. epidermidis. Resistant to:		
Methicillin	Vanco (+ RIF and gentamicin for prosthetic valve endocarditis)	
Methicillin, glycopeptides (EMID 48:137, 2004)	Quinu-dalfo (see comments on E. faecium)	Vanco more active than teicoplanin[NUS] (Clin Micro Rev 8:585, 1995). New FQs (levofloxacin, gatifloxacin, moxifloxacin) active in vitro, but development of resistance is a potential problem.
Methicillin, glycopeptides (JAC 49:203, 2005)		
S. pneumoniae. Resistant to:		
Penicillin G (MIC >0.1 ≤1.0)	Ceftriaxone or cefotaxime. High-dose penicillin (≥10 million units per day) or AMP (amox) likely effective for non-meningeal infection.	IMP, ERTA, cefepime, cefpodoxime, cefuroxime also active (IDCP 3:75, 1994). MER less active than IMP (AAC 38:898, 1994). Gati, gemi, levo, moxi also have good activity (AAC 38:898, 1994; DMID 37:45, 1998; Exp Open Invest Drugs 8:123, 1999).
Penicillin G (MIC ≥2.0)	(Vanco ± RIF). Alternatives if non-meningeal infection: ceftriaxone/cefotax., high-dose AMP, ERTA, IMP, MER, or an FQ with enhanced activity vs S. pneumo (gati, gemi, levo, moxi), telithro.	High-dose cefotaxime (300 mg per kg per day) effective in meningitis due to strains with cefotaxime MICs as high as 2 mcg per mL (AAC 40:218, 1996). Review IDCP 8:123, 1997.
Penicillin, erythro, tetracycline, chloram-phenicol, TMP-SMX	(Vanco ± RIF) (Gati, Gemi, Levo, Moxi), telithro (non-meningeal infections)	60–80% of strains susceptible to clindamycin (DMID 25:201, 1996)
Acinetobacter baumannii. Resistant to: IMP, AP Ceph 3, AP Pen, APAG, FQ	AM-SB (CID 34:1425, 2002). Subactam alone is active against some A. baumannii (JAC 42:793, 1998)	6/8 patients with A. baumannii meningitis (7 organisms resistant to IMP) cured with AM/SB (CID 24:932, 1997). Various combinations of FQs and AGs, IMP and AGs, IMP or RIF, or AP Pens or AP Ceph 3s with AGs may show activity against multiresistant strains in vitro (Ln:1268, 2000; AAC 42:2204, 2000; J Chemother 12:190, 2000; JAC 53:303, 2004). Active in vitro: triple drug combinations of polymyxin B, IMP, and RIF (AAC 48:753, 2004) & tigecycline (CID 41:S315, 2005)

[1] Guideline on prevention of resistance: CID 25:584, 1997

TABLE 5 (2)

ORGANISM/RESISTANCE	THERAPEUTIC OPTIONS	COMMENT
Campylobacter jejuni. Resistant to: FQs	Erythro, azithro, clarithro, doxy, clindamycin	Resistance to **both** FQs & macrolides reported (CID 22:868, 1996; EID 7:24, 2002; AAC 47:2358, 2003)
Klebsiella pneumoniae (producing ESBL) **Resistant to:** Ceftazidime & other 3° generation cephalosporins (see *Table 10C*), aztreonam	IMP, MER, ERTA (CID 39:31, 2004) (See Comment)	P Ceph 4, TC-CL, PIP-TZ show in vitro activity, but not proven entirely effective in animal models (JJAA 8:37, 1997); some strains which hyperproduce ESBLs are primarily resistant to TC-CL and PIP-TZ (J Clin Micro 34:358, 1996). Note: There are strains of ESBL-producing Klebsiella sensitive in vitro to P Ceph 3 but failed in animal models. PIP-TZ may be effective but response to P Ceph 2 or 3 (J Clin Micro 39:2206, 2001). FQ may be effective if susceptible. Note Klebsiella sp. with carbapenem resistance due to class A carbapenemase. Some of these organisms resistant to all antimicrobials except colistin (CID 39:55, 2004)
Pseudomonas aeruginosa. Resistant to: IMP, MER	CIP (check susceptibility), APAG (check susceptibility)	Many strains remain susceptible to aztreonam & ceftazidime or AP Pens (AAC 36:1037, 1995). Combinations of (AP Pen & APAG) or (AP Ceph 3 + APAG) may show in vitro activity (AAC 39:2411, 1995). IV colistin may have some utility (CID 28:1008, 1999)

TABLE 6: SUGGESTED MANAGEMENT OF SUSPECTED OR CULTURE-POSITIVE COMMUNITY-ACQUIRED PHENOTYPE OF METHICILLIN-RESISTANT S. AUREUS (CA-MRSA) INFECTIONS (See page 2 for abbreviations)

In the absence of definitive comparative efficacy studies, the Editors have generated the following guidelines. With the magnitude of the clinical problem and a number of new drugs, it is likely new data will require frequent revisions of the regimens suggested. Ref: CID 40:562, 2005.

CLINICAL ILLNESS	ABSCESS, AFEBRILE, & IMMUNOCOMPETENT: OUTPATIENT CARE	ABSCESS(ES) WITH FEVER: OUTPATIENT CARE	VENTILATOR-ASSOCIATED PNEUMONIA	BACTEREMIA OR POSSIBLE ENDOCARDITIS OR BACTEREMIC SHOCK	BLOOD CULTURES DRAWN ON DAY 7 OF VANCO ARE POSITIVE (See footnote)
Management (for drug doses, see footnote):	TMP-SMX-DS or **doxycycline or minocycline** (CID 40:1429, 2005) NOTE: for abscesses <5 cm diameter, I&D only sufficient (PIDJ 23:123, 2004)	TMP-SMX-DS or **rifampin**[1] or **linezolid**[1] dose of **dalbavancin**	**Vanco**[1] **telco**[2] IV or **linezolid**[1] IV Ref: Chest 124:1632, 2003	**Vanco**[1] or **linezolid**[1] IV or If vanco allergy, **Daptomycin.** Could start with **nafcillin (or oxacillin)** + **vanco**; DC inactive drug when suscept. data available	Switch to **daptomycin. Quinupristin-dalfopristin** (Q-D) 2nd alternative; it with vanco; ~70% effective in compassionate use trial (JAC 50:1017, 2002) No strong data that adding **rifampin** helps. Adding **gentamicin** to **vanco** ? risk of nephrotoxicity with little evidence of enhanced efficacy. Could try **Gati, Levo** or **Moxi** if isolate susceptible.
			Need quant. cultures to diagnosis; e.g., protect-ed specimen brush	Blood cultures. Target trough level of vanco 15 (range 10-20) mcg per mL.	In retrospective evaluation, linezolid & vanco equivalent efficacy—roughly 30% microbiologic failure with both drugs (JAC in press 10/2005)
Comments	Close followup. Fever should resolve quickly post I&D. Rarely S. pyogenes + MRSA. TMP-SMX not active vs S. pyogenes; **rifampin** active re and **Pen V-K**	If recurrent & post-rx decolonization desired, see page 39	**Linezolid** superior to **vanco** in retrospective subset analysis.	Can't rely on **clinda** without in vitro documentation of absence of inducible resistance (CID 40:280, 2005). **TMP-SMX** of limited efficacy vs bacteremic; S. aureus (NEJM 117:390, 1992)	If MRSA resistant to **erythro.** likely that Q-D will have bacteriostatic & not bactericidal activity. Interest in this drug, but no data. Do not add **linezolid** to **vanco;** no benefit & may be antagonistic. Linezolid successful in compassionate use (JAC 50:1017, 2002) & in pts with reduced vanco in vitro suscept. (CID 38:521, 2004). To date, no data for **dalbavancin** in vanco failures.

[1] Bacteremia may persist 7 days after starting vanco (AJM 115:674, 1991). Longer duration of bacteremia, greater likelihood of endocarditis (JID 190:1140, 2004)

[2] Before switching, look for undrained abscess(es) & infected foreign body. Recheck vanco MIC to exclude intermediate or high-level vanco resistance.

Dalbavancin: 1000 mg IV, then 500 mg IV 8 days later **Daptomycin:** 6 mg per kg IV q24h **Doxycycline or minocycline** 100 mg po bid **Linezolid:** 600 mg po/IV bid (expensive) **Nafcillin or oxacillin** 2 gm IV q4h **Quinupristin-dalfopristin (Q-D):** 7.5 mg per /kg IV q8h via central line. **Rifampin:** Long serum half-life justifies dosing 600 mg po q24h; however, frequency of nausea less with 300 mg po bid. **TMP-SMX-DS:** Standard dose 8–10 mg per kg per day. For 70 kg person = 700 mg TMP component per day. TMP-SMX-DS contains 160 mg TMP. Hence, suggest **2** TMP-SMX-DS po bid. 50% failure rate with one TMP-SMX-DS bid (J Am Acad Derm 50:854, 2004) **Vancomycin:** 1 gm IV q12h

TABLE 7: METHODS FOR PENICILLIN DESENSITIZATION (CID 35:26, 2002)
(See Table 10C, page 73, for TMP/SMX desensitization)

Perform in ICU setting. Discontinue all β-adrenergic antagonists. Have IV line, ECG and spirometer. Once desensitized, rx must not lapse or risk of allergic reactions ↑. A history of Stevens-Johnson syndrome, exfoliative dermatitis, erythroderma are nearly absolute contraindications (use only as an approach to desensitization [CCTID 13:131, 1993]).

Oral Route: If oral prep available and pt has functional GI tract, oral route is preferred. 1/3 pts will develop transient reaction during desensitization or treatment, usually mild.

Step	1	2	3	4	5	6	7	8	9	10	11	12	13	14
Drug (mg per mL)	0.5	0.5	0.5	0.5	0.5	0.5	5.0	5.0	5.0	50	50	50	50	50
Amount (mL)	0.1	0.2	0.4	0.8	1.6	3.2	0.64	1.2	2.4	0.48	0.96	2.0	4.0	8.0

* Interval between doses: 15 min. After Step 14, observe for 30 minutes.

Parenteral Route:

Step	1	2	3	4	5	6	7	8	9	10	11	12	13	14	15	16	17
Drug (mg per mL)	0.1	0.1	0.1	0.1	0.1	1.0	1.0	1.0	10	10	10	100	100	100	1000	1000	1000
Amount (mL)	0.1	0.2	0.4	0.8	1.6	0.32	0.64	1.2	0.24	0.48	1.0	0.2	0.4	0.8	0.16	0.32	0.64

** Interval between doses: 15 min. After Step 17, observe for 30 minutes, then 1.0 gm IV. [Adapted from Sullivan, T.J. in Allergy: Principles and Practice, C.V. Mosby, 1993, p. 1726, with permission]

TABLE 8: RISK CATEGORIES OF ANTIMICROBICS IN PREGNANCY

DRUG	FDA PREGNANCY RISK CATEGORIES
Antibacterial Agents	
Aminoglycosides	
Amikacin, gentamicin, isepamicin[NUS], netilmicin[NUS], streptomycin & tobramycin	D
Beta Lactams	
Penicillins, pens + BLI, cephalosporins, aztreonam	B
Imipenem/cilastatin	C
Meropenem, ertapenem	B
Chloramphenicol	C
Ciprofloxacin, ofloxacin, levofloxacin, gatiflox, gemiflox, moxiflox	C
Clindamycin	B
Colistin	C
Dalbavancin	C
Daptomycin	B
Fosfomycin	B
Linezolid	C
Macrolides:	
Erythromycins/azithromycin	B
Clarithromycin	C
Metronidazole	B
Nitrofurantoin	B
Rifaximin	C
Sulfonamides/trimethoprim	C
Tetracyclines, tigecycline	D
Tinidazole	C
Vancomycin	C
Antifungal Agents: (CID 27:1151, 1998)	
Amphotericin B preparations	B
Anidulafungin	C
Caspofungin	C
Fluconazole, itraconazole, ketoconazole, flucytosine	C
Antifungal Agents: (continued)	
Micafungin	C
Terbinafine	B
Voriconazole	D
Antiparasitic Agents:	
Albendazole/mebendazole	C
Atovaquone/proguanil; atovaquone alone	C
Chloroquine, eflornithine	C
Ivermectin	C
Mefloquine	C
Miltefosine	X
Nitazoxanide	B
Pentamidine	C
Praziquantel	B
Pyrimethamine/pyrisulfadoxine	C
Quinidine	C
Quinine	X
Antimycobacterial Agents:	
Capreomycin	C
Clofazimine/cycloserine	C
Dapsone	C
Ethambutol	B
Ethionamide	"avoid"
INH, pyrazinamide	C
Rifabutin	"safe"
Rifampin	C
Thalidomide	"do not use"
Antiviral Agents:	
Abacavir	C
Acyclovir	B
Adefovir	C
Amantadine	C
Antiviral Agents: (continued)	
Atazanavir	B
Cidofovir	C
Delavirdine	C
Didanosine (ddI)	B
Efavirenz	D
Emtricitabine	B
Enfuvirtide	B
Entecavir	C
Famciclovir	B
Fosamprenavir	C
Foscarnet	C
Ganciclovir	C
Indinavir	C
Interferons	C
Lamivudine	C
Lopinavir/ritonavir	C
Nelfinavir	B
Nevirapine	C
Oseltamivir	C
Ribavirin	X
Rimantadine	C
Ritonavir	B
Saquinavir	B
Stavudine	C
Tenofovir	B
Tipranavir	C
Valacyclovir	B
Valganciclovir	C
Zalcitabine	C
Zanamivir	C
Zidovudine	C

* FDA Pregnancy Categories: **A**—studies in pregnant women no risk; **B**—animal studies no risk, but human not adequate or animal toxicity but human studies show no risk; **C**—animal studies show toxicity, human studies inadequate but benefit of use may exceed risk; **D**—evidence of human risk, but benefits may outweigh; **X**—fetal abnormalities in humans, risk > benefit.

TABLE 9A: SELECTED PHARMACOLOGIC FEATURES OF ANTIMICROBIAL AGENTS

DRUG	DOSE, ROUTE OF ADMINISTRATION	FOR PO DOSING—Take Drug			% AB[1]	PEAK SERUM LEVEL mcg per mL[1]	PROTEIN BINDING, %	SERUM T½, HOURS[2]	BILIARY EXCRETION, %[3]	CSF[4]/BLOOD, %	CSF LEVEL POTENTIALLY THERAPEUTIC[5]
		WITH FOOD	WITHOUT FOOD	WITH OR WITHOUT FOOD							
PENICILLINS: Natural											
Benzathine Pen G	1.2 million units IM					0.15					
Penicillin G	2 million units IV					20			500	5-10	Yes for Pen-sens. S. pneumo
Penicillin V	500 mg po		X		60-73	5-6	65	0.5			
PENASE-RESISTANT PENICILLINS											
Clox/Diclox	500 mg po	X	X		50	10-15	95-98	0.5			
Nafcillin/Oxacillin	500 mg po	X	X		Erratic	10-15	90-94	0.5	>100/25	9-20	Yes-high-dose IV therapy
AMINOPENICILLINS											
Amoxicillin	250 mg po			X		4-5	17	1.2	100-3000	13-14	
AM-CL	875/125 mg po			X	75	11.6/2.2	20/30	1.4/1.1	100-3000		
AM-CL-ER		X				17/2.1	18/25	1.3/1.0			
Ampicillin	2 gm IV					47	18-22	1.2	100-3000	13-14	Yes
AM-SB	3 gm IV					109-150	28/38	1.2			
ANTIPSEUDOMONAL PENICILLINS											
Indanyl carb.	382 mg po			X	35	6.5	50	1.0	3000-6000	30	
Piperacillin	4 gm IV					400	16-48	1.0			Not for P. aeruginosa, marginal for coliforms
PIP-TZ	3/375 gm IV					209	16-48	1.0	>100		
Ticarcillin	3 gm IV					260	45	1.2		40	Not for P. aeruginosa, marginal for coliforms
TC-CL	3.1 gm IV					330	45/25	1.1			
CEPHALOSPORINS—1st Generation											
Cefadroxil	500 mg po			X	90	16	20	1.5	22		
Cefazolin	1 gm IV					188	73-87	1.9	29-300		
Cephalexin	500 mg po			X	90	18-38	5-15	1.0	216		
CEPHALOSPORINS—2nd Generation											
Cefaclor	500 mg po	X	X		93	9.3	22-25	0.8	≥60	1-4	No
Cefaclor-CD	500 mg po	X	X			8.4	22-25	0.8	≥60		
Cefotetan	1 gm IV					124	78-91	4.2	2-21		
Cefoxitin	1 gm IV					110	65-79	0.8	280		
Cefprozil	500 mg po	X				10.5	36	1.5		3	±
Cefuroxime	1.5 gm IV					100	33-50	1.3	35-80	17-88	Yes
Cefuroxime axetil	250 mg po	X				4.1	50	1.5			
Loracarbef	250 mg po		X		90	8	25	1.2			
CEPHALOSPORINS—3rd Generation											
Cefdinir	300 mg po			X	25	1.6	60-70	1.7			
Cefditoren pivoxil	400 mg po	X			16	4	88	1.6			

See page 63 for all footnotes; see page 2 for abbreviations

TABLE 9A (2)

DRUG	DOSE, ROUTE OF ADMINISTRATION	FOR PO DOSING—Take Drug			% AB[1]	PEAK SERUM LEVEL mcg per mL	PROTEIN BINDING, %	SERUM $T_{1/2}$, HOURS[2]	BILIARY EXCRETION, %[3]	CSF[4]/BLOOD, %	CSF LEVEL POTENTIALLY THERAPEUTIC[5]
		WITH FOOD	WITH OR WITHOUT FOOD	WITHOUT FOOD							
CEPHALOSPORINS—3rd Generation *(continued)*											
Cefixime	400 mg po		X		50	3-5	65	3.1	800		
Cefotaxime	1 gm IV					100	30-51	1.5	15-75	10	Yes
Cefpodoxime proxetil	200 mg po	X			46	2.9	40	2.3	115		
Ceftazidime	1 gm IV					60	<10	1.9	13-54	20-40	Yes
Ceftibuten	400 mg po			X	80	15	65	2.4	34-82		
Ceftizoxime	1 gm IV					132	30	1.7		8-16	Yes
Ceftriaxone	1 gm IV					150	85-95	8	200-500	10	Yes
CEPHALOSPORIN—4th Generation											
Cefepime	2 gm IV					193	20	2.0	≈5	10	Yes
CARBAPENEMS											
Ertapenem	1 gm IV					154	95	4	10	21	Yes
Imipenem	500 mg IV					40	15-25	1	minimal	8.5	+[9]
Meropenem	1 gm IV					49	2	1	3-300	Approx. 2	+
MONOBACTAM											
Aztreonam	1 gm IV					125	56	2	115-405	3-52	±
AMINOGLYCOSIDES											
Amikacin, gentamicin, kanamycin, tobramycin—see Table 10D, page 74, for dose & serum levels											
Neomycin	po				<3	0	0-10	2.5	10-60	0-30	No; intrathecal: 5-10 mg
FLUOROQUINOLONES[10]											
Ciprofloxacin	750 mg po		X		70	1.8-2.8	20-40	4	2800-4500	26	1 mcg per mL inadequate for Strep. species *(CID 31:1131, 2000)*.
	400 mg IV		X			4.6	20-40	4	2800-4500		
	500 mg ER po		X			1.6	20-40	6.6			
	1000 mg ER po		X			3.1	20-40	6.3			
Gatifloxacin	400 mg po/IV		X		96	4.2-4.6	20	7-8		36	
Gemifloxacin	320 mg po		X		71	0.7-2.6	55-73	7			
Levofloxacin	500 mg po/IV		X		98	5.7	24-38	7		30-50	
	750 mg po/IV		X		99	8.6	24-38	7			
Moxifloxacin	400 mg po/IV		X		89	4.5	50	10-14			
Ofloxacin	400 mg po/IV		X		98	4.6/6.2	32	9			
MACROLIDES, AZALIDES, LINCOSAMIDES, KETOLIDES											
Azithromycin	500 mg po		X		37	0.4	7-51	68	High.		
	500 mg IV					3.6	7-51	12/68			
Azithromycin-ER	2 gm po			X	≈30	0.8	7-50	7-50	6		
Clarithromycin	500 mg po				50	3-4	65-70	5-7			
	ER—500 mg po	X			≈50	2-3	65-70		7000		

See pages 62 for all footnotes, see page 2 for abbreviations

TABLE 9A (5)

DRUG	DOSE, ROUTE OF ADMINISTRATION	WITH FOOD	WITHOUT FOOD	WITH OR WITHOUT FOOD	% AB[1]	PEAK SERUM LEVEL mcg per mL[6]	PROTEIN BINDING, %	SERUM T½[2] HOURS	BILIARY EXCRETION, %[3]	CSF[7]/BLOOD, %	CSF LEVEL POTENTIALLY THERAPEUTIC[5]
MACROLIDES, AZALIDES, LINCOSAMIDES, KETOLIDES (continued)											
Dirithromycin	500 mg po	X			10	0.4	15-30	8			
Erythromycin Oral (various)	500 mg po		X		18-45	0.1-2 / 3-4	70-74 / 70-74	2-4 / 2-4			No
Lacto/glucep	500 mg iv					3-4					
Telithromycin	800 mg po			X	57	2.3	60-70	10	7	2-13	
Clindamycin	150 mg po / 600 mg iv			X	90	2.5 / 10	85-94 / 85-94	2.4 / 2.4	250-300 / 250-300		No / No
MISCELLANEOUS ANTIBACTERIALS											
Chloramphenicol	1 gm iv			X	High	11-18	25-50	4.1		45-89	Yes
Colistin	150 mg iv					5-7.5		2-3			No
Dalbavancin	1 gm, then 0.5 gm IV on day 8					240	93	168	0		
Daptomycin	4-6 mg per kg IV					58-99	92	8-9			No (26%)
Doxycycline	100 mg po			X		1.5-2.1	93	18	200-3200		
Fosfomycin	3 gm po		X			26	<10	5.7			
Linezolid	600 mg po/IV			X	100	15-20	31	5		60-70	
Metronidazole	500 mg po/IV			X		20-25	20	6-14	100	45-89	
Minocycline	200 mg po			X		2.0-3.5	76	16	200-3200		
Polymyxin B	20,000 units per kg IV					1-8		4.3-6			No
Quinu-Dalfo	7.5 mg per kg IV					5		1.5			
Rifaximin	600 mg po		X			4-32	80	2-5	10,000		
Rifaximin	200 mg po			X	<0.4	0.004-0.01		7-12			
Sulfamethoxazole (SMX)	2 gm po			X	70-90	50-120		8-15			
Trimethoprim (TMP)	100 mg po				80	1					
TMP-SMX-DS	160/800 mg po / 160/800 mg IV		X		85	1-2/40-60 / 9/105			100-200 / 40-70	50/40	Most meningococci resistant. Static vs coliforms
Tetracycline	250 mg po		X			1.5-2.2	71-89	6-12	200-3200		No (7%)
Tigecycline	50 mg IV q12h					0.63		42	138		
Vancomycin	1 gm IV q12h					20-50	<10-55	4-6	50	7-14	Need high doses. See Meningitis, Table 1, page 6
ANTIFUNGALS											
Amphotericin B											
Standard	0.4-0.7 mg per kg IV					0.5-3.5		24		0	
Ampho B lipid complex (ABLC)	5 mg per kg IV					1-2.5		24			
Ampho B cholesteryl complex	4 mg per kg IV					2.9		39			
Liposomal ampho B	5 mg per kg IV					58 ± 21		7-10/100			

See page 63 for all footnotes; see page 2 for abbreviations

TABLE 9A (4)

DRUG	DOSE, ROUTE OF ADMINISTRATION	WITH FOOD	WITHOUT FOOD[5]	WITH OR WITHOUT FOOD	% AB[1]	SERUM LEVEL mcg per mL	PROTEIN BINDING, %	SERUM T½, HOURS[4]	BILIARY EXCRETION, %	CSF[2]/BLOOD, %	CSF LEVEL POTENTIALLY THERAPEUTIC[3]
ANTIFUNGALS (continued)											
Azoles											
Fluconazole	400 mg po/IV			X	90	6.7		20-50		50-94	Yes
Itraconazole	800 mg po/IV			X	90	Approx. 14	99.8	20-50			
	Oral soln 200 mg po		X		Low			35		0	
Voriconazole	200 mg po		X		96	3	58	6		22-100	Yes (CID 37:728, 2003)
Caspofungin	70 mg IV x1, then 50 mg IV qd					9.9	97	9-11			
Flucytosine	2.5 gm po			X	78-90	30-40		3-6		60-100	Yes
Micafungin	150 mg IV					5-16	>99	15-17			
ANTIMYCOBACTERIALS											
Ethambutol	25 mg per kg po	X			80	2-6	10-30	4		25-50	No
Isoniazid	300 mg po		X		100	3-5	5-10	0.7-4		90	Yes
Pyrazinamide	20-25 mg per kg po			X	95	30-50		10-16		100	Yes
Rifampin	600 mg po		X		70-90	4-32	80	1.5-5	10,000	7-56	Yes
Streptomycin	1 gm IV (see Table 10D, page 74)					25-50	0-10	2.5	10-60	0-30	No. Intrathecal 5-10 mg
ANTIPARASITICS											
Albendazole	400 mg po	X				0.5-1.6	70				
Atovaquone suspension:	750 mg po	X			47	15	99.9	67		<1	No
Dapsone	100 mg po				100	1.1		10-50			
Ivermectin	12 mg po		X			0.05-0.08					
Mefloquine	1.25 gm po	X			"High"	0.5-1.2	98	13-24 **days**			
Nitazoxanide	200 mg po	X				3	99				
Proguanil[11]							75				
Pyrimethamine	25 mg po	X				0.1-0.3	87	96			
Praziquantel	20 mg per kg po	X			80	0.2-2.0		0.8-1.5			
Tinidazole	2 gm po	X			48		12	13	Chemically similar to metronidazole		
ANTIVIRAL DRUGS—NOT HIV											
Acyclovir	400 mg po			X	10-20	1.21	9-33	2.5-3.5			
Adefovir	10 mg po			X	59	0.02	≤4	7.5			
Entecavir	0.5 mg po		X		100	4.2 mg per mL	13	128-149			No
Famciclovir	500 mg po			X	77	3-4	<20	2-3			
Foscarnet	60 mg per kg IV					155		4			
Ganciclovir	5 mg per kg IV	X			75	8.3	1-2	3.5		<1	
Oseltamivir	75 mg po			X		0.650,5.5[12]	3	1-3			
Ribavirin	600 mg po	X			64	0.8		44			
Rimantadine	100 mg po			X		0.1-0.4	44	25			
Valacyclovir	1000 mg po			X	55	5.6	13-18	3			

See page 63 for all footnotes; see page 2 for abbreviations

TABLE 9A (5)

DRUG	DOSE, ROUTE OF ADMINISTRATION	FOR PO DOSING—Take Drug WITH FOOD⁵	WITHOUT FOOD⁵	WITH OR WITHOUT FOOD	% AB¹	PEAK SERUM LEVEL mcg per mL⁶	PROTEIN BINDING, %	INTRACELLULAR T½ HOURS²	SERUM T½ HOURS²	CYTOCHROME P450
ANTIVIRAL DRUGS—NOT HIV (continued)										
Valganciclovir	900 mg po	X			59	5.6	1-2	4	1.5	
ANTI-HIV DRUGS										
Abacavir	600 mg po			X	83	3.0	50	20.6	1.5	
Amprenavir	1200 mg po			X	No data	6-9	90		7-11	Inhibitor
Atazanavir	400 mg po	X			"Good"	2.3	86		7	Inhibitor
Delavirdine	400 mg po			X	85	19 ± 11	98		5.8	Inhibitor
Didanosine	400 mg EC¹³ po		X		30-40	?	<5	25-40	1.4	
Efavirenz	600 mg po			X	42	13 mcM	99		52-76	Inducer/inhibitor
Emtricitabine	200 mg po			X	93	1.8	<4	39	10	
Enfuvirtide	90 mg sc				84	5	92		4	
Fosamprenavir	1400 mg po			X	65	6	90		7.7	Inducer/inhibitor
Indinavir	800 mg po		X		No data	12.6 mcM	60		1.2-2	Inhibitor
Lamivudine	300 mg po			X	86	2.6	<36	18	5-7	
Lopinavir	400 mg po			X	No data	9.6	98-99		5-6	Inhibitor
Nelfinavir	1250 mg po	X			20-80	3-4	98		3.5-5	Inhibitor
Nevirapine	200 mg po			X	>90	2	60		25-30	Inducer
Ritonavir	300 mg po	X			65	7.8	98-99		3-5	Potent inhibitor
Saquinavir	1000 mg po (with 100 mg ritonavir)	X			4	3.1	97		1-2	Inhibitor
Stavudine	100 mg XR¹⁴ po			X	86	1.4	<5	3.5	1	
Tenofovir	300 mg po			X	39	0.12	<1-7	10->60	17	
Tipranavir	500 mg + 200 mg ritonavir	X				78-95 mcM	99.9		5.5-6	
Zalcitabine	0.75 mg po			X	85	0.03	<4	3	1.2	
Zidovudine	300 mg po			X	60	1-2	<38	11	0.5-3	

FOOTNOTES:
1. % absorbed under optimal conditions
2. Assumes CrCl >30 mL per min.
3. Peak concentration in blood/peak concentration in serum x 100.
4. If blank, no data.
5. CSF levels with inflammation
6. Judgment based on drug dose & organ susceptibility. CSF

6. concentration ideally ≥10 above MIC
7. Total drug; adjust for protein binding to determine free drug concentration.
8. For adult oral preps; not applicable for peds suspensions.
9. Food decreases rate and/or extent of absorption
10. Concern over seizure potential; see table 10

10. Take all po FQs 2-4 hours before sucralfate or any multivalent cations: Ca^{++}, Fe^{++}, Zn^{++}
11. Given with atovaquone as Malarone for malaria prophylaxis.
12. Oseltamivir/oseltamivir carboxylate
13. EC = enteric coated
14. XR = extended release

TABLE 9B: PHARMACODYNAMICS OF ANTIBACTERIALS*

BACTERIAL KILLING/PERSISTENT EFFECT	DRUGS	THERAPY GOAL	PK/PD MEASUREMENT
Concentration-dependent/Prolonged persistent effect	Aminoglycosides; daptomycin; ketolides; quinolones	High peak serum concentration	24-hr AUC/MIC
Time-dependent/No persistent effect	Penicillins; cephalosporins; carbapenems	Long duration of exposure	Time above MIC
Time-dependent/Moderate to long persistent effect	Clindamycin; erythro/azithro/clarithro; linezolid; tetracyclines; vancomycin	Enhanced amount of drug	24-hr AUC/MIC

* Adapted from Craig, WA. IDC No. Amer 17:479, 2003   ¹ AUC = area under drug concentration curve

See page 2 for abbreviations

TABLE 10A
SELECTED ANTIBACTERIAL AGENTS—ADVERSE REACTIONS—OVERVIEW

Adverse reactions in individual patients represent all-or-none occurrences, even if rare. After selection of an agent, the physician should read the manufacturer's package insert [statements in the product labeling (package insert) must be approved by the FDA].

Numbers = frequency of occurrence (%); + = occurs, incidence not available; ++ = significant adverse reaction; 0 = not reported; R = rare, defined as <1%. NOTE: Important reactions in bold print. A blank means no data found.

ADVERSE REACTIONS	Penicillin G,V	Dicloxacillin	Nafcillin	Oxacillin	Amoxicillin	Amox-Clav	Ampicillin	Amp-Sulb	Piperacillin	Pip-Taz	Ticarcillin	Ticar-Clav	Ertapenem	Imipenem	Meropenem	Aztreonam	Aminoglycosides (Amikacin, Gentamicin, Kanamycin, Netilmicin[NUS], Tobramycin)	Linezolid	Telithromycin
Rx stopped due to AE					2–4.4				3.2	3.2					1.2	<1			
Local, phlebitis	+		++	+				3	4	1		3	4	3	1	4			
Hypersensitivity														3	3				
Fever	+	+	+	+	+	+	+	+	+	2	+	+	+	+		2	+		
Rash	3	4	4	4	5	3	5	2	1	4	3	2	+	+	+	2			
Photosensitivity	0	0	0	0	0	0	0	0	0	0	0	0	0	0	0	+			
Anaphylaxis	R	0	R	R	0	R	R	0	0	+	+	+		+		+			
Serum sickness	4									+	+	+		+		+			
Hematologic																			
+ Coombs	3	0	R	R	+	0	+	0	+	+	0	+		2	+	R			
Neutropenia	R	0	+	R	+	+	+	+	6	+	0	+		+		+		1.1	
Eosinophilia	+	+	22	22	2	+	22	22	+	+	+	+	1	+		8			
Thrombocytopenia	R	0	R	R	R	R	R	R	+	+	R	R		+	+	+		3–10 (see 10C)	
↑ PT/PTT	R	0	+	0	+	0	+	0	+	+	+	+		R		R			
GI																			
Nausea/vomiting		+	0	0	2	3	2	+	+	7	+	1	3	2	4	R		3/1	7/2
Diarrhea		+	0	0	5	9	10	2	+	11	3	1	6	2	5	R		4	10
C. difficile colitis	R	0	R	R	+	R	+	R	+	+	+	+	+	+	+	+		+	+
Hepatic, LFTs	R	R	0	+	R	+	R	6	+	+	0	+	6	4	4	2			1.3
Hepatic failure	0	0	0	0	0	0	0	0	0	0	0	0		0					
Renal: ↑ BUN, Cr	R	0	0	0	R	0	R	R	+	+	0	0	+	0	0	+	5–25[1]		
CNS																			
Headache	R	0	R	R	0	+	R	R	R	8	R	R	2	+	3	+		2	2
Confusion	R	0	R	R	0	0	R	R	R	R	R	R		+		+			
Seizures	R	0	0		+	0	R	0	0	R	R	+	See footnote[2]			+			
Special Senses																			
Ototoxicity	0	0	0	0	0	0	0	0	0	0	0	0	0		R	0	3–14[1]		
Vestibular	0	0	0	0	0	0	0	0	0	0	0	0	0		0	0	4–6[1]		
Cardiac																			
Dysrhythmias	R	0			0		0	0	0		0			0		+			
Miscellaneous, Unique (Table 10C)	+	+	+	+	+	+	+	+		+		+		+	+				+
Drug/drug interactions, common (Table 22)	0	0	0	0	0	0	0	0	0	0	0	0		0			+	+	+

[1] Varies with criteria used

[2] **All β-lactams in high concentration can cause seizures** (JAC 45:5, 2000). In rabbit, IMP 10 times more neurotoxic than benzylpenicillin (JAC 22:687, 1988). In clinical trial of IMP for pediatric meningitis, trial stopped due to seizures in 7/25 IMP recipients; hard to interpret as purulent meningitis causes seizures (PIDJ 10:122, 1991). Risk with IMP less with careful attention to dosage (Epilepsia 42:1590, 2001).
Postulated mechanism: Drug binding to GABAA receptor. IMP binds with greater affinity than MER.
Package insert, percent seizures: ERTA 0.5, IMP 0.4, MER 0.7. However, in 3 clinical trials of MER for bacterial meningitis, no drug-related seizures (Scand J Inf Dis 31:3, 1999; Drug Safety 22:191, 2000). In febrile neutropenic cancer pts, IMP-related seizures reported at 2% (CID 32:381, 2001; Peds Hem Onc 17:585, 2000).

TABLE 10A (2)

CEPHALOSPORINS/CEPHAMYCINS

ADVERSE REACTIONS	Cefazolin	Cefotetan	Cefoxitin	Cefuroxime	Cefotaxime	Ceftazidime	Ceftizoxime	Ceftriaxone	Cefepime	Cefpirome^AUS	Cefaclor/Cef.ER/Loracarb	Cefadroxil	Cefdinir	Cefixime	Cefpodoxime	Cefprozil	Ceftibuten	Cefditoren pivoxil	Cefuroxime axetil	Cephalexin
Rx stopped due to AE									1.5				3	2.7	2	2	2	2.2		
Local, phlebitis	+	R	R	2	5	1	4	2	1											
Hypersensitivity	5	1				2			+		2									
Fever	+	+	+				R		R					R	+			R	R	
Rash	+		2	R	2	2	2	2	2	1	1	+	R	1	1	1	R	R	R	1
Photosensitivity	0	0	0	0	0	R	0	0												
Anaphylaxis	R	+				R					R			R						R
Serum sickness									≤0.5[2]	+										+
Hematologic																				
+ Coombs	3	+	2	R	6	4			14	3	R								R	R	+
Neutropenia	+		2	R	+	1	+	2	1		+	+	R	R	R	R			R	3
Eosinophilia			+	3	7	1	8	4	6	1			R	R	3	2	5	R	1	9
Thrombocytopenia	+					+	+		+		2		R	R	+	R				
↑ PT/PTT		++	+		+	+	+	+	+											
GI			2								3		3	13				6		2
Nausea/vomiting		1		R	R	R		R	1	+	2			7	4	4	2	6/1	3	
Diarrhea			4		R	1	1		3	1	+	1-4		15	16	7	3	3	1.4	4
C. difficile colitis	+	+	+	+	+	+	+	+	+	+	+	+	+	+	+	+	+	+	+	+
Hepatic, ↑ LFTs	+	1	3	4	1	6	4	3	+	+	3	+	1	R	4	2	R	R	2	+
Hepatic failure	0	0	0	0	0	0	0	0	0	0										
Renal: ↑ BUN, Cr	+		3			R		1	+		+		R		4	R	R	R		+
CNS																				
Headache	0				1			R	2		3		2		1	R	R	2	R	+
Confusion	0								+		+				R					
Seizures	0																			
Special Senses																				
Ototoxicity	0	0	0		0	0	0	0			0	0	0	0	0	0	0		0	0
Vestibular	0	0	0		0	0	0	0			0	0	0	0	0	0	0		0	0
Cardiac																				
Dysrhythmias	0	0	0	0	0	0	0	0			0	0	0	0	0	0	0		0	0
Miscellaneous, Unique (Table 10C)								+			+[2]							+		
Drug/drug interactions, common (Table 22)	0	0	0	0	0	0	0	0			0	0			0	0	0	0	0	0

[1] Cefaclor extended release tablets

[2] Serum sickness requires biotransformation of parent drug plus inherited defect in metabolism of reactive intermediates *(Ped Pharm & Therap 125:805, 1994)*

* See note at head of table, page 64

TABLE 10A (3)

ADVERSE REACTIONS (AE)	Azithromycin, Reg. & ER[2]	Clarithromycin, Reg. & ER[2]	Erythromycin	Ciprofloxacin/Cipro XR	Gatifloxacin	Gemifloxacin	Levofloxacin	Moxifloxacin	Ofloxacin	Chloramphenicol	Clindamycin	Colistimethate (Colistin)	Daptomycin	Metronidazole	Quinupristin-dalfopristin	Rifampin	Tetracycline/Doxy/Mino	Tigecycline	TMP-SMX	Vancomycin
Rx stopped due to AE	1	3		3.5	2.9	2.2	4	3.8	4				2.8					5		
Local, phlebitis					5						+	6	++			+	2		++	8
Hypersensitivity																	1	R	++	8
Fever				R	R		R			+	+	+	2			+	+	7	+	1
Rash	R		+	3	R	1-22[4]	1.7	R	2	+	+	+	4	+	R		+	2.4	+	3
Photosensitivity	R			R	R	R	R	R	R				4				+	+		0
Anaphylaxis			+	R			R		R											
Serum sickness											+									
Hematologic																				
Neutropenia	R	1		R	R				1	+	+		+		+		+			2
Eosinophilia				R					1	+	+						+		+	+
Thrombocytopenia	R	R		R						+	+				R		+		+	+
↑ PT/PTT		1																4		0
GI																				
Nausea/vomiting	3	3[9]	25	5	8/<3	2.7	7/2	7/2	7			+	6.3	**12**		+	30/20	+	+	
Diarrhea	5	3-6	8	2	4	3.6	1.2	6	4	+	**7**		5			+	13	3		
C. difficile colitis	+	+	+	**R**	**R**	**R**	**R**		**R**	+	++		+			R	+			+
Hepatic, LFTs	R	R	+	2	R		1.5	+	2		+			2	+	+	4			0
Hepatic failure	0	0												+	+					0
Renal																				
↑ BUN, Cr	+	4		1					R	0		R				+	+	2		5
CNS																				
Dizziness, lightheadedness				R	3	0.8	**2.5**	3	3									3.5		
Headache	R	2		1	4	1.2	5.4	2		+	+			5			+		+	
Confusion	+		+	+				+	R	+				+		+			+	
Seizures			+	+			+		R					+						
Special senses																				
Ototoxicity	+		+	0					0											R
Vestibular																	21[5]			
Cardiac																				
Dysrhythmias			+	R	+[1]	+[1]	+[1]	+[1]	+[1]		R									0
Miscellaneous, Unique (Table 10C)	+		+	+	+	+	+	+	+	+	+	+	+	+	+	+	+	+	+	+
Drug/drug interactions, common (Table 22)	+	+	+	+	+	+	+	+	+					+		++	+		+	+

[1] Fluoroquinolones as class assoc. **with QT$_c$ prolongation.** Ref.: *CID* 34:861, 2002.
[2] Regular and extended-release formulations
[3] Less GI upset/abnormal taste with ER formulation
[4] **Highest frequency:** females <40 years of age after 14 days of rx
[5] Minocycline has 21% vestibular toxicity

TABLE 10B: ANTIMICROBIAL AGENTS ASSOCIATED WITH PHOTOSENSITIVITY

The following drugs are known to cause photosensitivity in some individuals. There is no intent to indicate relative frequency or severity of reactions.
Source: 2005 Drug Topics Red Book, Medical Economics, Montvale, NJ. Listed in alphabetical order:
Amantadine, azithromycin, benznidazole, ciprofloxacin, clofazimine, dapsone, doxycycline, erythromycin ethyl succinate, flucytosine, ganciclovir, griseofulvin, interferons, levofloxacin, lomefloxacin, ofloxacin, pefloxacin, pyrazinamide, saquinavir, sulfonamides, tetracyclines, tigecycline, tretinoins, trimethoprim, voriconazole

* See note at head of table, page 64

TABLE 10C: SUMMARY OF CURRENT ANTIBIOTIC DOSAGE,* SIDE-EFFECTS, AND COST†

CLASS, AGENT, GENERIC NAME (TRADE NAME)	USUAL ADULT DOSAGE* (Cost§)	ADVERSE REACTIONS, COMMENTS (See Table 10A for Summary)
		Most common adverse reaction is hypersensitivity. Anaphylaxis in up to 0.05%, 5–10% total. Commercially available skin test antigen (penicillin/ polylysine) does not predict anaphylactic reactions. Hematologic, renal, CNS (seizures) reactions usually seen with high dose (>20 million units per day) and renal failure. With procaine pen G and benzathine pen G, an immediate but transient (5–30 min. after injection) toxic reaction with bizarre behavior and neurologic reactions can occur (Hoigné syndrome). Coombs test positive hemolytic anemias are rare but typically severe; in contrast, the Coombs test is often positive with cephalosporin therapy, but clinically significant hemolysis is rare. Penicillin allergy ref.: JAMA 278:1895, 1997
NATURAL PENICILLINS		
Benzathine penicillin G (Bicillin L-A)	600,000–1.2 million units IM q2–4 wks Cost: 1.2 million units $47	
Penicillin G	Low: 600,000–1.2 million units IM per day High: ≥20 million units IV q24h (=12 gm) Cost: 5 million units $42	
Penicillin V	0.25–0.5 gm po qid before meals & at bedtime Cost: 500 mg G $0.39	
PENICILLINASE-RESISTANT PENICILLINS		
Dicloxacillin (Dynapen)	0.125–0.5 gm po q6h ac. Cost: 500 mg G $0.20	Blood levels ~2 times greater than cloxacillin. Acute hemorrhagic cystitis reported. Acute abdominal pain with GI bleeding without antibiotic-associated colitis also reported.
Flucloxacillin^NUS (Floxapen, Lutropin, Staphcil)	0.25–0.5 gm po q6h	In Australia, cholestatic hepatitis (women predominate, age >65, rx ≥ mean 2 weeks, onset 3 weeks from starting rx) (Ln 339:679, 1992), 16 deaths since 1980, recommendation: use only in severe infection (Ln 344:676, 1994).
Nafcillin (Unipen, Nafcil)	1–2 gm IV q4h	Extravasation can result in tissue necrosis. With dosages of 200–300 mg per kg per day hypokalemia may occur
Oxacillin (Prostaphlin)	1–2 gm IV/IM q4h. Cost: 2 gm IV $20.11	Reversible neutropenia (over 10% with ≥21-day rx, occasionally WBC <1000 per mm³). Hepatic dysfunction with ≥12 gm per day, reversible 1 2–24 days after start of rx, more rash and liver toxicity with oxacillin as compared to nafcillin (CID 34:50, 2002).
	1–2 gm IV/IM q4h. Cost: 2 gm IV $20.11	
AMINOPENICILLINS		
Amoxicillin (Amoxil, Polymox)	250 mg·1 gm po tid. Cost: 500 mg G $0.13, NB $0.55	IV and Europe, UK amoxicillin rapidly converted to ampicillin. Rash with infectious mono—see Ampicillin.
Amoxicillin-clavulanate (Augmentin) AM-CL extra-strength peds suspension (ES-600) AM-CL ER extended release adult tabs	See Comment for adult products/cost Peds ES susp.: 600/42.9 per 5 mL. Dose: 90/6.4 mg per kg div bid. Cost: 75 mL $42.65. For adult formulations, see Comments	With bid regimen, less diarrhea. Clavulanic acid has reversible cholestatic hepatitis, esp. men >60 yrs, on rx >2 weeks (AIM 156:1327, 1996). 2 cases anaphylactic reaction to clavulanic acid (J All Clin Immun 95:748, 1995). **Comparison adult Augmentin product dosage regimens:**
			Cost for 10 days rx:
		Augmentin 500/125 1 tab po tid $114
		Augmentin 875/125 1 tab po bid $101
		Augmentin-XR 1000/62.5 2 tabs po bid $120
Ampicillin (Principen)	0.25–0.5 gm po q6h. Cost: 500 mg po G $0.30 150–200 mg per kg IV per day. Cost: 1 gm IV G $10.36	Rash with infectious mono, **not true penicillin allergy.** Rash occurs (not urticarial) in 65–100% pts with infectious mono, 90% with chronic lymphocytic leukemia, and 15–20% with allopurinol therapy.
Ampicillin-sulbactam (Unasyn)	1.5–3 gm IV q6h. Cost: 3 gm NB $14.15 (see Comment)	Supplied in vials: ampicillin 1 gm, sulbactam 0.5 gm or amp 2 gm, sulbactam 1 gm. Antibiotic is not active vs pseudomonas. Total daily dose subactam 4 gm.
ANTIPSEUDOMONAL PENICILLINS NOTE: Platelet dysfunction may occur with any of the antipseudomonal penicillins, esp. in renal failure patients.		
Piperacillin (Pipracil) (Canada only)	3–4 gm IV q4–6h (200–300 mg per kg per day up to 500 mg per kg per day). For urinary tract infection: 2	85 mEq Na⁺ per gm	
Piperacillin-tazobactam (Zosyn)	3.375 gm IV q6h or 4.5 gm IV q8h Cost: 3 gm NB $17.56 3.375 gm q6h reavailable 4.5 gm NB $21.81 For P. aeruginosa: 4.5 gm IV q6h + tobra	Supplied as: piperacillin 3 gm + tazobactam 0.375 gm. 1 2| similar to clavulanate, more active than subactam as β-lactamase inhibitor. Dose = pip-tazo given q6h-q8h as IV over pip or pip-tazo given q4h-q6h. If 4.5 gm q8h is **not adequate for serious pseudomonas infections,** for empiric treatment of P. aeruginosa, **4.5 gm q6h + tobramycin.** Rx longer than 10 d. may ↑ risk of neutropenia (CID 37:1508, 2003). Piperacillin can cause false-pos. test for galactomannan—a test for invasive aspergillosis.
Ticarcillin disodium (Ticar)	3 gm IV q4–6h. Cost: 3.0 gm NB $12.38	Coagulation abnormalities common with large doses, interferes with platelet function, ↑ bleeding times; may be clinically significant in pts with renal failure. (4.5 mEq Na⁺ per gm)
Ticarcillin-clavulanate (Timentin)	3.1 gm IV q4–6h. Cost: 3.1 gm NB $15.37	Supplied in vials: ticarcillin 3 gm, clavulanate 0.1 gm per vial. 4.5–5 mEq Na⁺ per gm. Diarrhea due to clavulanate. Rare reversible cholestatic hepatitis secondary to clavulanate (AIM 156:1327, 1996).

(See Page 2 for abbreviations)

* NOTE: all dosage recommendations are for adults (unless otherwise indicated) & assume normal renal/renal function.   § Cost = average wholesale price from 2005 Drug Topics Red Book, Medical Economics

TABLE 10C (2)

CLASS, AGENT, GENERIC NAME (TRADE NAME)	USUAL ADULT DOSAGE* (Cost)	ADVERSE REACTIONS, COMMENTS (See Table 10A for Summary)
CARBAPENEMS. NOTE: In pts with pen allergy, 11% had allergic reaction after imipenem or meropenem (CID 38:1102, 2004); 9% in a 2nd study (JAC 54:1155, 2004).		
Ertapenem (Invanz)	1 gm IV/IM q24h. Cost: 1 gm NB $51.39	Lidocaine diluent for IM use; ask about lidocaine allergy.
Imipenem + cilastatin (Primaxin)	0.5 gm IV q6h: for P. aeruginosa: 1 gm q6-8h (see Comment). Cost: 500 mg NB $32.64	For moderate or severe infection due to P. aeruginosa, dosage can be increased to 3 or 4 gm per day div. q6h or q8h, more efficacious & safer (J Clin Pharm 43:1116, 2003; AAC 49:1881, 2005). For seizure comment, see footnote 2, Table 10A, page 64.
Meropenem (Merrem)	0.5–1 gm IV q8h. Up to 2 gm IV q8h for meningitis. Cost: 1 gm NB $60	For seizure incidence comment, see Table 10A, page 64. Comments: Does not require a dehydropeptidase inhibitor (cilastatin). Activity vs aerobic gm-neg, slightly ↑ over IMP, activity vs staph & strep slightly ↓, anaerobes = to IMP. B. ovatus, B. distasonis more resistant to meropenem.
MONOBACTAMS		
Aztreonam (Azactam)	1 gm q8h–2 gm IV q6h. Cost: 1 gm NB $23.90	Can be used in pts with allergy to penicillins/cephalosporins. Animal data and a letter raise concern about cross-reactivity with ceftazidime (Rev Inf Dis 7:613, 1985); side-chains of aztreonam and ceftazidime are identical.
CEPHALOSPORINS (1st parenteral, then oral drugs).	**NOTE:** Prospective data demonstrate correlation between use of cephalosporins (esp. 3rd generation) and ↑ risk of C. difficile toxin-induced diarrhea. May also ↑ risk of colonization with vancomycin-resistant enterococci. For cross-allergenicity, see Oral, next page.	
1st Generation, Parenteral		
Cefazolin (Ancef, Kefzol)	0.25 gm q8h–1.5 gm IV/IM q6h. Cost: 1 gm G $1.20, NB $5.59	Do not give into lateral ventricles—seizures!
2nd Generation, Parenteral		
Cefotetan (Cefotan)	1–3 gm IV/IM q12h. (Max. dose not > 6 gm q24h). Cost: 1 gm NB $14	Increasing resistance of B. fragilis, Prevotella bivivus, Prevotella disiens (most common in pelvic infections). Ref.: CID 35(Suppl 1):S126, 2002. Methylthiotetrazole (MTT) side chain can inhibit vitamin K activation.
Cefoxitin (Mefoxin)	1 gm q6h–2 gm IV/IM q4h. Cost: 1 gm G $1.23, NB $15.29	In vitro may induce ↑ β-lactamase, esp. in Enterobacter sp.
Cefuroxime (Kefurox, Ceftin, Zinacef)	0.75–1.5 gm IV/IM q8h. Cost: 1.5 gm IV G $13.46	More stable vs staphylococcal β-lactamase than cefazolin.
3rd Generation, Parenteral	Use of P Ceph 3 drugs correlates with incidence of C. difficile toxin diarrhea, perhaps due to cephalosporin resistance of C. difficile (CID 38:646, 2004).	
Cefoperazone-sulbactam°°° (Sulperazon)	Usual dose 1–2 gm IV q12h; should use 2–3 gm IV q6h	Investigational in U.S. In SE Asia & elsewhere, used to treat intra-abdominal, biliary, & gyn. infections. Other uses due to broad spectrum of activity. Possible clotting problem due to side-chain. For dose logic: JAC 15:136, 1985.
Cefotaxime (Claforan)	1 gm q8-12h to 2 gm IV q4h. Cost: 2 gm G $22, NB $26.98	Maximum daily dose: 12 gm.
Ceftazidime (Fortaz, Tazicef, Tazidime)	1–2 gm IV/IM q8-12h. Cost: 2 gm NB $23.93–47.73	Excessive use may result in ↑ incidence of C. difficile-assoc. diarrhea and/or selection of vancomycin-resistant E. faecium. Ceftaz is susceptible to extended-spectrum cephalosporinases (CID 27:76 & 81, 1998).
Ceftizoxime (Cefizox)	1 gm q8–12h to 4 gm IV q8h. Cost: 2 gm NB $16.59	$24.64 Maximum daily dose: 12 gm.
Ceftriaxone (Rocephin)	Commonly used IV dosage in adults: < Age 65: 2 gm once daily > Age 65: 1 gm once daily; Purulent meningitis: 2 gm IV q12h. Can give IM in 1% lidocaine. Cost: 1 gm NB $51.16	Dosage: 2 gm IV q24h gives better tissue levels than 1 gm q12h (overcomes protein binding) (see footnote). "Pseudocholelithiasis" 2° to sludge in gallbladder by ultrasound (50%), symptomatic (9%) (NEJM 322:1821, 1990). More likely with 2 gm per day & pt on total parenteral nutrition and not eating (AnIM 115:712, 1991). Clinical significance still unclear but has led to cholecystectomy (JID 177:356, 1995) and gallstone pancreatitis (Ln 177:662, 1998).
4th Generation, Parenteral		
Cefepime (Maxipime)	1–2 gm IV q12h. Cost: 2 gm NB $36.59	Active vs P. aeruginosa and many strains of Enterobacter, serratia, C. freundii resistant to ceftazidime, cefotaxime, aztreonam (CID 20:56, 1995). More active vs S. aureus than 3rd generation cephalosporins.
Cefpirome°°° (HR 810)	1–2 gm IV q12h	Similar to cefepime; ↑ activity vs enterobacteriaceae, P. aeruginosa, Gm + organisms. Anaerobes: less active than cefotixin, more active than cefotax. or ceftaz.

* The age-related dosing of ceftriaxone is based on unpublished pharmacokinetic data that show an age-related reduction in hepatic clearance of ceftriaxone; hence, there is possible underdosing in younger pts, therefore the suggested 2 gm per day dose.
(See page 2 for abbreviations)
° NOTE: all dosage recommendations are for adults (unless otherwise indicated) & assume normal renal function. § Cost = average wholesale price from 2005 Drug Topics Red Book, Medical Economics Data.

TABLE 10C (3)

CLASS, AGENT, GENERIC NAME (TRADE NAME)	USUAL ADULT DOSAGE* (Cost†)	ADVERSE REACTIONS, COMMENTS (See Table 10A for Summary)
CEPHALOSPORINS (continued)		The oral cephalosporins are generally safe. **Patients with a history of IgE-mediated allergic reactions to a penicillin (e.g., anaphylaxis, angioedema, urticaria) should not receive a cephalosporin.** If the history is a "measles-like" rash to a penicillin, available data suggest a 5–10% risk of rash in such patients; there is no enhanced risk of anaphylaxis. Cephalosporin skin tests, if available, predictive of reaction (AnIM 141:16, 2004).
Oral Cephalosporins		
1st Generation, Oral		
Cefadroxil (Duricef)	0.5–1 gm po q12h. Cost: 0.5 gm G $2.48, NB $8.68	
Cephalexin (Keflex, Keftab, generic)	0.25–0.5 gm po q6h. Cost: 0.5 gm G $0.44, NB $23–4.85	Any of the cephalosporins can result in **C. difficile** toxin-mediated diarrhea/enterocolitis.
2nd Generation, Oral		The reported frequency of nausea/vomiting and non-C. difficile toxin diarrhea is summarized in Table 10A.
Cefaclor (Ceclor)	0.25–0.5 gm po q8h. Cost: 0.25 gm G $0.66, NB $2.40	**Cefaclor:** Serum sickness-like reaction 0.1–0.5%—arthralgia, rash, erythema multiforme but no adenopathy, proteinuria or demonstrable immune complexes. Anecdotal reports of similar reaction to loracarbef. Appear due to mixture of drug biotransformation and genetic susceptibility (Ped Pharm & Therap 125:805, 1994).
Cefaclor-ER (Ceclor CD)	0.375–0.5 gm po q12h. Cost: 0.5 gm $3.50	
Cefprozil (Cefzil)	0.25–0.5 gm po q12h. Cost: 0.5 gm NB $9.10	**Cefdinir:** Drug-iron complex causes red stools in roughly 1% of pts.
Cefuroxime axetil po (Ceftin)	0.125–0.5 gm po q12h. Cost: 0.5 gm NB $10.95	**Cefditoren pivoxil:** Hydrolysis yields pivalate. Pivalate absorbed (70%) & becomes pivaloylcarnitine which is renally excreted. In 4-wk study, **serum carnitine concentrations** decreased (up to 63%). In serum carnitine involved in fatty acid (FA) metabolism & FA transport into mitochondria. Effect transient & reversible. No clinical events documented to date (Med Lett 44:5, 2002). Also contains caseinate (milk protein): **avoid if milk allergy** (not same as lactose intolerance). Need gastric acid for optimal absorption.
3rd Generation, Oral		
Loracarbef (Lorabid)	0.4 gm po q12h. Cost: 0.4 gm NB $6.37	
Cefdinir (Omnicef)	300 mg po q12h or 600 mg q24h. Cost: 300 mg $4.75	**Cefpodoxime:** There are rare reports of acute liver injury, bloody diarrhea, pulmonary infiltrates with eosinophilia.
Cefditoren pivoxil (Spectracef)	200–400 mg po bid. Cost: 200 mg $2.08	**Cefixime:** Now available from Lupin Pharmaceuticals.
Cefixime (Suprax)		**Cephalexin:** Can cause false-neg. urine dipstick test for leukocytes.
Cefpodoxime proxetil (Vantin)	0.4 gm po q12–24h. Cost: 0.4 gm NB $10.26	
	0.1–0.2 gm po q12h. Cost: 0.2 gm G $4.44, NB $96.22	
Ceftibuten (Cedax)	0.4 gm po q24h. Cost: 0.4 gm NB $9.10	

AMINOGLYCOSIDES AND RELATED ANTIBIOTICS—See Table 10D, page 74, and Table 17, page 134

CLASS, AGENT, GENERIC NAME (TRADE NAME)	USUAL ADULT DOSAGE* (Cost†)	ADVERSE REACTIONS, COMMENTS (See Table 10A for Summary)
GLYCOPEPTIDES		
Dalbavancin (Trade name pending)	1 gm IV, then 0.5 gm IV on day 8. No cost data	Semi-synthetic lipoglycopeptide with very long serum half-life. As of 8/05, FDA approval pending. So far, 2 published clinical trials (CID 40:374, 2005 & 37:1298, 2003). No serious AEs. Drug fever described in 18% of a small patient sample.
Teicoplanin™¹ (Targocid)	For septic arthritis—maintenance dose 12 mg per kg per day.S. aureus endocarditis—trough serum levels >20 mcg per mL required.	S₁: Hypersensitivity: fever (al 3 mg per kg 2.2%, at 24 mg per kg 8.2%), skin reactions 2.4% (high dose 2t5 mg per kg per day). Red neck syndrome less common than with vancomycin.
	Use 12 mg per kg q12h 3 loading doses, then 12 mg per kg q24h)	
Vancomycin (Vancocin)	15 mg per kg IV q12h: 125 mg po q48–72h. Cost: 1 gm IV G $6, NB $20.35. Oral "Pulvule" 125 mg Cost $9.15	**Measure serum levels** if: planned dose ≥2 gm per day, rapidly changing renal function, chronic renal failure, or on hemodialysis Target levels: peak 20–50 mcg per mL, trough 5–10 mcg per mL.
	For other uses, see Comment.	Rapid infusion can cause non-specific histamine release manifest as angioneurotic edema, flushed skin ("red neck syndrome") or hypotension. Can continue vanco but infuse over 1–2 hrs.
	One report of safety & efficacy of once-daily vanco, 30 mg per kg (JAC 49:155, 2002).	**Ototoxicity and nephrotoxicity now** rare unless vanco given with an aminoglycoside; aminoglycoside amplifies the risk of nephrotoxicity. Neutropenia with linear dose/duration of dermatotoxin (CID 38:442, 2004).
		Intrathecal vanco too used for meningitis and/or shunt infections. **Initial** dosing ranges from 5–10 mg per day (infants) to 10–20 mg per mL; (children/adults) adjusted to achieve trough CSF conc. of 10–20 mcg per mL (AnPharmacotherapy 27:912, 1993).
		Critically ill pts: Safe & reasonable to give loading dose of 25 mg per kg at 500 mg per hr (JAC 47:246, 2001).

TABLE 10C (4)

CLASS, AGENT, GENERIC NAME (TRADE NAME)	USUAL ADULT DOSAGE* (Cost§)		ADVERSE REACTIONS, COMMENTS (See Table 10A for Summary)
CHLORAMPHENICOL, CLINDAMYCIN(S), ERYTHROMYCIN GROUP, KETOLIDES, OXAZOLIDINONES, QUINUPRISTIN-DALFOPRISTIN (SYNERCID)			
Chloramphenicol (Chloromycetin)	**0.25–1 gm po/IV q6h to max. of 4 gm per day.** Cost: IV $22.75; po $6.60		No oral drug distributed in U.S. Hematologic (↓ RBC −1/3 pts, aplastic anemia 1:21,600 courses). Gray baby syndrome in premature infants, anaphylactoid reactions, optic atrophy or neuropathy (very rare), digital paresthesias, minor disulfiram-like reactions.
Clindamycin (Cleocin)	**0.15–0.45 gm po q6h, 600–900 mg IV/IM q8h** Cost: IV $3.00, IM $8.55 po $8.57 G $3.3, 600 mg IV/IM NB $29.14, $4.31	Lincomycin (Lincocin) 0.6 gm IV/IM q8h Cost: 600 mg IV/IM $10.51	Based on number of exposed pts, these drugs are the most frequent cause of **C. difficile toxin-mediated diarrhea.** In most severe form can cause pseudomembranous colitis/toxic megacolon.
Erythromycin Group (Review drug interactions before use) Azithromycin (Zithromax) Azithromycin ER (ZMax)	IV preps: Tabs 250 & 600 mg. Peds suspension: 100 & 200 mg per 5 mL. Adult ER suspension: 2 gm. Dose varies with indication, e.g., see Table 1. Acute otitis media (page 9), acute exac. chronic bronchitis (page 28), Commun.-acq. pneumonia (pages 23–30), sinusitis (page 36). Cost: 250 mg G $7.53, NB $8.30. IV: 0.5 gm per day. Cost: $32.		**Motilin** is gastric hormone that activates duodenal/jejunal receptors to initiate peristalsis. Erythro (E) and E esters, both po and IV, activate motilin receptors and cause uncoordinated peristalsis with resultant 20–25% incidence of anorexia, nausea or vomiting (Gut 33:397, 1992). Less binding and GI distress with azithromycin/clarithromycin. Systemic erythro in 1st 2 wks of life associated with **infantile hypertrophic pyloric stenosis** (J Ped 139:380, 2001).
Base and esters (Erythro, Ilosone) IV name: E. lactobionate	**0.25 gm q6h–0.5 gm po/IV q6h: 15–20 mg per kg up to 4 gm q24h. Infuse over 30 or more minutes.** Cost: NB $7.50, stearate $0.18, estolate $0.31, ESS $0.23. IV 1 gm NB $7.73		**Frequent GI distress** (see Table 22, page 148. Major concern is prolonged QTc interval on EKG. **Prolonged QTc:** Mutations in 9 genes (LQT 1–6) produce abnormal cardiac K+/Na+ channels. Variable penetrance: no symptoms, reported syncope, to sudden death. Females (♀) > (♂). **Risk amplified by drugs** [macrolides, antiarrhythmics, & drug-drug interactions (see Table, pages 77–72 for list)]. Can result in torsades de pointes (ventricular tachycardia) and/or cardiac arrest. Refs.: NEJM 348:1837 & 1866, 2003; 351:1053 & 1089, 2004. www.qtdrugs.org.
Clarithromycin (Biaxin) or clarithro extended release (Biaxin XL)	**0.5 gm po q12h.** Cost: 500 mg $55. **Extended release: Two 0.5 gm tabs po per day.** Cost: 500 mg ER $4.93		Cholestatic hepatitis in approx. 1:1000 adults (not children) given E estolate.
Dirithromycin (Dynabac)	**0.5 gm po q24h.** Cost 250 mg po $4.25		**Transient reversible tinnitus or deafness** with high doses of erythro IV in pts with renal or hepatic impairment. Reported with ≥500 mg per day of azithro (Ann Pharmacother 28:76, 1994). Dosages of oral erythro preparations expressed as base equivalents. With differences in absorption/biotransformation, variable amounts of erythro required to achieve same free erythro serum level, e.g., 400 mg E ethyl succinate = 250 mg E base. Dirithromycin available as once-daily macrolide. **Very low serum levels; do not use if potential for bacteremic disease.**
Ketolides Telithromycin (Ketek) (Med Lett 46:66, 2004)	**PO dose: 800 mg po q24h.** Cost: 400 mg tabs. 300 mg tabs available		1° ketolide (similar to erythro). **Common:** diarrhea 10%, nausea 7%, vomiting 2.4%. **Uncommon: blurred vision 2°** slow accommodation, occurs in 1% (women 2%, men 0.8%) Am J Ophthal 139:114, 2004). Potential QTc prolongation. Several **drug-drug interactions** (Table 22, pages 150–151).
Linezolid (Zyvox)	**PO or IV dose: 600 mg q12h all indications except uncomplicated skin infections.** Available as 400 & 600 mg tabs, oral suspension (100 mg per 5 mL) & IV solution. 600 mg po $65, 600 mg IV $82.		**Reversible myelosuppression:** thrombocytopenia, anemia, & neutropenia reported. Not see if incidence of thrombocytopenia greater after 2 wks of rx: 7/20 osteomyelitis pts; 5/7 pts treated with vanco & lin. Refs.: CID 37:1609, 2003 & 38:1058 & 1065, 2004. **Other serious adverse effects:** Lactic acidosis (NV, low HCO₃), toxic neuropathy (reported after prolonged rx, peripheral and/or optic neuropathy) (CID 42:1111–1117, 2006; AnIM 142:1153/114, 2005). **Inhibitor of monoamine oxidase** (risk of severe hypertension if taken with tyramine-rich foods rich in tyramine. Be careful with drugs containing pseudoephedrine, phenylpropanolamine or if taking SSRIs¹. **Serotonin syndrome** (fever, agitation, mental status changes, tremors) reported (CID 36:1197, 2003 & 37:1274, 2003).
Quinupristin + dalfopristin (Synercid) (CID 36:473, 2003)	**7.5 mg per kg IV q8h via central line** Cost: 350 mg=150 mg IV $122		Venous irritation (5%); none with central vein. Asymptomatic ↑ in unconjugated bilirubin. **Arthralgia 2%–50%** (CID 36:476, 2003). **Drug-drug interactions:** Cyclosporine, nifedipine, midazolam, many more—see Table 22.

¹ **SSRI** = selective serotonin reuptake inhibitors, e.g. fluoxetine (Prozac).
(See page 2 for abbreviations)
* NOTE: all dosage recommendations are for adults (unless otherwise indicated) & assume normal renal function.
§ Cost = average wholesale price from 2005 DRUG TOPICS RED BOOK, Medical Economics

TABLE 10C (5)

CLASS, AGENT, GENERIC NAME (TRADE NAME)	USUAL ADULT DOSAGE* (Cost*)	ADVERSE REACTIONS, COMMENTS (See Table 10A for Summary)
TETRACYCLINES		
Doxycycline (Vibramycin, Doryx, Monodox, Adoxa)	**0.1 gm po/IV q12h.** Cost: 100 mg po G $0.08–0.11, NB $5.10; 100 mg IV NB $14.16	Similar to other tetracyclines. ↑ nausea on empty stomach. Erosive esophagitis, esp. if taken at bedtime. Phototoxicity + but less than with tetracycline. Deposition in teeth less. Can be used in patients with renal failure. *Comments:* Effective in treatment and prophylaxes for malaria, leptospirosis, typhus fevers.
Minocycline (Minocin, Dynacin)	**0.1 gm po q12h.** Cost: 100 mg G $1.80, NB $3.88	Similar to other tetracyclines. **Vestibular symptoms** (30–90% in some groups; none in others): vertigo 33%, ataxia 43%; nausea 50%, vomiting 3%, women more frequently than men. Hypersensitivity pneumonitis, reversible, ~34 cases reported (*BMJ* 310:1520, 1995). *Comments:* More effective than other tetracyclines vs staph and in prophylaxis of meningococcal disease. P. acnes: many resistant to other tetracyclines, not to mino. Active vs Nocardia asteroides, Mycobacterium marinum.
Tetracycline, Oxytetracycline (Sumycin) *(CID 36:462, 2003)*	**0.25–0.5 gm po q6h, 0.5–1 gm IV q12h.** Cost: 250 mg po $0.06	GI (oxy 19%, tetra 4%), anaphylactoid reaction (rare), deposition in teeth, negative N balance, hepatotoxicity, enamel agenesis, pseudotumor cerebri/encephalopathy. Outdated drug: Fanconi syndrome. See *drug-drug interactions, Table 22*. **Contraindicated in pregnancy, hepatotoxicity to fetus.** *Comments:* IV dosage over 2.0 gm may be associated with fatal hepatotoxicity. False-neg urine dipstick for leukocytes.
Tigecycline (Tygacil)	**100 mg IV initially, then 50 mg IV q12h.** *If severe liver dis. (Child Pugh C):* 100 mg IV initially, then 25 mg IV q12h	Derivative of tetracycline. High incidence of nausea (25%), vomiting (20%) but only 1% of pts discontinued therapy due to an adverse event. Pregnancy Category D. Do not use in children under age 18. Like other tetracyclines, may cause photosensitivity, pseudotumor cerebri, pancreatitis, & a catabolic state (elevated BUN).
FLUOROQUINOLONES (FQs)		
Ciprofloxacin (Cipro) **and Ciprofloxacin-extended release** (Cipro XR)	**500–750 mg po bid. Urinary tract infection: 250 mg po bid or Cipro XR 500 mg po q24h.** **Parenteral** rx 200–400 mg IV q12h. Cost: 500 mg po $5.80, Cipro XR 500 mg IV $8.66, 400 mg IV $30	**Children:** No FQ approved for use under age 16 based on joint cartilage injury in immature animals. Articular SEs in children est. at 2–3% (*LnID* 3:537, 2003). **CNS toxicity:** Poorly understood. Varies from mild (lightheadedness) to moderate (confusion) to severe (seizures). May be aggravated by NSAIDs.
Gatifloxacin (Tequin)	**200–400 mg IV/po q24h.** Cost: 400 mg po/IV $39.84, 400 mg IV q24h	**Gemi skin rash:** Maculer rash after 8–10 d. of rx. Frequency higher in females. < age 40, treated 14 d. (22.6%). In men, < age 40, treated 14 d., frequency 7.7%. Mechanism unclear. Indication to DC therapy.
Gemifloxacin (Factive)	**320 mg po q24h.** Cost: 320 mg po $18.78	**Hypoglycemia/hyperglycemia** (*Med Lett* 45:64, 2003): Data based on case reports only. Various FQs ↑ insulin release in rats. No known drug-drug interactions; most pts reported have type 2 diabetes; no interaction with oral hypoglycemic drugs found. No data to allow comparative frequency between FQs.
Levofloxacin (Levaquin)	**250–750 mg. po/IV q24h.** Cost: 750 mg po $21; 750 mg IV $58	**Opiate screen false-positives:** FQs can cause false-positive urine assay for opiates (*JAMA* 286:3115, 2001: *Ar Pharmacotherapy* 38:1525, 2004).
Moxifloxacin (Avelox)	**400 mg po/IV q24h.** Cost: 400 mg po/IV $44	**Photosensitivity.** *See Table 10B, page 66* **QTc (corrected QT) interval prolongation:** ↑ QTc (>500 msec or >60 msec over baseline) is considered possible with any FQ. ↑ QTc can lead to torsades de pointes and ventricular fibrillation. Risk low with current marketed drugs). Risk ↑ in women, ↓ K+, ↓ Mg²⁺, brady-cardia. (Refs.: *NEJM* 348: 1837 & 1966, 2003). Major problem is ↑ risk with concomitant drugs.

(continued on next page)

TABLE 10C (6)

CLASS, AGENT, GENERIC NAME (TRADE NAME)	USUAL ADULT DOSAGE* (Cost§)	ADVERSE REACTIONS, COMMENTS (See Table 10A for Summary)

FLUOROQUINOLONES (FQs) (continued)

Ofloxacin (Floxin)	200–400 mg po bid. Cost: 400 mg po $6.80	(continued from previous page) Avoid concomitant drugs with potential to prolong QT$_c$:

Antiarrhythmics: Amiodarone, Disopyramide, Dofetilide, Ibutilide, Flecainide, Procainamide, Quinidine, Sotalol

Anti-Infectives: Clarithro, Erythro, Foscarnet, Mefloquine, Pentamidine

Anti-Hypertensives: Bepridil, Isradipine, Nicardipine, Moexipril

CNS Drugs: Fluoxetine, Sertraline, Tricyclics, Venlafaxine, Haloperidol, Phenothiazines, Pimozide, Quetiapine, Ziprasidone, Risperidone

Misc. Salmeterol, Naratriptan, Sumatriptan, Dolasetron, Droperidol, Fosphenytoin, Indapamide, Tamoxifen, Tizanidine

Updates online: www.qtdrugs.org; www.torsades.org.
Tendinopathy: Over age 60, approx. 2–6% of all Achilles tendon ruptures attributable to use of FQ (ArIM 163:1801, 2003). ↑ risk with concomitant steroid or renal disease (CID 36:1404, 2003)

POLYMYXINS

Polymyxin B (Poly-Rx)	Rarely used parenterally in U.S. Use colistin for parenteral therapy	‖ Used as/for: bladder irrigation, intrathecal, ophthalmic. Source: Bedford Labs, Bedford, OH
Polymyxin E = colistin Colistin sulfate used po or topical; IV form is colisti-methate (Coly-Mycin M) (CID 40:1333, 2005)	**Inhalation dose:** 80 mg q12h. **Intrathecal:** not standardized. Reports range from 1.6 mg to 20 mg intraventricularly; usually 10 mg. ↑ colistin = 12,500 units U.S.: 2.5–5 mg per kg per day div. in 2–4 equal doses. Cost: 150 mg IV $64.34 U.K.: >60 kg: 80–160 mg q8h <60 kg: 4–6 mg per kg per day div. q8h	**Nephrotoxicity** (tubular necrosis): Reports vary from 14–20%. Reversible. **Neurotoxicity** (frequency?): Vertigo, facial paresthesia, abnormal vision, confusion, ataxia, & neuromuscular blockade → respiratory failure. Dose-dependent; paresthesia, 29% experienced paresthesia, ataxia or both.

MISCELLANEOUS AGENTS

Daptomycin (Cubicin) (Med Let 46:11, 2004; CID 38:994, 2004)	**Skin/soft tissue: 4 mg per kg IV q24h** **Bacteremia/endocarditis: 6 mg per kg IV q24h** (See Comment). Cost: 4 mg/kg $177.88	FDA approved skin/soft tissue infections. Bacteremia/endocarditis trials ongoing. **Potential muscle toxicity:** At 4 mg per kg per day, ↑ CPK in 2.8% dapto pts & 1.8% comparator-treated pts. In very small study, no CPK ↑ in pts taking a statin drug given dapto/month (manufacturer suggests stopping statins during dapto rx).
Fosfomycin (Monurol)	3 gm with water po times 1 dose. Cost: $38.77	Diarrhea in 9%, compared to 6% of pts given nitrofurantoin and 2.3% given TMP-SMX.
Fusidic acid*NUS (Fucidin)	500 mg po IV tid (Leo Laboratories, Denmark)	Mild GI upset, jaundice (17% with IV, 6% with po). (None in CSF; <1% in urine).
Immune globulin IV therapy	**Dosage, frequency vary with the indication.** At least 7 manufacturers. Cost for 10–12 gm ranges from $500–$1100.	Reported adverse effects range from 1–15%. Fever, headache, myalgia, N/V related to rate of infusion; mild, & self-limited. **More serious:** anaphylactoid reactions, thromboembolic, aseptic meningitis, & renal injury in 6.7% (QJM 93:751, 2000).
Methenamine hippurate (Hiprex, Urex)	**1 gm po q6h.** Cost: 1 gm $1.23 1 gm = 460 mg methenamine	Nausea and vomiting, skin rash or dysuria. Overall ~3%. Methenamine requires (pH ≤5) urine to liberate formaldehyde. Useful in suppressive therapy after infecting organisms cleared; do not use for pyelonephritis. **Comment:** Do not force fluids; may dilute formaldehyde. Of no value in pts with chronic Foley. If urine pH >5.0, co-administer ascorbic acid (1–2 gm q4h) to acidify the urine; cranberry juice (1200–4000 mL per day) has been used, results ±.
Methenamine mandelate (Mandelamine)	**1 gm po q6h (480 mg methenamine)** 1 gm NB $0.29	

(See page 2 for abbreviations)
* NOTE: all dosage recommendations are for adults (unless otherwise indicated) & assume normal renal/renal function.
§ Cost = average wholesale price from 2005 DRUG TOPICS RED BOOK, Medical Economics

TABLE 10C (7)

CLASS, AGENT, GENERIC NAME (TRADE NAME)	USUAL ADULT DOSAGE* (Cost§)	ADVERSE REACTIONS, COMMENTS (See Table 10A for Summary)
MISCELLANEOUS AGENTS *(continued)*		
Metronidazole (Flagyl) Ref.: Mayo Clin Proc 74:825, 1999	**Anaerobic infections:** usually IV, 7.5 mg per kg (~500 mg) q6h (not to exceed 4 gm q24hr). **With long t½, can use IV at 15 mg per kg loading dose, then 7.5 mg per kg q6h.** Alt: can use IV at 15 mg/kg load then 7.5 mg per kg q6h. **Oral dose: 500 mg qid.** Cost: 500 mg tab \$0.21; NB \$4.56; 500 mg IV G \$2.80, NB \$26.16; 70 gm vaginal gel \$63.24, ext release 750 mg \$9.50	Can be given rectally (enema or suppository). In pts with decompensated liver disease (manifest by ≥2 L of ascites, encephalopathy, ↑ prothrombin time, ↓ serum albumin) t½ prolonged; unless dose ↓ by approx. ⅓, side-effects ↑. Absorbed into serum from vaginal gel. **Neurol.:** headache, rare paresthesias of peripheral neuropathy, ataxia, seizures, aseptic meningitis, reversible confusion. Rare: pancreatitis (AnIM 120:445, 1994); reversible encephalopathy during & 48 hrs after (disulfiram-like reaction). Very dark urine (common but harmless). Skin: urticaria. Mutagenic in Ames test. Tumorigenic in animals (high dose over lifetime). No evidence of risk in man. No teratogenicity.
Mupirocin (Bactroban)	**Skin cream or ointment 2%:** Apply tid times 10 days. 15 gm \$31.48 **Nasal ointment 2%:** Apply bid times 5 days. 22 gm NB \$49.90	Skin cream: itch, burning, stinging 1-1.5%. Nasal: headache 9%, rhinitis 6%, respiratory congestion 5%.
Nitrofurantoin macrocrystals (Macrodantin, Furadantin)	**For long-term UTI suppression:** 50-100 mg at bedtime	Nausea and vomiting, much reduced if taken after food. Not effective in endstage renal disease (JAC 33[Suppl A]:121, 1994). Pulmonary reactions (with chronic rx): acute ARDS type. Hemolytic anemia in G6PD deficiency. **Contraindicated in renal failure.** Should not be used in infants <1 month of age.
monohydrate/macrocrystals (Macrobid)	100 mg po bid Cost: 100 mg \$2.44	acute desquamative interstitial pneumonia with fibrosis. Intrahepatic cholestasis & hepatitis similar to chronic active hepatitis. Efficacy of Macrobid 100 mg bid = Macrodantin 50 mg qid. Adverse effects 5.6%, less nausea than with Macrodantin.
Rifaximin (Xifaxan)	200 mg tab tid times 3 days. Cost: 200 mg \$3.60	For traveler's diarrhea. In general, adverse events equal to or less than placebo.
Sulfonamides [e.g., sulfisoxazole (Gantrisin), sulfamethoxazole (Gantanol)]	Sulfisoxazole (Gantrisin) peds suspension: Cost 500 mg per 5 mL 480 mL \$46.02	**Short-acting are best:** high urine concentration and good solubility at acid pH. More active in alkaline urine. **Allergic reactions:** Rash, drug fever, pruritus, photosensitization. Periarteritis nodosa & SLE, Stevens-Johnson syndrome, serum sickness syndrome, myocarditis. Crystalluria. Nausea & vomiting, headache, dizziness, lassitude, mental depression, acidosis, sulfhemoglobinemia. **Hematol.:** Anemia (hemolytic, aplastic), agranulocytosis (psychosis, neuritis), hepatic toxicity. Blood dyscrasias, usually agranulocytosis. Hemolysis (G6PD deficient & unstable hemoglobins (Hb Zurich, H, etc.). Do not use in newborn infants or at term in pregnancy (kernicterus from displacement of bilirubin from albumin).
Tinidazole (Tindamax)	2 gm po times 1 with food. Cost 2 gm \$18.24	**Adverse reactions:** metallic taste 3.7%, nausea 3.2%, anorexia/vomiting 1.5%. All higher with multi-day dosing.
Trimethoprim (Trimpex, Proloprim, and others)	**100 mg po q12h or 200 mg po q24h.** Cost: 100 mg NB \$0.90, G \$0.15	Rash in 3% at 100 mg bid, 6.7% at 200 mg q24h. Rare reports of photosensitivity, exfoliative dermatitis, Stevens-Johnson syndrome, toxic epidermal necrolysis, and aseptic meningitis (CID 19-431, 1994). Check drug interaction with phenytoin. Increases serum K⁺ (see TMP-SMX Comments). TMP can ↑ homocysteine blood levels (JJn 352:1827, 1998).
Trimethoprim (TMP)/ Sulfamethoxazole (SMX) (Bactrim, Septra) Single-strength (SS) is 80 TMP/400 SMX, double-strength (DS) 160 TMP/800 SMX. Ref.: AnIM 163:402, 2003	**Standard po rx (UTI, otitis media): DS tab bid. For Pneumocystis (PCP): 15-20 mg per kg per day div in 3-4 doses IV or po (base on TMP component); standard 8-10 mg per kg per day divided q6h, q8h, or q12h. For shigellosis: 2.5-10 mg per kg q12h.** 160/800 IV G \$11.21 160/800 SS po G \$0.15; NB \$2; 160/800 DS \$0.15, NB \$2;	Adverse reactions in 10%: GI: nausea, vomiting, anorexia. Skin: Rash, urticaria, photosensitivity. More serious (1-10%): Stevens-Johnson syndrome & toxic epidermal necrolysis. Skin reactions may represent host metabolite of SMX rather than allergy (AJ-Pharmacotherapy (JAIDS 36:1045-2004). TMP competes with creatinine for tubular secretion, serum creatinine can ↑. TMP also blocks distal renal tubule secretion of K⁺. ↑ serum K⁺ in 21% of pts (AnIM 124:316, 1996). TMP suspected etiology of aseptic meningitis (CID 19-431, 1994). TMP-SMX can cause thrombocytopenia (AnIM 129:886, 1998).

Rapid Oral TMP-SMX Desensitization:

Hour	Dose TMP-SMX (mg)
0	0.004/0.02
1	0.04/0.2
2	0.4/2

Hour	Dose TMP-SMX (mg)
3	4/20
4	40/200
5	160/180

Comment: Perform in hospital or clinic. Use oral suspension (40 mg TMP/ 200 mg SMX per 5 mL (tsp)). Take 6 oz water after each dose. Corticosteroids, anti-histaminics NOT used. Refs.: CID 20:849, 1995; AIDS 5:311, 1991

(See page 2 for abbreviations)
* NOTE: all dosage recommendations are for adults (unless otherwise indicated) & assume normal renal function.
§ Cost = average wholesale price from 2005 DRUG TOPICS RED BOOK, Medical Economic

TABLE 10D
AMINOGLYCOSIDE ONCE-DAILY AND MULTIPLE DAILY DOSING REGIMENS
(See Table 17, page 134, if estimated creatinine clearance <90 mL per min.)

General: Dosage given as both once-daily (OD) and multiple daily dose (MDD) regimens.

Pertinent formulae: (1) Estimated creatinine clearance (CrCl): [(140–age)/ideal body weight in kg] = CrCl for men in ml per min; multiply answer times 0.85 for CrCl of women

$$\frac{(140-age)/ideal\ body\ weight\ in\ kg}{(72)(serum\ creatinine)}$$

(2) Ideal body weight (IBW)—Females: 45.5 kg + 2.3 kg per inch over 5' = weight in kg
Males: 50 kg + 2.3 kg per inch over 5' = weight in kg

(3) Obesity adjustment: use if actual body weight (ABW) is >30% above IBW. To calculate adjusted dosing weight in kg: IBW + 0.4(ABW–IBW) = adjusted weight (CID 25:112, 1997)

DRUG	MDD AND OD REGIMENS/ TARGETED PEAK (P) AND TROUGH (T) SERUM LEVELS	COST$ Name Brand (NB), Generic (G)	COMMENTS For more data on once-daily dosing, see AJM 105:182, 1998, and Table 17, page 134
Gentamicin (Garamycin), **Tobramycin** (Nebcin)	MDD: 2 mg per kg load, then 1.7 mg per kg q8h P 4–10 mcg/ml, T 1–2 mcg per ml	Gentamicin: 80 mg $5.75 Tobramycin: 80 mg NB $7.28, G $4.20	All aminoglycosides have potential to cause tubular necrosis and renal failure, deafness due to cochlear toxicity, vertigo due to damage to vestibular organs, and rarely neuromuscular blockade. Risk minimal with oral or topical application due to small % absorption unless tissues altered by disease.
	OD: 5.1 (? if critically ill) mg per kg q24h P 16–24 mcg per ml, T < 1 mcg per ml		
Kanamycin (Kantrex), **Amikacin** (Amikin), Streptomycin	MDD: 7.5 mg per kg q12h P 15–30 mcg per ml, T 5–10 mcg per ml	Kanamycin: 1 gm $9.60 Amikacin: 500 mg NB $34.26, G $7.80 Streptomycin: 1 gm $9.75	Risk of nephrotoxicity ↑ with concomitant administration of cyclosporine, vancomycin, ampho B, radiocontrast. Risk of nephrotoxicity ↓ by once-daily dosing method and perhaps by once-daily dosing method (especially if baseline renal function normal).
	OD: 15 mg per kg q24h P 56–64 mcg per ml, T < 1 mcg per ml		
Netilmicin^{NUS}	MDD: 2 mg per kg q8h P 4–10 mcg per ml, T 1–2 mcg per ml		In general, same factors influence risk of ototoxicity. **NOTE: There is no known method to eliminate risk of aminoglycoside nephro/ototoxicity. Proper rx attempts to ↓ the % risk.**
	OD: 6.5 mg per kg q24h P 22–30 mcg per ml, T < 1 mcg per ml		The clinical trial data of OD aminoglycosides have been reviewed extensively by meta-analysis (CID 24:816, 1997). Serum levels: Collect serum for a peak serum level (PSL) exactly 1 hr after the start of the infusion of the 3rd dose. In critically ill pts, it is reasonable to measure the PSL after the 1st dose as well as later doses as volume of distribution and renal function may change rapidly.
Isepamicin^{NUS}	Only OD: Severe infections 15 mg per kg q24h; less severe 8 mg per kg q24h		Other dosing methods and references: For once-daily 7 mg per kg per day of gentamicin—Hartford Hospital method, see AAC 39:650, 1995.
Spectinomycin (Trobicin)	2 gm IM times 1—gonococcal infections	2 gm NB $34.06	
Neomycin—oral	Prophylaxis GI surgery: 1 gm po times 3 with erythro, see Table 15B, page 125 For hepatic coma, 4–12 gm per day po	500 mg G $1.24	
Tobramycin—inhaled (Tobi). See Cystic fibrosis, Table 1, page 32. Adverse effects: few, transient voice alteration (13%) and transient tinnitus (3%). Cost: 300 mg $57.23		500 mg G $1.24	
Paromomycin—oral: See Entamoeba and Cryptosporidia, Table 13, page 95. Cost: 250 mg $2.72			

† Estimated CrCl invalid if serum creatinine < 0.6 mg per dL. Consultation suggested.

$ Cost = average wholesale price from 2005 DRUG TOPICS RED BOOK, Medical Economics.

TABLE 11A: TREATMENT OF FUNGAL, ACTINOMYCOTIC, AND NOCARDIAL INFECTIONS—ANTIMICROBIAL AGENTS OF CHOICE*
(See Table 11B for Amphotericin B Preparations and Adverse Effects)

TYPE OF INFECTION/ORGANISM/ SITE OF INFECTION	ANTIMICROBIAL AGENTS OF CHOICE		COMMENTS
	PRIMARY	ALTERNATIVE	
Actinomycosis (A. israelii most common, also A. naeslundii, A. viscosus, A. odontolyticus, A. meyeri, & A. gerencseriae) Cervicofacial, pulmonary, abdominal, cerebral, & rarely pericarditis (Dis Mon 29:1, 1983). Classically abdominal actino presents as interabdominal or pubic mass abscess, fistula tract (Dis Colon Rectum 48:575, 2005) years after surgery & may mimic cancer (World J Gastro 11:1722, 2005). Fine needle aspirate of cervicofacial actino established dx in 15 pts in Spain (AJM 112:183)	**Ampicillin** 50 mg per kg per day IV times 4-6 wks, then 0.5 gm **amoxicillin** po 4x/d OR **Penicillin G** 10-20 million units per day IV times 4-6 wks, then **penicillin V** 2-4 gm per day po; (oral penicillin individualized, duration 3-6 mos. total duration 3-6 mos. usually adequate for thoracic & abdominal dz).	**Doxycycline** or **ceftriaxone** or **clindamycin** or **erythromycin**. **Chloramphenicol** 12.5–15 mg per kg IV/po q6h has been recommended in CNS infection in pen-allergic pts.	Tuboovarian abscesses may complicate IUDs. Removal of IUD is primary rx. When abscesses, inflammatory mass or fistulae, surgery often required. While penicillins + tetracyclines have been effective, others in IV infusion agents given q24h, e.g., ceftriaxone, are more practical (CID 38-444, 2004). Surgery may be necessary for hemoptysis (An Thor Surg 74:185, 2002).
Aspergillosis (A. fumigatus most common, also A. flavus and others) (CID 30:696, 2000)			
Allergic bronchopulmonary aspergillosis (ABPA) ABPA found in 1–2% of pts with asthma & ~15% with cystic fibrosis (CID 37 (Suppl.3):S37, 2003). Clinical manifestations: wheezing, pulmonary infiltrates, bronchiectasis & fibrosis. Airway colonization assoc. with ↑ blood eosinophils, ↑ serum IgE.	Rx of ABPA: **Itraconazole**[1] 200 mg po q24h times16 wks or longer (Allergy 60:1004, 2005)	In 2 PRCTs[1], itra ↓ number of exacerbations requiring corticosteroids (p <0.03), improved immunological markers (eosinophils in sputum & ↓ serum IgE levels), & in 1 study improved lung function & exercise tolerance (NEJM 342:756, 2000; Cochrane Database Syst Rev 3:CD001108, 2004).	
Allergic fungal sinusitis ABPA-like syndrome: relapsing chronic sinusitis; nasal polyps without bony invasion; asthma, eczema or allergic rhinitis; ↑ IgE levels and isolation of Aspergillus sp. or other dematiaceous sp. (Alternaria, Cladosporium, etc.)	Rx controversial: systemic corticosteroids + surgical debridement (80% respond but 2/3 relapse) (Otolaryn Head Neck Surg 131:704, 2004)	Rx of ABPA: **Itraconazole** (po) benefit reported sporadically (J Am Acad Derm 23:607, 1990).	In 1 report, fungal elements identified by histopathology in 93% of cases of "chronic sinusitis" & in a DBRCT in 24 pts, intranasal ampho was superior, with a ↓ in mucosal thickening of 8.8% by CT scan vs 2.5% in placebo (LnID 4:257, 2004) in controversial area.
Aspergilloma (fungus ball) (J Resp Dis 23:300, 2002)	Efficacy of antimicrobial agents not proven. Itraconazole (po) reported sporadically (J Am Acad Derm 23:607, 1990).		Aspergillus may complicate pulmonary sequestration (Eur J Cardio Thor Surg 27:28, 2005).
Invasive, pulmonary (IPA) or extrapulmonary: (See COID 18:314, 2005) Post-transplantation and post-chemotherapy in neutropenic pts (PMN <500 per mm³) but may also present in patients without obvious immunosuppression. (Mayo Clin Proc 159:181, 2005). Most common manifestation is pneumonia in transplant recipients. Usually a late (≥100 days) complication in allogeneic bone marrow & the complication in allogeneic bone marrow transplantation: median survival 36 days; but even all mortality rates very high (Clin Micro Inf 11:427, 2005). **Typical x-ray/CT lung lesions** (halo sign, cavitation & air-crescent sign) suggest dz, but diagnosis is difficult in many pts without invasive dz (e.g., positive culture value in Aspergillus sp. in invasive malignancies (Abstracts in Heme & Onc 6:11, 2005). An immunologic test that detects circulating galactomannan (Platelia) is in 15-18 minute-dx of aspergillosis. A recent article reviews the strengths & weaknesses of the test (CID 41(Suppl. 6):S3B) (continued on next page)	**Voriconazole** 6 mg per kg IV q12h x2, then either (4 mg per kg IV q12h) or (200 mg po q12h for body weight ≥40 kg, or 100 mg po q12h for body weight <40 kg). **OR Lipid-based ampho B** as effective as less expensive than standard ampho B but much more expensive (see footnote* for dosages). Some authorities now prefer lipid-based ampho B over standard ampho B as initial rx (CID 32:415, 2003). **OR Ampho B** (dosage footnote*, pg 76): Rapid increase to 1 mg per kg IV (q12h) or (200 mg po q12h for neutropenic pts or for body weight ≥40 kg. Total dose of 2–2.5 gm by some. Check data and mg/kg per dosing (see footnote* in above dosages) **+ caspo** (dosage below) are currently being used in compassionate use program 44% (J Inf 50:196, 2005). Minimal favorably reported (Transpl Inf Dis 1:25, 2002). (continued on next page)	Voriconazole more effective than ampho B in randomized trial of 277 immunosuppressed pts with IPA. 53% responded to vori with ampho B. Overall survival better (71 vs 58%) (NEJM 347: 408, 2002). Appears particularly advantageous in cerebral aspergillosis (CID 37:S52, 2003). Among 81 pts with refractory infection (Eur J Haematol 79:330, 2004) 48 of 81 pts survived with vori alone. Vori reported satisfactory results in 11/20 pts with bone involvement (18 for salvage), follow-up average of 3 mos. (CID 40:1141, 2005). **Ampho B overall success rate 34–42%** (CID 32:358, 2001) in pulmonary aspergillosis in pts rx 214 days. Success depended on underlying disease: 83% heart/lung transplants, 54% neutropenic leukemia pts, 33% bone marrow transplant (CID 23:608, 1996). 44% of 398 pts receiving **ampho B lipid complex (ABLC)** were cured or improved & 21% stabilized; most had failed to respond to prior antifungal rx (CID 40:S392, 2005). **A. terreus infections particularly resistant to ampho B: in 83 cases, 73.4% mortality with ampho B rx vs 55.8% with voriconazole** (CID 39:192, 2004). **Combination therapy:** To date no controlled clinical trials, and they are not needed (CID 39:803, 2004). No antagonism between triazoles (vori & itra), echinocandins (caspo), & ampho B. Synergy (continued on next page)

* See page 2 for abbreviations. All dosage recommendations are for adults (unless otherwise indicated) and assume normal renal function

** PRCTs = Prospective randomized controlled trials
*** Oral solution preferred to tablets because of ↑ absorption (see Table 11B, page 83)
**** Dosages: **ABLC** 5 mg per kg per day IV over 2 hrs; **ABCD** 3–4 mg per kg per day IV over 2 hrs; **liposomal Ampho B** 3–5 mg per kg per hr.

TABLE 11A (2)

TYPE OF INFECTION/ORGANISM/SITE OF INFECTION	ANTIMICROBIAL AGENTS OF CHOICE		COMMENTS
	PRIMARY	ALTERNATIVE	
Aspergillosis/invasive, pulmonary (IPA) or extrapulmonary (continued from previous page)	(continued from previous page) **Alternative: Caspofungin** 70 mg IV on day 1, then 50 mg IV q24h (reduce to 35 mg/day with moderate hepatic insufficiency). Can change to oral antifungal rx and may switch to oral **vori** after 2–3 wks (See previous page) **Micafungin**^NFDA 150 mg IV q24h	(continued from previous page) demonstrated vs aspergillus in vitro &/or animal models between triazoles & caspo (AAC 47:1416, 2003) & ampho B plus caspo (AAC 46:245 & 2564, 2005; JID 187:1834, 2003). Some failures to show synergy (AAC 56:166, 2005). **Resistance:** A. fumigatus isolates from stem cell transplants showed ↓ susceptibility to vori, caspo & some to ampho B.	
Blastomycosis (CID 30:679, 2000) (Blastomyces dermatitidis) Cutaneous, pulmonary or extrapulmonary For bloodtype antigen, call 1-866-647-2847	**Itraconazole**^b oral solution 200–400 mg po bid po for 6 mos. **OR Ampho B** 0.7–1 mg per kg per day to a total dose of 1.5 gm for very sick pts	**Fluconazole** 400–800 mg per day for at least 6 mos. 89% effective for non-life-threatening disease (CID 25:200, 1997)	Itra (in patients treated for 22 months, 95% cure (AJM 93:489, 1992). Ampho B successful in >95% (CID 22:S102, 1996). Vori not successful in rx of 1 pt with cerebral blastomycosis (CID 40:e69, 2005).

Candidiasis: A decrease in C. albicans & increase in non-albicans species continues. The latter show ↓ susceptibility to antifungal agents. These changes predominantly in immunocompromised pts wherein antifungal prophylaxis (esp. fluconazole) is widely used (JCM 43:2729, 2005; CID 18:490, 2005). In vitro susceptibility testing for antifungal drugs has not undergone in vivo validation studies; clinical outcomes often more dependent on host factors (AJM 112:380, 2002). Susceptibility profiles help predict empiric antifungal rx. The table summarizes current published reports of frequency of candida isolates, & interpretation as to whether a drug is clinically effective (**S** = susceptible, **S-DD** = susceptible with dose escalation), may require dose escalation (IDSA Guidelines, CID 38:161, 2004). In vitro testing for caspo not standardized. (**R** = resistant) **S-I** = less activity in vitro but clinically effective: only rare failures reported (IDSA Guidelines, 2004). In clinical studies of candida infections, MIC of caspo did not correlate with treatment outcome following caspofungin therapy (AAC 49:3616, 2005).

% of Candida Isolates		Risk Factors	% Sensitive In Vitro				Caspofungin	Micafungin/ Anidulafungin	Rx if species known
			Fluconazole	Voriconazole	Itraconazole	Ampho B			
C. albicans	45–63	HIV/AIDS, surgery	97% (S)	99% (S)	93% (S)	>95% (S)	S	S	Flu, caspo, or ampho B
C. glabrata	12–24	Heme malignancies, azole prophylaxis	85–90% (S-DD)	92% (S)	50% (S-DD)	>95% (S-I)	S	S	Caspo, ampho B, or vori
C. parapsilosis	11–29	Heme malignancies, neonates, foreign bodies	99% (S)	99% (S)	4% (R)	>95% (S)	S-I	S-I	Flu, caspo, or ampho B
C. tropicalis	6–19	Neutropenia	98% (S)	99% (R)	58% (S)	>95% (S)	S	S	Flu, caspo, or ampho B
C. krusei	1–5	Heme malignancies, azole prophylaxis	5% (R)	69% (R)	69% (R)	>95% (S-I)	S	S	Caspo, ampho B, or vori^f
C. guilliermondi	1	Azole prophylaxis, previous ampho rx	>95% (S)	?	?	? (R)	S	S	Flu, caspo, or ampho B
C. lusitaniae	1	Previous ampho rx	>95% (S)	>95% (S)	?	? (R)	S	S	Flu, caspo, or vori

† Int Med 21:S17, 2004   ‡ If patient had prior fecal exposure, use ampho B or caspo (CID 35:1073, 2002; 36:1497, 2003)   ⁹ JAC 35:188, 2005

	PRIMARY	ALTERNATIVE	COMMENTS
Bloodstream: clinically stable with or without venous catheter^†	**Fluconazole** 26 mg per kg per day or 400 mg IV q24h (IV or po times 7 days then po) for 14 days after last blood culture (for non-neutropenic: mortality 21% vs 4% if catheter not removed). **or Caspofungin** 70 mg IV on day 1 followed by 50 mg IV q24h (reduce to 35 mg/day with moderate hepatic insufficiency). Would use in place of azoles (i.e. flu or itra prophylaxis) **OR** (continued on next page)	use **ampho B** 0.6–1 mg per kg per day **OR fluconazole** 800 mg/day IV q24h for 14 days. **Be sure catheter is removed.** **or Voriconazole** 6 mg per kg IV q12h times 2 doses, then maintenance dose of 3 mg per kg IV q12h or 200 mg po q12h; after at least 3 days of IV therapy (continued on next page)	Observational studies suggest flu & ampho B are similarly effective in neutropenic patients (IDSA Guidelines, 2003). A randomized study (277 pts, 10% were neutropenic) found caspofungin equivalent to ampho B. For candidemia 71.7% rx with caspo vs 62.8% with ampho B had successful outcomes but caspo had significantly less toxicity (NEJM 347:2020, 2002). Caspo also favorable response vs 50% for ampho B in 58 cancer pts with candidemia (J Infect 49:443, 2005). In 119 pts with candidemia, micafungin effective in 88% with new infection, 76% with (continued on next page)

- **All positive blood cultures require therapy!**
- Remove &/or replace venous catheter^‡ (not over a guidewire), add/test blood culture 48 hrs after last blood culture.
- Option B has been recommended so all pts with candidemia.
- Treat for 2 wks after last pos. blood culture and resolution of signs & symptoms of infection.

---

1 Hydration before and after an infusion with 500 cc saline has been shown to reduce renal toxicity.
2 Oral solution preferred due to better absorption (see Table 11B, page 83).

See page 2 for abbreviations. All dosage recommendations are for adults (unless otherwise indicated) and assume normal renal/renal function

TABLE 11A (3)

TYPE OF INFECTION/ORGANISM/SITE OF INFECTION	ANTIMICROBIAL AGENTS OF CHOICE		COMMENTS
	PRIMARY	**ALTERNATIVE**	
Candidiasis/ Bloodstream: clinically stable with or without venous catheter (continued)	(continued from previous page) **Micafungin** 50 mg IV q24h for C. albicans, 100 mg IV q24h for non-albicans Candida **Ampho B** 0.6 mg per kg IV q24h, total dose 5–7 mg per kg or lipid-based ampho B[2]	(continued from previous page) **or** **Anidulafungin** 200 mg IV times 1, then 100 mg q24h (no dosage adjustments for renal or hepatic insufficiency) (Pending FDA label)	(continued from previous page) reinfection (Eur J Clin Inf Dis, in press). Preliminary data from a double-blind study (n=245) suggests anidula-fungin was superior to flu for invasive candidiasis/candidemia. Global response (clinical + micro) at end of IV rx, 75.6% vs 60.2% with flu (non-inferior at least). Toler-ability was comparable (ICAAC 2005; IDSA 2005)
Bloodstream: unstable, deteriorating ± neutropenia OR stable disseminated (pulmonary, eye, hepatosplenic) IDSA Guidelines: CID 38:161, 2004) For endophthalmitis, see below	**Ampho B** 0.8–1 mg per kg per day IV ± 5FC 37.5 mg per kg po q6h or lipid-based ampho B (ABLC) 5 mg per kg per day **OR** **Fluconazole** 800 mg po/IV (or 6 mg per kg po day) IV q24h. If start ampho B, switch to flucon 400 mg po q24h times 14 days after last positive blood culture, resolution of signs/ symptoms of candidal infection. **OR** **Combination of fluconazole** 800 mg per day + ampho B 0.7 mg per kg per day for first 5–6 days, then switch to flu 400 mg per day po	**Voriconazole** 6 mg per kg IV q12h times 2 doses, then maintenance doses of 3 mg per kg IV q12h or 200 mg po q12h, after at least 3 days of IV therapy. **or** **Caspofungin** 70 mg IV on day 1 followed by 50 mg IV q24h (reduce to 35 mg IV q24h with moderate hepatic insufficiency)	In a randomized trial of 219 pts with non-neutropenic candidemia, fluconazole (800 mg per day) + ampho B (0.7 mg per kg per day for the 1st 5 days) was slightly better than flu alone: Primary analysis, success rate on day 30 was 69% vs 57% (p = .08) respectively, overall success rate 69% vs 56% (p = .045) respectively. Duration of fungemia 94% vs 83% (p = .02), & renal toxicity in combination greater (23% vs 3%, p = .001) CID 36:1221, 2003). Given difficulty with interpretation of this study, the editors reserve combination of flu + ampho B for only the sickest candidemic patient. Voriconazole may have a role in this clinical setting.
Cutaneous (including paronychia, Table 1, page 21)	Apply topical ampho B, clotrimazole, econazole, miconazole, or nystatin 3-4 times daily for 7–14 days, or ketoconazole 400 mg once daily times 14 days.		Cost (30 gm tube cream): Clo $13, Eco $28, Mic $50, Nys $4.
Endocarditis Causes: C. albicans 24%, non-albicans Candida sp. 24%, Aspergillus sp. 24%, others 27% (CID 32:50, 2001) Surgery may not always be required (Scand J Inf Dis 32:86, 2000 & 37:320, 2001)	(Ampho B 1 mg per kg IV per day, then 0.8 mg every other day for 30 days, or lipid-based ampho B 5 mg per kg per day. Continue 6–8 weeks after surgery + surgical resection	**Fluconazole** 200–400 mg per day for chronic suppression may be of value when valve cannot be replaced (Chest 122:302, 2002) + Surgical resection	Cic $19 **adjust flucyt dose and interval to produce serum levels; peak 70–80 mg per L, trough 30–40 mg per L Caspofungin** initial vs caspofungin: several reports of cure (CID 39:1093–6, 2004; CID 40:e-72, 2005). Cure of refractory candidal meningitis with caspo (J Clin Micro 42:5949, 2004).
Endophthalmitis (IDSA Guidelines: CID 38:161, 2004) • Occurs in 10% of candidemia (PIDJ 23:635, 2004), thus ophthalmological consult for all pts • Diagnosis: typical white exudates on retinal exam/dx confirmed by vitrectomy	**Ampho B** or lipid-based ampho B (ABLC 4.5 mg per kg per day) IV 0.8 mg per kg per day) or follow-up ampho B 0.8 mg per kg IV po or IV either as initial rx or Role of intravitreal ampho B not well defined but commonly used in pts with substantial vision loss (CID 27:1130, 1998). Treat 6–12 weeks.	**Fluconazole** 6 mg per kg per day) OR fluconazole 400 + **Clotrimazole** 1 troche (10 mg) 5 times per day times 14 days.	Treatment results mixed in small series: Fluconazole (CID 26:657, 1995), ABLC (J Inf 40:192, 2000), and vitrectomy (CID 27:1130, 1998). Vori successful alone or with caspo (Korean J Ophthal 19:73, 2005; Am J Ophthal 139:135, 2005).
Oral (thrush)—not AIDS patient (See below for vaginitis)	**Fluconazole** 200 mg single dose or 100 mg per day po times 14 days or **Itraconazole** oral solution 200 mg q24h without food times 7 days.	**Nystatin pastilles** (200,000 units) lozenge qid, 1 per day (swish & swallow) qid 2 x (500,000 units) tabs tid for 14 days **OR Clotrimazole** 1 troche (10 mg) 5 times per day times 14 days.	Maintenance not required in non-AIDS pts. Usually improves in 3–4 days, longer rx ± relapse. Fluconazole-resistant C. krusei fungemia reported in flucon-rx pts (NEJM 325:1315, 1991).

[1] ABLC or liposomal ampho B recommended for pts intolerant of or refractory to ampho B, i.e. failure of 500 mg ampho B, initial renal insufficiency (creatinine >2.5 mg per dL or CrCl <25 mL per min), a sig. ↑ in serum Cr (to >2.5 mg per dL for adults or 1.5 mg per dL for children) or severe acute administration-related toxicity (CID 26:1383, 1998). Since efficacy similar and toxicity less, some now recommend lipid-based preps in place of ampho B as initial rx (CID 32:415, 2003).

[2] Some experts reduce dose of 5FC to 25 mg per kg q6h.

See page 2 for abbreviations. All dosage recommendations are for adults (unless otherwise indicated) and assume normal renal function

TABLE 11A (4)

TYPE OF INFECTION/ORGANISM/SITE OF INFECTION	ANTIMICROBIAL AGENTS OF CHOICE		COMMENTS
	PRIMARY	**ALTERNATIVE**	
Candidiasis (continued) **AIDS patient** **Stomatitis, esophagitis** (adult) has ↑ in prevalence of oropharyngeal & esophageal candidiasis in HIV-infected pts in relationship to ↓ in prevalence of oropharyngeal & esophageal candidiasis in relationship to disease. *MMWR 53(RR-15):97, 2004* Oral candidiasis is a strong clinical marker of immunodeficiency in pts receiving HAART *AIDS Pt Care STDs 19:70, 2005*.	**Oropharyngeal:** initial episodes (7–14 day rx): • **Fluconazole** 100 mg po q24h; or • **itraconazole** oral solution 200 mg po q24h; or • **clotrimazole** troches 10 mg po 5 times per day; or **nystatin** suspension 4-6 mL q6h; or flavored pastilles 1-2 q4-5 times per day. **Esophageal (14-21 days):** • **Flucon** 100 mg (up to 400 mg) po or IV q24h; or • **itra** oral solution 200 mg po q24h; or • **vori** 200 mg po q12h; or • **caspofungin** 50 mg IV q24h; or • **micafungin** 150 mg IV q24h for 14 days. Suppressive rx is generally not recommended unless pts have frequent or severe recurrences. • **Oropharyngeal:** **fluconazole** 100 mg po 3 times per week. • **Vulvovaginal:** **fluconazole** daily.	**Fluconazole-refractory oropharyngeal:** • **itra** oral solution ≥200 mg po q24h; or • **ampho B** suspension 100 mg per mL (not U.S.), 1 mL q6h; or • **ampho B** 0.3 mg per kg IV q24h **Fluconazole-refractory esophageal:** • **Caspofungin** 50 mg IV q24h; or • **vori** 200 mg po or IV q12h; or • **ampho B** 0.3-0.7 mg per kg IV q24h; or • **ampho B liposomal** 3-5 mg per kg IV q24h; or **ampho B lipid complex** 5 mg per kg IV q24h. • **Esophageal:** **Vori po q24h.** Chronic or prolonged use of azoles might promote development of resistance.	**Fluconazole-refractory disease remains uncommon** (4% in ACTG 816). As is seen in pts with low CD4 counts (<50 per mm³). **Flu** superior to oral suspension of **nystatin** (4% in ACTG 816). **Flu** superior to oral suspension of nystatin (4% in ACTG 816). **Itra** 100 mg bid times 14 days achieved clinical response in 41/74 (55%) pts unresponsive to flu. *(AIDS Res Hum Retrovir 15:1413, 1999)*. **Ampho B** suspension may be useful in refractory cases *(J AIDS 14:845, 2001)*. For esophagitis, **caspofungin** as effective as **ampho B IV** but less toxic *(CID 33:1529, 2001)*. **Voriconazole** as effective as flucon with similar toxicity profile *(AJM 113:294, 2002)*. **Micafungin** 100 mg or 150 mg IV per day equal to flucon po per day *(CID 39:842, 2004; Aliment Pharmacol 21:899, 2005)*. **Anidulafungin** 100 mg IV per day followed by 50 mg per day — in oral flu: cure rate 97% vs 98.8% *(CID 39:770, 2004)*. Pending FDA labeling.
Post-treatment chronic suppression (secondary prophylaxis) for recurrent candidiasis, most would do: if CD4 count ↑ (>200 per mm³).			**Fluconazole** 200 mg q24h does reduce risk of candida esophagitis & cryptococcosis *(NEJM 332:700, 1995)*. Concern with enhanced risk of emergence of fluconazole (azole)-resistant Candida species.
Peritonitis (Chronic Ambulatory Peritoneal Dialysis) *See Table 19, page 139*	**Fluconazole** 400 mg po q24h times 4-7 wks or **caspofungin** 70 mg IV on day 1 followed by 50 mg IV q24h for 14 days	**Ampho B**, continuous IP dosing at 1.5 mg per L of dialysis fluid times 4-6 weeks	Remove cath immediately or in 4-7 days. In 1 study, all 8 pts with candida peritonitis who received caspo responded favorably (as compared to 7/8 pts on ampho B) *NEJM 347:2020, 2002*.
Urinary. Candiduria • Usually colonization of urinary catheter, a benign event • Rarely may be source of dissemination if pt has obstructive uropathy or marker of acute hematogenous dissemination Persistent candiduria in immunocompromised pt warrants ultrasound or CT of kidneys	Remove urinary catheter or stent. 40% will clear but only 20% if antifungal *(CID 30:14, 2000)*. Antifungal rx not indicated unless pt has symptoms of UTI, neutropenic, low-birth-weight infant, has renal allograft or is undergoing urologic manipulation. Then: **fluconazole** 200 mg per day po or IV times 7-14 days OR **ampho B** 0.5 mg per kg per day IV times 1-7 days	**Fluconazole**. In a placebo controlled study, candiduria was cleared more rapidly in pts treated with flucon 200 mg per day times 14 days; 2 weeks after completion, clearance was not different than placebo group *(CID 30:15, 2000)*. **Bladder washout** with ampho B not recommended; will not treat upper tract infection. 5FC may be of value in non-albicans UTI but resistance develops rapidly. **Caspofungin** was effective in clearing candiduria in 12 pts (most with candidemia) but urine levels low *(IDSA 2003, Abst. 155)*. **NOTE:** Vori still not in active form.	
Vaginitis—Non-AIDS patients *Review article: MMWR 51(RR-6), 2002* (Candida vaginitis in AIDS patients: see *Stomatitis, vaginitis above*). *(See Table 1, page 19)* **Sporadic/infrequent**	**Oral: Fluconazole** 150 mg po times 1 **OR** itraconazole 200 mg po bid times 1 day ** For over-the-counter preparations, see below in footnote¹	**Intravaginal:** **Azoles** with 85-95% efficacy. See cure rates. See footnote¹	**In general, oral & vaginal azoles are similarly effective.** Rx aided by avoiding tight clothing, e.g., pantyhose. Oral drugs ↓ rectal candida & may ↓ relapses. **Ampho B** vaginal 50 mg suppository effective in non-albicans candida infection when other rx failed *(Am J Ob Gyn 192:2009 & 2012, 2005)*.
Chronic, recurrent (5-8%) 2-4 episodes per yr *Ref.: NEJM 351:876, 2004*	**Fluconazole** 150 mg po times 3 & then 150 mg po q wk	After 6 mos., ~90% of disease vs 36% of 173 receiving placebo. By 6 mos., off rx, 42.9% free of disease vs 21.9% who received placebo *(p <0.001)*. Significance: *NEJM 351:2554, 2004*. Only 76.9% cured 1 mo. following 3-day rx with itra *(Mycosis 48:165, 2005)*.	

¹ **Butoconazole** 2% cream (5 gm) q24h at bedtime times 3 days** or 2% cream SR 5 gm times1; or **clotrimazole** 1% cream (5 gm) at bedtime times 3 days or 1% cream (5 gm) at bedtime times 7 days (14 days may ↑ cure rate) or 100 mg vaginal tab times 7 days or 500 mg vaginal tab times 1; or **miconazole** 200 mg vaginal suppos. (1 at bedtime times 3 days**) or 100 mg vaginal suppos. q24h times 7 days or 2% cream (5 gm) at bedtime times 7 days; or **terconazole** 80 mg vaginal suppos (1 at bedtime times 3 days) or 0.4% cream (5 gm) at bedtime times 7 days or 0.8% cream 5 gm intravaginal q24h times 3 days; or **tioconazole** 6.5% vag. ointment times 1 dose²**. ** = over-the-counter product

See page 2 for abbreviations. All dosage recommendations are for adults (unless otherwise indicated) and assume normal renal function

TABLE 11A (5)

TYPE OF INFECTION/ORGANISM/ SITE OF INFECTION	ANTIMICROBIAL AGENTS OF CHOICE		COMMENTS
	PRIMARY	**ALTERNATIVE**	
Chromoblastomycosis (*J Am Acad Derm* 44:585, 2001) (*Cladosporium* or *Fonsecaea*); Cutaneous (usually feet, legs); raised scaly lesions, most common in tropical climate	If lesions small and few, **surgical excision or cryosurgery with liquid nitrogen** (*Int J Dermatol* 42:408, 2003)]. If lesions chronic, extensive, burrowing: **itraconazole.**	**Itraconazole** 100 mg po q24h times 18 months (or until response). **Terbinafine** experience disappointing.	**Terbinafine**[*plus* *itra* impressive in 35 pts rx for 12 mos. (800 mg per day)—86% mycologic cure; 12 mths dzs. over 12 (*Med Mycol* 40:258, 1998). In vitro terbinafine developed on rx chromoblastomycosis (*Mycoses* 47:216, 2004). 5/6 responded to **posaconazole** (*Drugs* 65:1560, 2005).
Coccidioidomycosis (*Coccidioides immitis*) (*ID Clin Review* 17:41, 2003; *Medicine* 83:149, 2004) (IDSA Guidelines 2005: *CID* 41:1217, 2005)			
Primary pulmonary (San Joaquin or Valley Fever). Rx low risk persistence/complication	**Antifungal rx not generally recommended.** Treat if fever, wt loss, and/or fatigue do not resolve within several wks to 2 months (see below).	Uncomplicated pulmonary in normal host. Influenza-like illness of 1–2 wks duration.	13/13 patients rx responded (*CID* 15:553, 1992).
Primary pulmonary in pts with ↑ risk for complications or dissemination.		Mild to moderate illness: **Itraconazole** solution 200 mg po q12h OR **Fluconazole** 400 mg po q24h for 3–12 months	**Ampho B cure rate 50–70%. Responses to azoles are similar. Itra may have slight advantage esp. in soft tissue infection. Relapse rates after rx 40%. Relapse rate 1 if ↑ CF titer ≥ 1:256** (*RR+ - 4.7*) (*CID* 25:1205, 1997). Following CF titers after completion of rx important; rising titers
• Immunosuppressive disease, AIDS, post-transplantation.			
• hematological malignancies (*AnM* 165:113, 2005), or therapies (steroids, TNF-α antagonists) (*Arth Rheum* 50:1959, 2004)	**Locally severe or disseminated disease:** **Ampho B** 0.6–1 mg per kg per day times 7 days then 0.8 mg per kg every other day. Total dose 2.5 gm or more, followed by **itra** or **flu.**		warrant readministration of rx (*CID* 25:1271, 1994). In an RDBS[1] of 198 pts with chronic non-meningeal cocci, **57% responded to itra** vs **72% to flu** (*p=0.05*) (*AnIM* 133:676, 2000). **Vori** effective in 1 case of widely disseminated cocci (*CID* 39:e74, 2004).
• Pregnancy in 3rd trimester			
• CF antibody >1:16	**Consultation with specialist recommended:** surgery may be required.		**Caspofungin** successful in a renal transplant pt (*CID* 39:879, 2004).
• pulmonary infiltrates			**Posaconazole**, oral suspension 800 mg per day, successful in 5/6 pts with refractory non-meningeal cocci (*CID* 40:1770, 2005) & 11/16 cases successful reported overall (*Drugs* 65:1559, 2005).
• Dissemination (identification of spherules or culture of organism from ulcer, joint effusion, pus from abscess or bone fx, etc.)	Lifetime suppression in HIV+ patients, flu 200 mg po q24h or itra 200 mg po q24h (see Comment)		
Meningitis occurs in 1/3 to 1/2 of pts with disseminated coccidioidomycosis			
Adult	**Fluconazole** 400–800 mg po q24h	**Ampho B** IV as for pulmonary (above) + (0.1–0.3 mg daily) intrathecal (intraventricular-cisternal) via reservoir device. **OR Itra** 400–800 mg po q24h **OR voriconazole** (see Comment)	**80% relapse rate, continue flucon indefinitely. Voriconazole** successful in high doses (6 mg per kg IV q12h) followed by oral suppression (400 mg po q12h) (*CID* 36:1619, 2003; failed in another case *CID* 39:879, 2004).
Child	**Fluconazole** [po] (*Pediatric dose not well established*, 6 mg per kg q24h used)	**Itra** 6–10 mg per kg per day OR **caspo** (see Comment)	**Caspofungin** also used (*JAC* 54:292, 2004) & (*CID* 39:879, 2004).
Cryptococcosis (*CID* 30:710, 2000). Excellent review: *Brit Med J* 72:99, 2005. Non-meningeal (non-AIDS)	**Fluconazole** 400 mg po or IV times 6–8 wks to 6 mos	**Itraconazole** 200–400 mg po solution q24h for 6–12 mos OR	**Flucon alone 90% effective for meningeal and non-meningeal forms.** Fluconazole as effective as ampho B (*CID* 32:E14, 2001). Addition of **interferon-γ** (IFN-γ·1b 50 mcg per
Risk: >57% organ transplant (*Transpl Inf Dis* 4:183, 2002 & *CID* 40:1756, 2005) & those receiving other forms of immunosuppressive agents (e.g. alemtuzumab—*Transplant Proc* 37:934, 2005).	**For more severe disease:** **Ampho B** 0.5–0.8 mg per kg per day IV till response then change to **fluconazole** 400 mg po q24h for 8–10 week course	**flucytosine** 37.5 mg per kg po qid times 6 wks.	M[1] subcut. 3 times per wk times 9 wks) to liposomal ampho B assoc. with response in pt failing antifungal rx (*CID* 38: 910, 2004).
Meningitis (non-AIDS)	**Ampho B** 0.5–0.8 mg per kg per day IV + **flucytosine** 37.5 mg per kg po q6h until pt afebrile and cultures negative (~6 weeks); then **fluconazole**. B/flucyt, start fluconazole 400 mg po q24h times 8–10 weeks then reduce (see CID 28:297, 1999).		**Fluconazole alone used successfully**, comparative clinical trials lacking (*NEJM* 330:263, 1994). Hydrocephalus may be successfully rx with VP[2] or VA[2] shunting (*CID* 28:629, 1999); poor response if pts encephalitis (*CID* 37:673, 2003).
HIV+/AIDS: Cryptococcosis and/or Meningitis			
Treatment (see *CID* 30:710, 2000) ↓ in incid w HAART (see p.288) but still common when pt presents w AIDS & HIV status unknown (*AIDS* 18:555, 2004). (continued on next page)	**Ampho B** 0.7 mg per kg IV q24h + **flucyto- sine** 25 mg per kg po q6h (continued on next page)	[**Fluconazole** 400–800 mg po or IV q24h for less severe disease **or** **voriconazole** (continued on next page)	If normal mental status, >20 cells per mm³ CSF, and CSF crypto antigen <1:1024, flucon alone is reasonable (*CID* 22:322, 1996). Serum cryptococcal antigen useful in dx (95% sens), no help in monitoring therapy.

[1] Some experts would reduce to 25 mg per kg q8h
[2] **VP** = ventriculoperitoneal, **VA** = ventriculoatrial.
[3] **Flucytosine** = 5-FC

See page 2 for abbreviations. All dosage recommendations are for adults (unless otherwise indicated) and assume normal renal function

TABLE 11A (6)

TYPE OF INFECTION/ORGANISM/ SITE OF INFECTION	ANTIMICROBIAL AGENTS OF CHOICE		COMMENTS
	PRIMARY	ALTERNATIVE	

Cryptococcosis/HIV+/AIDS: Cryptococcemia and/or Meningitis	**Treatment** (continued) (*data continued from previous page*)	(*continued from previous page*) If ↑ CSF pressure, lower with CSF removal (*CID 38:134, 2004*). If frequent LPs not possible, ventriculoperitoneal shunts an option (*Surg Neurol 63:529 & 531, 2005*). Higher levels assoc. with bone marrow toxicity. Ampho B does not penetrate CSF (*CID 22:S2, 1996*). In study of 230 pts (*Ln 363:1764, 2004*) pts treated with ampho B & 5FC (26%) by 2 wks; ampho alone (39%). When amb still alive & culture-neg. at 10 wks (*CID 28:82, 1999*) by combination of all 3 drugs (*p <0.001*). In 64 pts, only 12% (55%) when alive & culture-neg at 10 wks (*CID 28:82, 1999*). Successful outcomes were observed in 14/29 (48%) subjects with crypto-coccal meningitis treated with posaconazole (*AAC 56:745, 2005*). Must monitor 5-FC levels: peak 70-80 mg per L, trough 30-40 mg per L.	
With HAART, symptoms of acute meningitis may return: Immune Reconstitution Inflammatory Syndrome (IRIS), in study of 59 cryptomeningitis (CM) pts started on HAART, 18 (30%) IRIS or 17.9 events per 100 pt years. Symptoms were recrudescent CM, lymphadenitis (*CID 40:1049, 2005*). When to start HAART in pt with acute crypto pres-sure. ↑ WBC, & glucose level in pts with CM, but cultures were negative. Median time to symptoms following HAART was 30 days, but pts who received HAART within 30 days of dx & rx of CM were more likely to develop IRIS (RR 11-3 p=0.04) (*CID 40:1049, 2005*). In some, decision to start HAART 2-10 wks after treatment initiated. HAART 10-30 days after rx for CM would seem prudent albeit in 1 study, most clinicians initiate ART after 2 wks (*AIDS 19:535, 2005*).	**Fluconazole** 400-800 mg po or IV q24h + **flucytosine** 25 mg per kg po q6h times 4-6 wks or **Ampho B** 0.7 mg per kg IV times 4-6 wks **Then** **Consolidation therapy: Fluconazole** 400 mg po q24h to complete a 10-week course or until CSF culture sterile, then suppression (see below) Start Highly Active Antiretroviral Therapy (HAART) if possible.		
Suppression (chronic maintenance therapy)			
Discontinuation of antifungal rx considered if pts asymp-tomatic, with CD4 > 100–200 per mm³ for ≥6 months (*www.hivatis.org*). Must have culture-neg. CSF	**Fluconazole** 200 mg po per day	**Itraconazole** 200 mg po bid (if flu intolerant or failure)	

Dermatophytosis (See *Superficial fungal infections, Derm Ther 17:517, 2004; Brit J Derm 149:402, 2003; Am J Clin Derm 5:225, 2004; Cutis 74:516, 2004*)			
Onychomycosis (Tinea unguium) A typical nail lacquer (ciclopirox) approved in 2000; ↓ effec-tiveness after 48 wks of use, only 5-8% of pts cured in another study (*Cutis 73:81, 2004*). May enhance oral rx (*Cutis 74:55, 2004; Eur J Acad Dermatol Venereol 19:21, 2005*). Itraconazole appears to be most cost-effective rx (*J Manag Care 12:47, 2006; Manag Care Interface 18:55, 2005*). Mean cure time from 18 randomized control trials is 76% (*J Drugs Derm 4:302, 2005*).	**Fingernail Rx Options:** **Terbinafine** 250 mg po q24h times 6 wks. **Itraconazole** 200 mg po q24h times 2 mos. or **Itraconazole** 200 mg po bid times 1 wk per mo. times 2 mos. **NOTE:** *For side-effects, see footnotes 1 & 2*	**Toenail Rx Options:** **Terbinafine** 250 mg po q24h (children <20 kg: 67.5 mg per day; 20-40 kg: 125 mg per day; >40 kg: 250 mg per day) times 12 wks (76% effective)[MFDA-I] or **Itraconazole** 200 mg po q24h times 3 mos (59% effective) or **Fluconazole**[MFDA-I] 150-300 mg po q wk times 6-12 mos (48% effective)[MFDA-I] [Data reflect cure in meta-analysis of all randomized controlled trials (*Brit J Derm 150:537, 2004*)]	**Terbinafine** 250 mg po q24h (children <20 kg: 67.5 mg or >40 kg: 125 mg per day, >40 kg 250 mg per day) times 12 wks (76% effective)[MFDA-I] or **Itraconazole** 200 mg po q24h times 3 mos (59% effective) or **Fluconazole**[MFDA-I] 150-300 mg po q wk times 6-12 mos (63% effective)[MFDA-I]
Tinea capitis ("ringworm") (*Trichophyton tonsurans, Microsporum canis.* In N. America; other sp. elsewhere) (*PIDJ 18:191, 1999*)	**Terbinafine** 250 mg po q24h times 4 wks¹ for *T. tonsurans*, 4-8 wks for Microsporum canis. Children 125 mg (or 6-12 mg per kg per day) (*CID 17:97, 2004; Exp Opin Pharm Ther 5:219, 2004; J Eur Acad Dermatol Venereol 18:155, 2004*)	**Itraconazole¹** 3-5 mg per kg q24h times 4-6 wks for Microsporum canis[MFDA-I] **Itraconazole** 8 mg per kg q wk times 8-12 days[MFDA-I] or **Griseofulvin** adults 500 mg q24h times 4-6 wks, children 10-20 mg per kg per day times 6-8 wks.	All agents with similar cure rates (60-100% in clinical studies (*Ped Derm 17:304, 2000*). Griseofulvin considered drug of choice by some although concerns for resistance and toxicities. Addition of topical ketoconazole or selenium sulfate shampoo reduces transmissibility (*J Am Acad Derm 39:261, 2000*)
Tinea corporis, cruris, or pedis (*Trichophyton rubrum, T. mentagrophytes, Epidermophyton floccosum*) "Athlete's foot, jock itch," and ringworm	**Topical rx:** Generally applied 2 times per day. Available as creams, ointments, sprays, solutions. Apply 2 times per day over the counter. Apply 1 time per day for 2-3 wks. See footnote³ for names and prices. Recommend: Lomitrin Ultra or Lamisil AT, con-tain butenafine & terbinafine—both are fungicidal	**Terbinafine** 250 mg po q24h times 2 wks[MFDA-I] OR **ketoconazole** 200 mg po q24h times 4 wks or **Itraconazole** 200 mg po q24h 1 time per mo times 4 wks[MFDA-I] or **Griseofulvin** 150 mg po 1 time per day times 2-4 wks for pedis	Keto or clotrim effective in severe recalcitrant infection. Follow for hepatotoxicity. terbinafine: 87% achieved mycological cure in double-blind study (32 pts) (*J Med Assn Thai 76:388, 1993; Brit J Derm 130(543):22, 1994*) and fluconazole 78% (*J Am Acad Derm 40:31, 1999*).

¹ **Serious but rare cases of hepatic failure** have been reported in pts receiving terbinafine & should not be used in those with chronic or active liver disease. (*See Table 11B, page 83*). Suggest checking ALT & AST before prescribing (*Am J Health Sys Pharm 58:1076, 2001*).

² Use of itraconazole has been associated with onset of congestive heart failure (*see Ln 357:1766, 2001*).

³ **Drug name** (trade name) & wholesale price for 15 gm. All are applied to affected area bid. **Prescription drugs:** butenafine (Mentax) $40, ciclopirox (Loprox) $23, clotrimazole (Lotrimin) $19, Mycelex $11),
(*continued on next page*) See page 2 for abbreviations. All dosage recommendations are for adults (unless otherwise indicated) and assume normal renal function

TABLE 11A (7)

TYPE OF INFECTION/ORGANISM/ SITE OF INFECTION	ANTIMICROBIAL AGENTS OF CHOICE		COMMENTS
	PRIMARY	ALTERNATIVE	
Dermatophytosis (continued)			
Tinea versicolor (Malassezia furfur or Pityrosporum orbiculare) Rule out erythrasma—see Table 1, page 40	**Ketoconazole** (400 mg po single dose)[super NFDA] or (200 mg po q24h times 7 days) or (2% cream applied 1 time q24h times 2 wks)	Fluconazole 400 mg po single dose or Itraconazole 400 mg po q24h times 3–7 days	Keto (po) times 1 97% effective in 1 study. Another alternative: Selenium sulfide (Selsun), 2.5% lotion, apply as lather, leave on 10 min then wash off, 1 time per day times 7 day or 3–5 times per week times 2–4 weeks
Fusariosis Infections in eye, skin, sinus & disseminated diseases—↑ in transplant & cancer pts (Clin Micro Inf 10:499 & 567, 2004; COID 17:527, 2004)	**Voriconazole** 6 mg per kg IV q12h on day 1, then either (4 mg per kg q12h) or (200 mg po q12h for body weight ≥40 kg), but 100 mg po q12h for body weight <40 kg)	Ampho B 1–1.2 mg per kg or lipid-associated ampho B	Voriconazole successful in 9/21 4 eye, 2 bloodstream, 2 sinus & 1 skin (CID 35:909, 2002; 36:1122, 2003; 37:311, 2003).
Histoplasmosis (Histoplasma capsulatum) See CID 30:688, 2005; ID Clin No. Amer 17:1, 2003. Best diagnostic test 2nd generation urine, serum, or CSF histoplasma antigen. MiraVista Diagnostics (1-866-647-2847)			
Immunocompetent patient: Pulmonary, localized, disseminated Definition of severe—Temp >39.5°C, Karnofsky <60, albumin <3 gm per dL, hepatic enzymes >5 times normal, WBC <500, platelets <50,000, creatinine >6 mg per dL.	**Minimal disease: No rx** **Moderate:** Itraconazole 200 mg po solution po for 9 months. If life-threatening 200 mg po bid times 3 days; then 200 mg po bid until response. **Severe, including meningitis: Liposomal ampho B** 3 mg per kg every other day IV up to 1 gm, then switch to **itra** 200 mg per day for 9 months. **Itra not recommended for meningitis** (See CID 38:463, 2004)	Moderate: Itraconazole 200 mg per day solution po for 9 months. If life-threatening 200 mg po bid until response. If IV rx necessary: Dose 200 mg IV bid times 4 doses followed by 200 mg IV q24h (see Table 11B). Severe, including meningitis: Ampho B 4 mg per kg per day IV times 7 days, then 0.8 mg per kg every other day IV	**With ≥2 months itra rx, 86% success in chronic pulmonary & extrapulmonary** (AJM 93:489, 1992). Meningitis ↑ difficult to rx & no prospective studies. **Liposomal ampho B** recommended because of ↑ CSF levels vs ampho B. Histo antigen in CSF should fall to undetectable levels before rx dc (see CID 40:844, 2005). **Flu less effective than itra.**
Immunocompromised patient (AIDS) (CID 30:688, 2000, & 32:1215, 2001) Risk factors for death: dyspnea, platelet count <100,000 per mm³ & LDH >2 times upper limit normal (CID 38:134, 2004). In 1 study suppression was safely dc after 12 mos. of antifungal & 6 mos. of HAART with CD4 >150; 0 relapses after 2 yrs follow-up in 32 pts (CID 38:1485, 2004).	**Primary prophylaxis:** Consider for pts from endemic areas with CD4 <150 per mcL. If used: itraconazole 200 mg po q24h. **Severe disseminated: Acute phase** (3–10 days or until clinically improved) • **Ampho B** 0.7 mg per kg IV q24h; or • **liposomal ampho B** 4 mg per kg IV q24h **Continuation phase** (12 wks): Itra 200 mg po q12h **Less severe disseminated:** Itra 200 mg po q8h times 3 days, then 200 mg po q12h times 12 wks. **Meningitis:** Ampho B or liposomal ampho B times 12–16 wks. **Suppression:** Insufficient data to rec. dc with ↑ CD4 from HAART but probably OK— Itraconazole 200 mg po q24h indefinitely	**Acute phase:** Itra 400 mg po q24h **Continuation phase • Itra** oral solution 200 mg q12h; or • **flucon** 800 mg po q24h **Mild disseminated: Fluconazole** 800 mg po q24h **Amphotericin B** 1 mg per kg IV weekly or biweekly indefinitely	**Acute pulmonary histoplasmosis among HIV-1 infected pts with CD4 counts >300** per mm³ might not require rx. **Liposomal ampho B** superior at 2 wks vs ampho B (88% vs 64% clinical success) in 81 pts with ↓ nephrotoxicity (97% vs 37%) (AnIM 137:105, 2002). **Itra** (ACTG 120) 50/59 (85%) pts responded, cleared fungemia with only 5% toxicity. Avoid rifampin; reduces itra serum concentration (AJM 98:336, 1995). Mortality 12.5% in 110 cases of disseminated histo + AIDS receiving itra 300 mg po q24h for suppression at 200 mg q24h but 3/46 had probable hepatic toxicity (J AIDS & HR 16:100, 1997). Itra best drug for suppression. Itra followed by itra in Panama (CID 40:1199, 2005). Itra induces flu resistance (CID 37:1910, 2001). There are no prospective studies addressing the management of CNS histoplasmosis (CID 40:844, 2005).
Madura foot (See Nocardia & Scedosporium, below)			

econazole (Spectazole) $22, ketoconazole (Nizoral) $22, miconazole (Monistat-Derm) $25, naftifine (Naftin) $21, naftifine (Naftin) $27, oxiconazole (Oxistat) $26, sulconazole (Exelderm) $13, terconazole (Terazol) $30, sertaconazole (Ertaczo) $47. **Non-prescription (over-the-counter):** Tolnaftate (Tinactin $5, Ting or Tolnate $2), undecylenic acid (Cruex $5, Desenex $5), Lotrimin 1% 12 gm $6.17, Lamisil AT 1%, 12 gm $6.79.

¹ **Oral solution preferred to tablets because of ↑ absorption** (see Table 11B, page 83).

See page 2 for abbreviations. All dosage recommendations are for adults (unless otherwise indicated) and assume normal renal function.

TABLE 11A (8)

TYPE OF INFECTION/ORGANISM/ SITE OF INFECTION	ANTIMICROBIAL AGENTS OF CHOICE		COMMENTS
	PRIMARY	ALTERNATIVE	
Mucormycosis Zygomycetes—Rhizopus, Rhizomucor, Absidia) Rhinocerebral, pulmonary (AJM 159:1301, 1999) Key to successful rx: early dx with symptoms suggestive of sinusitis (or lateral facial pain or numbness): think mucor with palatal ulcers, &/or black exudate, unilateral blindness in immunocompromised (Ophthalmol 34:1166, 2005). Rapidly fatal without dx. Dx by biopsy of tissue or stain: wide ribbon-like, non-septated with variation in diameter & right angle branching (A-n J Clin Micro Inf Dis 24:142, 2004).	**Ampho B** Increase rapidly to 0.8–1.5 mg per kg per day, by then, when improving, then every other day. Total dose usually 2.5–3 gm. **Lipid-based Ampho B** or **Posaconazole** 200 mg qid (when available will be drug of choice)		Cure dependent on: (1) surgical debridement, (2) rx of hyperglycemia, acidosis, neutropenia, or reduction of immunosuppression (3) correction of neutropenia and use of lipid amphotericin (CID 43:2012, 2005)—striking improvement reported; 54–70% overall success in refractory zygomycosis vs 25% or less with amphotericin or lipid ampho B (Drugs 65:1553, 2005).
Nocardiosis (N. asteroides & N. brasiliensis) Culture & sensitivities may be valuable in refractory cases: Reference Labs, R.J. Wallace (903) 877-7680 or CDC (404) 639-3158 (IDCP 8:27, 1999) **Cutaneous and lymphocutaneous** (sporotrichoid)	**TMP-SMX**—5–10 mg per kg per day of SMX. TMP & 25–50 mg per kg per day of SMX in 2–4 div. doses per day, (see Comment)	**Sulfisoxazole** 2 gm po qid or **minocycline** 100–200 mg po bid	Linezolid 300–600 mg po bid times 3–24 mos. successful in 6/6 pts; 4 with disseminated disease of whom 2 had brain abscesses (CID 36: 313, 2003; Eur J Neurol 12:536, 2005)
Pulmonary, disseminated, brain abscess Duration of rx generally 3 mos. for immunocompetent host (36% & 6 mos. for immunocompromised (62% organ transplant, malignancy, chronic lung disease, diabetes, ETOH use, steroid rx, AIDS, & infliximab rx (Canad Med J 171:1063, 2004).	**TMP-SMX** 15 mg per kg per day of SMX IV or po, div. in 2–4 doses. After 3–4 wks, ↓ dose to 10 mg per kg per day as TMP, in 2–4 doses. (see Comment)	**IMP** 500 mg IV q6h⁺ (amikacin ⁻7.5 mg per kg per day q12h) times 3–4 wks & then po regimen	Survival improved when sulfa-containing regimen used (Medicine 68:38, 1999). Prosthetic valve endocarditis cured by TMP & + amikacin times 2 mos. followed by TMP-SMX times 4 mos. (A-M 115:330, 2003). Measure sulfonamide blood levels: Peak of 100–150 mcg per mL. 2 hrs post-po dose. Increasing sulfa resistance—recommend sensitivity testing (Eur J Clin Micro Inf Dis 24:142, 2005; AAC 48:632, 2004).
Paracoccidioidomycosis (South American blastomycosis)/P. brasiliensis	**Itraconazole** 200 mg per day po times 6 months or **Ketoconazole** 400 mg per day for 6–18 months	**Ampho B** 0.4–0.5 mg per kg per day IV to total dose of 1.5–2.5 gm followed by sulfonamides (dose: see Comment)	Improvement >90% pts on itra or keto. Sulfa: 4–6 gm per day for 3 weeks, then 500 mg per day for 3–5 yrs also used (CID 14 (Suppl):S-68, 1992). Low-dose itra (50–100 mg per day), keto (200–400 mg per day) and sulfadiazine (up to 6 mg per day) showed similar clinical responses in 4–6 mos. in a randomized study (Med Mycol 40: 411, 2002). HIV+: TMP-SMX suppressive rx indefinitely (CID 21:1275, 1995).
Lobomycosis (keloidal blastomycosis)/ P. loboi	**Surgical excision**, clofazimine⁺ or ampho B		
Penicilliosis (Penicillium marneffei) Common disseminated fungal infection in AIDS pts in SE Asia (esp. Thailand & Vietnam) (CID 24:1080, 1997; Int J Inf Dis 3:48, 1998)	**Ampho B** 0.5–1 mg per kg per day times 2 wks followed by **itraconazole** 400 mg per day po indefinitely for HIV-infected pts (CID 26:1107, 1998). See Comment	**Itra** 200 mg po bid times 3 days, then 200 mg bid times 12 wks. (IV if unable to take po.) For less sick patients	3rd most common in AIDS pts in SE Asia following TB: and cryptococcosis. Prolonged fever, lymphadenopathy, hepatomegaly. Skin nodules are umbilicated (mimic cryptococcal infection or molluscum contagiosum). In AIDS pts, suppressive rx with itra effective in preventing relapses (NEJM 339:1739, 1998).
Phaeohyphomycosis (black molds/ dematiaceous fungi) (See CID 41:1521, 2005) Sinuses, skin, bone, brain abscess, endocarditis **Species: Scedosporium** (see above), Bipolaris, Wangiella, Curvularia, Exophiala, Phialophora, Scytalidium, Alternaria	**Surgery + itraconazole** 400 mg per day po, duration not defined, probably 6 months⁺	**Voriconazole** has in vitro activity, but clinical experience limited vs S. prolificans (CID 37:221, 2003). **Itraconazole + terbinafine** synergistic against S. prolificans (AAC 44:470, 2000). No clinical data that combination could show toxicity (see Table 11B, page 85)	
Scedosporium apiospermum (Pseudallescheria boydii) (not considered a true dematiaceous mold) (Medicine 81:333, 2002); Mycoses (Madura foot), brain abscess, Spain. Chemotherapy (CID 25:1080, 2002, Med Mycos 44: 295, 2002). May appear after near-drowning incidents.	**Voriconazole** 6 mg per kg IV q12h (or 4 mg per kg IV q12h) day 1, then either 4 mg per kg IV q12h (>40 kg body weight ≥40 kg), but 100 mg po q12h for body weight <40 kg) (PID 21:240, 2002)		Notoriously resistant to antifungal drugs including amphotericin. In vitro voriconazole more active than itra (J Clin Micro 39: 954, 2001). Case reports of successful rx of disseminated and CNS disease with voriconazole (Clin Micro Inf 9:750, 2003; EJCMID 22:408, 2003).

⁺ **Oral solution preferred to tablets because of ↑ absorption** (see Table 11B, page 85).

See page 2 for abbreviations. All dosage recommendations are for adults (unless otherwise indicated) and assume normal renal function

TABLE 11A (9)
ANTIMICROBIAL AGENTS OF CHOICE

TYPE OF INFECTION/ORGANISM/ SITE OF INFECTION	PRIMARY	ALTERNATIVE	COMMENTS
Sporotrichosis **Cutaneous/Lymphonodular**	Itraconazole 100–200 mg per day po solution times 3–6 mos. (then 200 mg po bid long-term)" for HIV-infected pts	Fluconazole 400 mg po q24h times 6 mos. SSKI soln. 1 gm per mL, start 5–10 drops tid (max 40–50 drops tid) with 5–10 drops bid. Take after meals.	Itra ref.: CID 17:59, 2003; Derm Ther 17:523, 2004. Some authorities use ampho B po times 3–6 mos. (then 200 mg po bid long-term)" for HIV-infected pts. Resistant strains described (CID 23: 394, 1996). SSKI side-effects: nausea, rash, fever, metallic taste, salivary gland swelling.
Extraarticular: Osteoarticular, pulmonary, disseminated, meningeal	Osteoarticular, pulmonary: Itraconazole 300 mg po bid times 6–12 mos	Disseminated, meningeal: **Ampho B** 0.5 mg per kg per day to total of 1–2 gm, followed by itra 200 mg bid or flu 800 mg q24h	

TABLE 11B: ANTIFUNGAL DRUGS: ADVERSE EFFECTS, COMMENTS, COST

DRUG NAME, GENERIC (TRADE)/ USUAL DOSAGE/COST*	ADVERSE EFFECTS, COMMENTS/COMMENTS
Non-lipid amphotericin B deoxycholate (Fungizone): 0.3–1 mg per kg per day as single infusion 50 mg $36.55	**Admin.:** Ampho B is a colloidal suspension that must be prepared in electrolyte-free D5W at 0.1 mg per mL to avoid precipitation. No need to protect drug suspensions from light. Ampho B infusions cause chills/fever, myalgia, anorexia, nausea, rarely hemodynamic collapse/hypotension. Postulated due to proinflammatory cytokines but does not appear to be histamine release (Pharmacol 34:1402, 1982) Several recommends a test dose of 1 mg, but often not done (1st few mL of 1st dose is a test dose). Duration of infusion usually 4 or more hrs. No difference found in 1- vs 4-hr infusions (severe dyspnea and focal infiltrates suggesting pulmonary edema) associated with rapid infusion (CID 33:75, 2001). Rare pulmonary reactions (severe dyspnea and focal infiltrates suggesting pulmonary edema) associated with rapid infusion (CID 33:75, 2001). Severe rigors respond to meperidine (25–50 mg) IV. Premedication with acetaminophen, diphenhydramine, hydrocortisone (25–50 mg) and heparin (1000 units) had no influence on rigors/fever (CID 10:755, 1995). If cytokine postulate correct, NSAIDs or high-dose steroids may prove efficacious but their use may risk worsening infection under rx or increased risk of nephrotoxicity (i.e., NSAIDs). Clinical side-effects: ↓ with ↑ age (CID 26:334, 1998). **Toxicity:** Major concern is nephrotoxicity. Rapid fall in GFR (15% of 102 pts in one study; CID 29:1402, 1999). Manifest by kaliuresis and hypokalemia, then fall in serum creatinine. With high initial creatinine, may proceed to renal tubular acidosis (RTA) and renal failure, with rising BUN/serum creatinine. Hypomagnesemia may occur. Can reduce risk of renal injury by **(a) pre- and post-infusion hydration with 500 mL saline (if clinical status will allow salt load), (b)** avoidance of other nephrotoxins, e.g., radiocontrast, aminoglycosides, cis-platinum, **(c)** use of lipid prep of ampho B. Use of low-dose dopamine did not significantly reduce renal toxicity (AAC 42:3163, 1998). In a single randomized controlled trial of 80 neutropenic pts with refractory fever & suspected or proven invasive fungal infection, ampho B deoxycholate over 24 hrs, compared to the classical rapid infusion of 0.95 mg per kg per day, 4-hr **infused over 4 hrs.** Continuous infusion produced less nephrotoxicity (8 vs 41%) in max. serum Cr (p=0.005), a reduction in fever, chills & vomiting (p <0.05, 0.0003) & appeared as effective as rapid infusion but in very low proven fungal infections (7 & 3, respectively) (BMJ 322:1, 2001). Continuous infusion also allows a dramatic ↑ in administered dosage without sig. toxicity (CID 36:943, 2003). It is disturbing that these exciting observations have not led to controlled trials examining efficacy in rx of life-threatening fungal infections (CID 36:952, 2003). Await trials of efficacy in larger number of proven fungal infections!
¹ **Oral solution preferred to tablets because of ↑ absorption** (see Table 11B, page 82).	
Lipid-based ampho B products: **amphotericin B lipid complex (ABLC) (Abelcet):** 5 mg per kg per day as single infusion 100 mg IV $240	**Admin.:** Consists of ampho B complexed with lipid bilayer ribbons. Compared to standard ampho B, larger volume of distribution, rapid blood clearance and high tissue concentration (liver, spleen, lung). **Dosage: 5 mg per kg per day.** Infuse at 2.5 mg per kg per hr; adult and ped. dose the same. Do NOT use an in-line filter. Do not dilute with saline or mix with other drugs! **Toxicity:** Fever and chills ↑ in 1st infusion. Nausea 9%, vomiting 8%, serum creatinine ↑ in 11%, renal failure 5%, anemia 4%, ↓ K 5%; rash 4%. A fatal case of fat embolism reported following ABLC infusion (Exp Mol Path 177:246, 2004).
² Published data from patients intolerant of or refractory to conventional ampho B deoxycholate (Am J Med 137:105, 2002; Clin Micro 37:415, 2003). **None of the lipid ampho B preps has shown superior efficacy compared to ampho B in prospective trials (except lipid liposomal ampho B in Rx of disseminated histoplasmosis at 2 wks** (AnIM 137:105, 2002; Clin Micro 37:415, 2003). **Dosage equivalency has not been established** (CID 36:1500, 2003). Nephrotoxicity ↑ with all lipid preps of ampho B preps (NEJM 340:764, 1998).	
³ Comparisons between Abelcet & AmBisome suggest higher infusion-assoc. toxicity with Abelcet (70% vs 36%) but a higher frequency of mild hepatic toxicity with AmBisome (59% vs 38%, p=0.05). Mild elevations in serum creatinine were observed in 1/3 of both (BJ Haemat 103:198, 1998; Focus on Fungal Inf #9, 1999; Bone Marrow Tx 20:39, 1997; CID 26:1383, 1998).	

TABLE 11B (2)

DRUG NAME GENERIC (TRADE)/ USUAL DOSAGE/COST*	ADVERSE EFFECTS/COMMENTS
Liposomal amphotericin B (L-AmB, AmBisome): 1–5 mg/kg per day IV as single infusion. 50 mg/day $188	**Admin.:** Consists of vesicular bilayer liposome with ampho B intercalated within the membrane. Dosage: **3–5 mg per kg per day** IV as single dose; infusion time can be reduced to 60 min. (see footnote 3, page 83). 1 mg per kg per day as effective as 4 mg per kg per day (6 mos. survival rates 43% vs 37%), especially in pts with invasive aspergillosis complicating bone marrow transplant and/or neutropenia from malignancy (CID 27:1406, 1998). Tolerated well in elderly pts (J Inf 56:47, 2005). **Major Toxicity:** With ampho B. Nephrotoxicity less with liposomal ampho B: Cr ↑ in 18.7% vs 33.7%; renal function deterioration 48.7% vs 56.7%; chills 47% vs 75%, nausea 39.7% vs 38.7%, vomiting 31.8% vs 43.9%, and 24% for both. Ca 18.4% vs 20.9%, ↓ K 20.4% vs 25.6%, ↓ Mg 20.4% vs 25.6%. Acute infusion-related reactions are common with liposomal ampho B. 20–40%, 86% occurred with 5 min. of infusion, including chest pain, dyspnea & hypoxia or severe abdominal, flank or leg pain; 14% developed flushing & urticaria near the end of 4-hr infusion. All responded to diphenhydramine (1 mg per kg) & interruption of L-AmB infusion. These reactions may be due to complement activation by the liposome (CID 36:1213, 2003).
Amphotericin B cholesteryl complex (Amphotec) or **Amphotericin B colloidal dispersion, ABCD, Amphotec):** 3–4 mg per kg per day as single infusion. 100 mg $160	**Admin.:** Consists of ampho B deoxycholate stabilized with cholesteryl sulfate resulting in a disc-shaped colloidal complex. Compared to standard ampho B, largely distributes into reticuloendothelial system, rapid blood clearance. **Dosage:** Initial dose for adults & children: **3–4 mg per kg per day** IV over 2 hrs. Can ↑ to 6 mg per kg/day. Dilute in D5W & infuse at 1 mg per kg per hr. Do NOT use in-line filter. **Toxicity:** Chills 50%, fever 33%, ↑ serum creatinine 12–20%, ↓ Ca 6% & ↑ K 17% with continuing rx. Hepatotoxicity more common (incidence 1.5) in bone marrow transplant pts when ampho B (inc. 0.78/100 pt days) (CID 41:301, 2005) & ↑ with continuing rx.
Caspofungin (Cancidas) 70 mg IV day 1 followed by 50 mg IV q24h (reduce to 35 mg IV q24h with moderate hepatic insufficiency). 70 mg $424.44, 50 mg $329.47 or $485.26 for 21-day course	An echinocandin which inhibits synthesis of β-(1,3)-D-glucan. Fungicidal against candida (MIC <2 mcg per mL) including those resistant to other antifungals & active against aspergillus (MIC 0.4–2.7 mcg per mL). Interestingly, in some preclinical studies very high drug concentrations found to be less effective (AAC 48:3407, 2004), but this has not been demonstrated clinically. Approved indications for caspo include: empirical rx for febrile neutropenic pts; rx of candidemia, candida intra-abdominal abscesses, peritonitis, & pleural space infections; esophageal candidiasis; & invasive aspergillosis in pts refractory to or intolerant of other therapies. Serum levels on rec. dosages = peak 12, trough 1.3 (24 hrs) mcg per mL. **Toxicity:** remarkably non-toxic (Mycoses 48:227, 2005). Only 2% of 263 pts in double-blind trial of candidemia/invasive candida stopped rx due to drug-related adverse event (Transpl Int Dis 7:225, 2005). Most common adverse effect: phlebitis at infusion site & headache, fever, chills, vomiting, & diarrhea associated with infusion. ↑ serum creatinine in 8% on caspo vs 21% short-course ampho B in 422 pts with candidemia (Ln, Oct. 12, 2005, online). Drug metabolized in liver & dosage ↓ to 35 mg in moderate to severe hepatic failure. Class C for pregnancy (embryotoxic in rats & rabbits). See Table 22, page 146 for drug-drug interactions. See cyclosporine (hepatic toxicity) & tacrolimus (drug level monitoring recommended) interactions reported (Pharmacotherapie 24:1408, 2004).
Micafungin (Mycamine) 50 mg IV for prophylaxis post-bone marrow stem cell transplant; $95 per day. 150 mg IV per day for rx; $280.50 per day (50 mg vials). $5580.30 for 150 mg IV q24h for 21 days.	Active against most strains of candida & aspergillus sp., including those resistant to fluconazole such as C. glabrata & C. krusei. No antagonism seen when combined with other antifungal drugs & occ. synergism with ampho B (AAC 49:2994, 2005). No dosage adjustment for severe renal failure or moderate hepatic impairment. Watch for drug-drug interactions with sirolimus or nifedipine. Micafungin is well tolerated & common adverse events include nausea 2.8%, vomiting 2.4%, & headache 2.4%. Transient ↑ LFTs, BUN, creatinine reported; rare cases of significant hepatitis (see Table 22).
Anidulafungin 200 mg IV on day 1 followed by 100 mg per day for invasive candidiasis/candidemia; 100 mg IV followed by 50 mg IV q24h for esophageal candidiasis. IV (FDA approval pending) 100 mg IV day 1, then 50 mg IV q24h. (no cost data available)	An echinocandin with broad antifungal activity (cidal) against candida sp. & aspergillus sp. including ampho B- & azole-resistant strains. Effective in clinical trials of esophageal candidiasis & in 1 trial was superior to fluconazole for rx of invasive candidiasis/candidemia in 245 pts (75.6% vs 60.2%) (CMAC 2005). Like other echinocandins, remarkably non-toxic; most common side-effects: nausea, vomiting, ↓ Mg, ↓ K & headache in 11–13% of pts. Few drug-drug interactions (see Table 22). No dose adjustments for renal or hepatic insufficiency.
Fluconazole (Diflucan) 100 mg tabs NB $9.80, G $1.73 150 mg tabs NB $16, G $7 200 mg tabs NB $16, G $5 400 mg IV $123.94, G $24.42 Oral suspension: 50 mg per 5 mL, $40/35 mL; $40/35 mL bottle—NB	[IV=oral dose; for excellent bioavailability.] **Pharmacology:** absorbed po, water solubility enables IV. Peak serum levels (see Table 9, page 62). $T_{1/2}$ 30 hrs (range 20–50 hrs). 12% protein bound. CSF levels 50–90% of serum in normals. ↑ in meningitis. No effect on mammalian sterol metabolism. **Drug-drug interactions common, see Table 22.** Side-effects overall 16% [more common in HIV+ pts (21%)]. Nausea 3.7%, headache 1.9%, skin rash 1.8%, abdominal pain 1.7%, vomiting 1.7%, diarrhea 1.5%, ↑ SGOT 25%. Rare: severe hepatocellular necrosis, anaphylaxis, exfoliative dermatitis. Alopecia (scalp, pubic crest) 12–20% with higher doses (400–800 mg per day) (AnIM 123:354, 1995). Reversible (BMJ 3(2:1341, 1991). Ref: AnIM 330:263, 1994.
Flucytosine (Ancobon) 500 mg cap $9	**AEs:** Overall 30%. GI 6% (diarrhea, anorexia, nausea, vomiting). Hematologic 22% (leukopenia, thrombocytopenia ↑ with serum level >100 mcg per mL, esp. in azotemic pts.) Hepatotoxicity (asymptomatic ↑ SGOT, reversible), rash 7%, aplastic anemia (rare—2 or 3 cases). False ↑ in serum creatinine on EKTACHEM analyzer. (JAC 26:171, 2000)
Griseofulvin (Fulvicin, Grifulvin, Grisactin) 500 mg G $3.45, susp 125 mg per mL $52	Photosensitivity, urticaria, GI upset, fatigue, leukopenia (rare). Increases blood and urine porphyrins, should not be used in patients with porphyria. Minor disulfiram-like reactions. Exacerbation of systemic lupus erythematosus.
Imidazoles Topical: for vaginal use see Table 1 & Table 15A Applies broadly to topical use in terms of toxicity. Apply minimal amount to lesions twice daily.	Local reactions: 0.5–1.5%: dyspareunia, mild vaginal or vulvar erythema, burning, pruritus, urticaria, rash. Rarely, similar symptoms in sexual partner.

* From 2005 Drug Topics Red Book, Medical Economics Data and Hospital Formulary Pricing Guide. **Price is average wholesale price (AWP).**
See page 2 for abbreviations. All dosage recommendations are for adults (unless otherwise indicated) and assume normal renal function

TABLE 11B (3)

DRUG NAME: GENERIC (TRADE)/ USUAL DOSAGE/COST*	ADVERSE EFFECTS/COMMENTS
Itraconazole (Sporanox) 100 mg cap $10 10 mg per mL oral solution (fasting state) (150 mL: $141) (AAC 42:1862, 1998) IV usual dose 200 mg bid times 4 doses followed by 200 mg q24h for a maximum of 14 days ($213/250 mg)	**Itraconazole tablet and solution forms are not interchangeable. Solution preferred.** Many authorities recommend measuring drug serum concentration after 2 wks to ensure adequate absorption. To obtain the highest plasma concentration, the tablet is given with food and acidic drinks (e.g., cola) while the solution is taken in the fasted state; under these conditions, the peak conc. of the capsule is approx. 3 mcg per mL and of the solution 5.4 mcg per mL. Peak levels are reached faster (2.2 vs 5 hrs) with the solution. **Food improves the absorption of the capsule (200 mg); improves the absorption of the solution 30%. IV form (do not use in renal failure) and oral solution only contraindicated in the fasted state (200 mg); drug exposure of oral solution at steady-state 30% higher than the capsule. Liver toxicity—rare. 14% of 50 pts developed hepatitis. Oral solution contains the virtual gamma of retinoids into the CSF (do not use to treat meningitis)** Most common adverse effects are dose-related nausea 10%, diarrhea 9%, vomiting 6%, and abdominal discomfort 5.7%. Allergic rash 8.6%, bilirubin 6%, edema 3.5%, and hepatitis 2.7% reported. ↑ doses may produce hypokalemia 8% and ↑ blood pressure 3.2%. Delirium & peripheral neuropathy reported (Psychosomatics 44:260, 2003; Diabetes Care 28:225, 2005). **Reported to produce impairment in cardiac function** (see footnote 2 page 80). Severe liver failure requiring transplant in pts receiving pulse rx for onychomycosis. FDA reports 24 cases with 11 deaths out of 50 million pts who received the drug prior to warning (N Engl J Med & Werner & Werner 9/26, 2004). **Some interactions can be life-threatening.** Other concern, as with fluconazole and ketoconazole, is **drug-drug interactions; see Table 22.** Some interactions reported.
Ketoconazole (Nizoral) 200 mg tab $2.25	Gastric acid required for absorption—cimetidine, omeprazole, antacids block absorption. In achlorhydria, dissolve tablet in 4 mL 0.2N HCl, drink with a straw. Coca-Cola ↑ absorption by 65% (AAC 39:1671, 1995). CSF levels "none". **Drug-drug interactions important, see Table 22.** Some interactions can be life-threatening. **Dose-dependent nausea and vomiting.** Liver toxicity of hepatocellular type reported in about 1:10,000 exposed—usually after several days to weeks of exposure. At doses of ≥800 mg per day serum testosterone and plasma cortisol levels fall. With high doses, adrenal (Addisonian) crisis reported.
Miconazole (Monistat 7) 200 mg—not available in U.S.	IV miconazole indicated in patient critically ill with Scedosporium (Pseudallescheria boydii) infection. Very toxic due to vehicle needed to put drug into solution.
Nystatin (Mycostatin) 30 gm cream NF $8, G $2.30 500,000 units oral tab $0.70	Topical. Clinically virtually no adverse effects. PO: large doses may cause occasional GI distress and diarrhea.
Posaconazole (FDA approval pending) 200 mg po qid or 400 mg po qid with chronobblastomycosis. Clinical (See Drugs 65:1552, 2005)	An oral triazole with activity against a wide range of fungi refractory to other antifungal rx including: aspergillosis, fusariosis, Scedosporium species, zygomycosis, candidiasis, refractory coccidioidomycosis, refractory cryptococcosis, & refractory chronobblastomycosis. Clinical response in 75% of 176 AIDS pts with azole-refractory oral/esophageal candidiasis. Posaconazole has similar toxicities as other triazoles: nausea 9%, vomiting 6%, abd. pain 5%, headache 5%, diarrhea, ↑ ALT, AST, & rash (3% each). ↑ QTc interval prolongation. 12/112 pts included adrenal insufficiency, neurotoxicity, & QTc interval prolongation. Inhibits CYP3A4 (see Table 22). Significant drug-drug interactions.
Terbinafine (Lamisil) 250 mg tab $10.50	In pts receiving terbinafine for onychomycosis, rare cases (8) of idiosyncratic & symptomatic hepatic injury and more rarely liver failure leading to death or liver transplantation. The drug is **not recommended** for pts with **chronic or active liver disease**. Hepatotoxicity occurs in pts with or without pre-existing disease. Pretreatment serum transaminases (ALT & AST) advised & alternate rx used for those with abnormal levels. If symptoms develop, drug should be discontinued & liver function immediately evaluated. In controlled trials, changes in crystalline lens and retina reported—clinical significance unknown. Major drug-drug interaction is 100% ↑ in rate of clearance by rifampin. AEs: usually mild (headache, GI upset). Rare AE: neutropenia, severe skin reactions (e.g. erythema multiforme vs Stevens-Johnson). Taste disturbance (dysgeusia) 0.8 vs 0.7. Inhibits CYP2D6 enzymes (see Table 22). An acute generalized exanthematous pustulosis has been reported in 13 cases (Brit J Derm 152:780, 2005) & 5 cases of subacute cutaneous lupus erythematosus (Acta Derm Venereol 84:472, 2004).
Voriconazole (Vfend) IV: Loading dose 6 mg per kg q12h times 1 day, then 4 mg per kg IV q12h for serious aspergillosis & serious mold infections; 3 mg per kg IV q12h for serious candida infections Oral: Body weight ≥40 kg: 400 mg po q12h times 1 day, then 200 mg po q12h <40 kg body weight: 200 mg po q12h times 1 day, then 100 mg po q12h Take 1 hour before or 1 hour after eating. Oral suspension (40 mg per mL) $36.49/200 mg dose. Oral suspension dosing: Same as for oral tabs. Reduce to ½ maintenance dose for moderate hepatic insufficiency	A triazole with activity against Aspergillus sp. **including Ampho resistant strains of A. terreus** (J Clin Micro 37:2343, 1999). Active vs Candida sp. (including krusei), Fusarium sp. & various molds. Steady state serum levels reach 2.5-4 mcg per mL. Toxicity similar to other azole/triazoles including uncommon serious hepatic toxicity (hepatitis, cholestasis & fulminant hepatic failure). Liver function tests should be monitored. Most pts (≈30%) with significant ↑ in bilirubin, AST, or ALT had other serious co-morbidities & rare fever and hypertension (CID 39:884, 2004). 1 case of QT prolongation with ventricular tachycardia in a 15 y/o with ALL reported (CID 39:884, 2004). **Approx. 21% experience a transient visual disturbance** following IV or po ("altered/enhanced visual perception", "blurred vision", "color vision change" or photophobia). Visual disturbance onset within 30-60 min. after initiation of drug & lasts ≈30 min. No persistence of effect reported. Cause unknown. In patients with ClCr <50 mL per min., the drug should be given orally, not IV, since the intravenous vehicle (SBECD-sulfobutylether β-cyclodextrin) may accumulate. Hallucinations, electrolyte disturbance & pancreatitis attributed to drug concentrations (CID 39:1241, 2004). Potential for drug-drug interactions high—see Table 22 (CID 36:630, 1087, 1122, 2003). **NOTE:** Not in urine via active form. **Cost:** 50 mg tab $9, 200 mg tab $35, 200 mg IV $109

*From 2005 Drug Topics Red Book, Medical Economics Data and Hospital Formulary Pricing Guide. Price is **average wholesale price (AWP).**
See page 2 for abbreviations. All dosage recommendations are for adults (unless otherwise indicated) and assume normal renal function

TABLE 12A: TREATMENT OF MYCOBACTERIAL INFECTIONS*

Tuberculin skin test (TST). Same as PPD [MMWR 52(RR-2):15, 2003].
Criteria for positive TST after 5 tuberculin units (intermediate PPD) read at 48-72 hours:
≥5 mm induration: + HIV; immunosuppressed; ≥15 mg prednisone per day; recent close contact
≥10 mm induration: foreign-born; countries with high prevalence; IVDUsers; low income, NH residents; chronic illness; silicosis
≥15 mm induration: otherwise healthy
Two-stage test to detect sluggish positivity: If 1st PPD pos. but <10 mm, repeat intermediate PPD in 1 week. Response to 2nd PPD.
BCG vaccine: as child: If ≥10 mm induration, & from country with TBc, should be attributed to M. tuberculosis. In areas of low TB prevalence, TST reactions of ≤18 mm more likely from BCG than TB [CID 34:1457, 2002]. Routine use and ongoing no longer favored [CID 34:1449, 1457, 2002]. CDC recommends for TB suspects & pts at ↑ risk for progression to active TB & suggests either TST or QFT for individuals at ↑ risk for latent TB (LTBI). For persons who warrant testing but are deemed at low risk for LTBI [MMWR 54:49, 2005].
Whole blood interferon-gamma release assay (QuantiFERON-TB GOLD) approved by U.S. FDA as diagnostic test for TB [JAMA 286:1740, 2001; CID 34:1449, 1457, 2002]. A more sensitive assay based on M. tbc-specific antigens (QuantiFERON-TB GOLD) and an enzyme-linked immunospot method (ELISpot) using antigens specific for MTB [MMWR 52(RR-2):15, 2003; & look promising (QuantiFERON-TB GOLD) [Ln 140:769, 2004; Ln 4761, 2005; CID 40:246, 2005; JAMA 293:2756, 2005].

CAUSATIVE AGENT/DISEASE	CIRCUMSTANCES	SUGGESTED REGIMENS	
		INITIAL THERAPY	CONTINUATION PHASE OF THERAPY
I. Mycobacterium tuberculosis but TST negative (household members & other close contacts of potentially infectious cases)	Neonate—Rx essential	INH (10 mg per kg per day for 3 months)	Repeat tuberculin skin test (TST) in 3 mos. If mother's smear negative & infant's TST negative & chest x-ray (CXR) normal, stop INH. In UK, BCG is then given [Ln 21:479, 1990], unless mother HIV+. If repeat TST positive &/or CXR abnormal (hilar adenopathy &/or infiltrate), INH + RIF ... 20 mg per kg per day (or SM). Total rx 6 months. (see Category I below)
	Children <5 years of age—Rx indicated	As for neonate for 1st 3 months. Risk 2–4% 1st year	If mother is being rx, separation of infant from mother not indicated. If infant's TST positive, stop. If negative, repeat TST at 3 mos. If positive rx with INH for 9 mos.
	Older children & adults—	No rx	

CAUSATIVE AGENT/DISEASE	MODIFYING CIRCUMSTANCES	SUGGESTED REGIMENS		
		INITIAL THERAPY	ALTERNATIVE	COMMENTS
II. Treatment of latent tuberculosis infection (formerly known as "prophylaxis") [NEJM 347:1860, 2004; NEJM 350:2060, 2004; JAMA 293:2776, 2005]	(1) + tuberculin reactor & HIV+ (risk of active disease 10% per yr, AIDS 170 times ↑ due to reinfection, not INH failure)	INH (5 mg per kg per day, maximum 300 mg per day for adults; 10 mg per kg per day for children). May use twice weekly INH with DOT [MMWR 52:735, 2003]. Optimal duration 9 mos. (includes children, HIV+, & old fibrotic lesions on chest x-ray). In some cases, 6 mos. may be given for cost-effectiveness [AJRCCM 161:S221, 2000]. Do not use 6 mos. regimens in pts <18 yrs or old, or those with fibrotic lesions on chest film [NEJM 345:189, 2001]	If compliance problem: INH by DOT 15 mg per kg 2× per week times 9 mos. INH + RIF for 3 mos. effective in HIV- and HIV+ [AJRCCM 161:S221, 2000; JAMA 283:1445, 2000]. **However, there are several reports of severe & fatal hepatitis in immunocompetent pts on RIF + PZA** [MMWR 50:289, 2001]. Therefore, this regimen is no longer recommended for LTBI [MMWR 52:735, 2003; CID 39:488, 2004]. The risk appears lower in HIV+ pts [CID 39-561, 2004]. RIF 600 mg per day for 4 mos. (HIV- and HIV+). Meta-analysis suggests 3 months of INH + RIF equivalent to 'standard' (6–12 mos.) INH therapy [CID 40:670, 2005]	Reanalysis of earlier studies favors INH prophylaxis (if INH related, hepatitis case fatality rate <1% as the case) [AJM 150:2517, 1990]. Recent data suggest INH prophylaxis less hepatotoxic than previously thought [Annals IM 127:1051, 1997]. Overall risk of hepatotoxicity 0.1–0.15% [JAMA 281:1014, 1999]. Risk of INH hepatitis may be ↑ [Ln 346:199, 1995].
A. INH indicated due to high-risk (Assumes INH susceptibility likely. INH 54–88% effective in preventing active TB) for ≥20 years.	(2) Newly infected persons (TST conversion in past 2 yrs— risk 3.3% 1st yr)			
	(3) (4) + tuberculin reactors with CXR consistent with non-progressive tuberculous			
	(5) + tuberculin reactors with specific predisposing conditions; illicit drug use [MMWR 38:236, 1989], silicosis, diabetes mellitus, immunosuppressive rx, hematologic disease (Hodgkin's, leukemia), end-stage renal disease, clinical condition with substantial rapid weight loss or chronic under-nutrition, previous gastrectomy [ARRD 134: 355, 1986]			
	• NOTE: For HIV, see SANFORD GUIDE TO HIV/AIDS THERAPY and/or MMWR 48:RR-10, 1999			

CAUSATIVE AGENT/DISEASE	MODIFYING CIRCUMSTANCES	SUGGESTED REGIMENS		
		INITIAL THERAPY	ALTERNATIVE	COMMENTS
B. TST positive (organisms likely to be INH-susceptible)	Age no longer considered modifying factor (see Comments)	INH (5 mg per kg per day, max. 300 mg per day for adults; 300 mg per day for children). INH as effective at 12 mos. (65% vs 75% reduction in disease) or more as current recommendation. See II.A above for details and alternate rx.	INH (5 mg per kg per day for adults, max. 300 mg per day; 10 mg per kg per day for children). Begin INH after delivery unless HIV+ or recently infected. For women at risk for progression of latent to active disease, INH should not be delayed even during the first trimester.	
	Pregnancy—Any risk factors (II.A above)			

See page 2 for abbreviations, page 90 for footnotes

* Dosages are for adults (unless otherwise indicated) and assume normal renal/renal function   † DOT = directly observed therapy

TABLE 12A (2)

II. Treatment of latent infection with M. tuberculosis ("prophylaxis") TST positive (organisms likely to be INH-susceptible) (continued)

CAUSATIVE AGENT/DISEASE	MODIFYING CIRCUMSTANCES	SUGGESTED REGIMENS — INITIAL THERAPY	SUGGESTED REGIMENS — ALTERNATIVE	COMMENTS
TST positive & drug resistance likely (For data on worldwide prevalence of resistance, see NEJM 344:1294, 2001; JID 185:1197, 2002)	Pregnancy—No risk factors (see Comment)			Delay rx until after delivery (AJRCCM 149:1359, 1994)
	INH-resistant (or adverse reaction to INH), RIF-sensitive organisms likely	RIF 600 mg per day po for 4 mos. (HIV+ or HIV−)	IDSA guideline lists rifabutin in 600 mg per day dose as another alternative; however, current recommended max. dose of rifabutin is 300 mg per day. Estimate RIF alone has protective effect of 56%, 26% of pts reported adverse effects (only 2/157 ...) (AJRCCM 155:1735, 1997).	
	INH- and RIF-resistant organisms likely	Efficacy of all regimens unproven. (PZA 25-30 mg per kg per day to max. of 2 gm per day + ETB 15-25 mg per kg per day po) times 6-12 mos.	(PZA 25-30 mg per kg per day + levoflox 500 mg per day) or (PZA 25-30 mg per kg per day + oflox 400 mg po bid), all po. times 6-12 mos.	PZA + oflox has been associated with asymptomatic hepatitis (CID 21:1264, 1997).

III. Mycobacterium tuberculosis — Pulmonary TB

CAUSATIVE AGENT/DISEASE: III. Mycobacterium tuberculosis: Pulmonary TB [General reference on rx in adults & children: Ln 362: 887, 2003; MMWR 52(RR-11):1, 2003]

MODIFYING CIRCUMSTANCES: Rate of INH resistance known to be <4% (drug-susceptible organisms) [Modified from MMWR 52 (RR-11) 1, 2003]

Isolation essential. Pts with active TB should be isolated in single rooms, not cohorted. Older observations on relatively susceptible M. tbc before and after rx (ARRD 85:5111, 1962) may be individual. Extended isolation may be appropriate.

See footnotes, page 90
USE DOT REGIMENS IF POSSIBLE
(continued on next page)

SUGGESTED REGIMENS FOR DOSAGE AND DIRECTLY OBSERVED THERAPY (DOT) REGIMENS — SEE COMMENTS FOR DOSAGE (in vitro susceptibility known)

INITIAL PHASE

Regimen (in order of preference)	Drugs	Interval/Doses[a] (min. duration)
1 (See Fig. 1, page 89)	INH RIF PZA ETB	7 days per wk times 56 doses (8 wk) or 5 days per wk times 40 doses (8 wk)[a]
2 (See Fig. 1, page 89)	INH RIF PZA ETB	7 days per wk times 14 doses (2 wk), then 2 times per wk times 12 doses (6 wk) or 5 days per wk times 10 doses (2 wk)[a] then 2 times per wk times 12 doses (6 wk)
3 (See Fig. 1, page 89)	INH RIF PZA ETB	3 times per wk times 24 doses (8 wk)
4 (See Fig. 1, page 89)	INH RIF ETB	7 days per wk times 56 doses (8 wk) or 5 days per wk times 40 doses (8 wk)[a]

CONTINUATION PHASE OF THERAPY

Regimen	Drugs	Interval/Doses[a] (min. duration)	Range of Total Doses (min. duration)
1a	INH/RIF	7 days per wk times 126 doses (18 wk) or 5 days per wk times 90 doses (18 wk)[a]	182-130 (26 wk)
1b	INH/RIF	2 times per wk times 36 doses (18 wk)	92-76 (26 wk)
1c[c]	INH/RPT	1 time per wk times 18 doses (18 wk)	74-58 (26 wk)
2a	INH/RIF	2 times per wk times 36 doses (18 wk)	62-58 (26 wk)
2b[c]	INH/RPT	1 time per wk times 18 doses (18 wk)	44-40 (26 wk)
3a	INH/RIF	3 times per wk times 54 doses (18 wk)	78 (26 wk)
4a	INH/RIF	7 days per wk times 217 doses (31 wk) or 5 days per wk times 155 doses[a]	273-195 (39 wk)
4b	INH[3]/RIF[3]	2 times per wk times 62 doses (31 wk)	118-102 (39 wk)

Dosage — Dose in mg per kg (max. q24h dose)

Regimen* Q24h:	INH	RIF	PZA	ETB	SM	RFB
Child	10-20 (300)	10-20 (600)	15-30 (2000)	15-25	20-40 (1000)	10-20 (300)
Adult	5 (300)	10 (600)	20-25 (2000)	15-25	15 (1000)	5 (300)
2 times per wk — Child	20-40 (900)	10-20 (600)	50-70 (4000)	50	25-30 (1500)	10-20 (300)
2 times per wk — Adult	15 (900)	10 (600)	50-70 (4000)	50	25-30 (1500)	5 (300)
3 times per wk — Child	20-40 (900)	10-20 (600)	50-70 (3000)	25-35	25-30 (1500)	NA
3 times per wk — Adult	15 (900)	10 (600)	50-70 (3000)	25-35	25-30 (1500)	NA

COMMENTS: Second-line anti-TB agents can be dosed as follows to facilitate DOT: Cycloserine 500-750 mg po q24h (3-5 times per wk). Ethionamide 500-750 mg po q24h. Kanamycin or capreomycin 15 mg per kg IM/IV q24h (5 times per wk). Ciprofloxacin 750 mg po q24h (5 times per wk). Ofloxacin 600-800 mg po q24h (5 times per wk). Levofloxacin 750 mg po q24h (5 times per wk) (CID 21:1245, 1995).

COMMENTS: Risk factors for drug-resistant TB: Recent immigration from Latin America or Asia or living in area of ↑ resistance (≥4%) or previous rx without RIF; exposure to known MDR-TB. Incidence of MDR-TB in U.S. appears to have stabilized and may be slightly decreasing in early 1990s (JAMA 278:833, 1997). Incidence of primary drug resistance is particularly high (>25%) in parts of China, Thailand, Russia, Estonia & Latvia (NEJM 344:1294, 2001; NEJM 347:1850, 2002). (continued on next page)

* Dosages are for adults (unless otherwise indicated) and assume normal renal function

[a] DOT = directly observed therapy

See page 2 for abbreviations, page 90 for footnotes

TABLE 12A (3)

CAUSATIVE AGENT/DISEASE	MODIFYING CIRCUMSTANCES	SUGGESTED REGIMEN	DURATION OF TREATMENT (mo.)*	SPECIFIC COMMENTS*	COMMENTS
III. Mycobacterium tuberculosis A. Pulmonary TB (continued from previous page) REFERENCE: AAC 47:683, 1996	INH (± SM) resistance	RIF, PZA, ETB (an FQ may strengthen the regimen in pts with extensive disease). Emergence of FQ resistance a concern (LnID 3:432, 2003)	6	(continued from previous page) In British Medical Research Council trials, 6-mo. regimens have yielded ≥95% success rates provided resistance to INH if 4 drugs were used in the initial phase & RIF + ETB or SM were used throughout (ARRD 133: 423, 1986). Additional studies suggested that results were best if PZA was also used throughout the 6 mos (ARRD 136:1339, 1987). TCs were not universally used, but may strengthen the regimen for pts with more extensive disease. INH should be stopped in cases of INH resistance [see MMWR 52(RR-11):1, 2003 for additional discussion]	(continued from previous page) For MDR TB regimens (~30% RIF-resistant strains are rifabutin-susceptible). Note that CIP not as effective as PZA + ETB in multidrug regimen for susceptible TB (CID 22:287, 1996). Moxifloxacin, gatifloxacin and levofloxacin have enhanced activity vs tuberculosis (AAC 46: 1022, 2002; AAC 47:2242, 2003; AAC 47:3117, 2003; JAC 53:441, 2004; AAC 48:780, 2004). FQ resistance has been seen in pts previously treated with FQ (CID 37:1448, 2003). Linezolid has activity in vitro, including MDR strains (AAC 47: 416, 2003). Mortality reviewed: Ln 349:71, 1997
Multidrug-Resistant Tuberculosis (MDR TB) Defined as resistant to at least 2 drugs. P clusters with high mortality (AnIM 119:17, 1993; ECMID 23: 174, 2004) **See footnotes, page 90** Reviews of therapy for MDR TB: JAC 54:593, 2004; Med Lett 2:83, 2004	Resistance to INH & RIF (± SM)	FQ, PZA, ETB, IA ± alternative agent[7]	18-24	In such cases, extended rx is needed to ↓ the risk of relapse. In cases with extensive disease, the use of an additional agent (alternative agents) may be prudent to ↓ the risk of failure & acquired drug resistance. Resectional surgery may be appropriate.	Rapid (24-hr) diagnostic tests for M. tuberculosis: (1) the Amplified Mycobacterium tuberculosis Direct Test amplifies and detects the ribosomal RNA; (2) the AMPLICOR Mycobacterium tuberculosis Test amplifies and detects M. tuberculosis DNA. Both tests have sensitivities & specificities >95% in sputum samples that are AFB-positive. In AFB-negative samples, the specificity remains >95% but sensitivity is 40-77% (AJRCCM 155:1497, 1997). Note that MTB may grow out on standard blood agar plates in 1-2 wks (J Clin Micro 41: 1710, 2003).
	Resistance to INH, RIF (± SM), & ETB (or PZA)	FQ [ETB or PZA if active], IA, & 2 alternative agents[7]	24	Use the first-line agents to which there is susceptibility. Add 2 or more alternative agents in case of extensive disease. Surgery should be considered. Survival ↑ in pts receiving active FQ & surgical intervention (AJRCCM 169:1103, 2004).	
	Resistance to RIF	INH, ETB, FQ, supplemented with PZA (for first 2 mos) IA may be included for the first 2-3 mos. for pts with extensive disease)	12-18	Q24i & 3 times per wk regimens of INH, PZA, & SM given for 9 mos. were effective in a BMRC trial (ARRD 115:727, 1977). However, INH & RIF could not be tested in this regimen. If ETB was used instead of PZA, INH, ETB & SM would be as effective as SM for 9 mos. An all-oral regimen of INH, ETB, & FQ times 12-18 mos. should be effective. But for more extensive disease &/or to shorten the duration (e.g., to 12 mos.) IA may be added in the initial 2 mos. of rx.	

CAUSATIVE AGENT/DISEASE; MODIFYING CIRCUMSTANCES	SUGGESTED REGIMENS (In vitro susceptibility known)		DURATION OF TREATMENT (mo.)	COMMENTS
	INITIAL THERAPY	**CONTINUATION PHASE OF THERAPY**		
B. Extrapulmonary TB	INH + RIF (or RFB) + PZA q24h times 2 months. Authors add pyridoxine	INH + RIF	6	6-month regimens probably effective. Most experience with 9-12 mo. regimens. Am Acad Ped (1994) recommends 6 mos. rx for isolated cervical adenitis, renal and 12 mos for meningitis, miliary, bone/joint. DOT useful here as well as for pulmonary tuberculosis. IDSA recommends 6 mos for lymph node, pleural, pericarditis, disseminated disease, genitourinary & abdominal TBc; 6-9 mos. for bone & joint; 9-12 mos. for CNS (including meningioma) TBc. Corticosteroids recommended only for pericarditis & meningeal TBc [MMWR 52(RR-11):1, 2003].
C. Tuberculosis meningitis For critical appraisal of adjunctive steroids: CID 25:872, 1997	INH + RIF + ETB + PZA	May add INH + RIF when susceptibility to INH and RIF established. See Table 9, page 62, for CSF drug penetration.	9-12 months	INH is drug of choice for TB. Infection with MDR TB ↑ mortality & morbidity (CID 38:851, 2004). Dexamethasone (for 1st month) has been shown to ↓ complications (Pediatrics 99:226, 1997) & ↑ survival in pts >14 yrs old (NEJM 351:1741, 2004). PCR of CSF markedly increases diagnostic sensitivity and provides rapid (1 day) diagnosis (J Neuro 45:2228, 1995; J Neuro 53:771, 1996) but could be considerable variability in sensitivity depending on method used (LnID 3:633, 2003).
D. Tuberculosis during pregnancy	INH + RIF + ETB (or) 9 months	PZA not recommended: teratogenicity data inadequate. SM should not be used unless drugs contraindicated. Add pyridoxine 25 mg/day or per kg per day for pregnant women on INH. Breast-feeding should not be discouraged in pts on first-line drugs [MMWR 52(RR-11):1, 2003]		
E. Treatment failure or relapse: Usually due to poor compliance or resistant organisms [AJM 102:164, 1997]	Directly observed therapy (DOT). Check susceptibility of original isolates and obtain susceptibility on current isolates. Add ≥2-3 agents not previously given. See Table III-A, page 87 & above)	Pts whose sputum has not converted after 5-6 mos. = treatment failures. Failures may be due to non-compliance or resistant isolates. Non-compliance common; resistant organisms common, modify regimen to include at least 2 effective agents, preferably ones which pt has not received. Surgery may be necessary. In HIV+, reinfection is a possible cause of "failure"		**DOT** = directly observed therapy

* Dosages are for adults (unless otherwise indicated) and assume normal renal function

See page 2 for abbreviations, page 90 for footnotes

TABLE 12A (4)

FIGURE 1: TREATMENT ALGORITHM FOR TUBERCULOSIS *(Modified from MMWR 52(RR-11):1, 2003)*

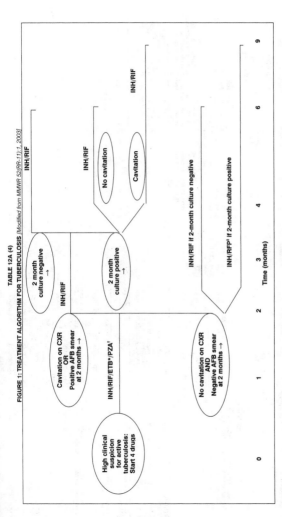

If the pt has HIV infection & the CD4 cell count is <100 per mcL, the continuation phase should consist of q24h or 3 times per wk INH & RIF for 4–7 months.
* ETB may be discontinued in <2 months if drug susceptibility testing indicate no drug resistance. † PZA may be discontinued after 2 months (56 doses). ‡ RFP should not be used in HIV patients with tuberculosis or in patients with extrapulmonary tuberculosis.

See page 2 for abbreviations

TABLE 12A (5)

CAUSATIVE AGENT/DISEASE	MODIFYING CIRCUMSTANCES	SUGGESTED REGIMENS PRIMARY/ALTERNATIVE		COMMENTS

III. Mycobacterium tuberculosis (continued)

F. HIV infection or AIDS pulmonary or extrapulmonary

	INH + RIF (or RFB) + PZA		1. Because of the possibility of developing resistance to RIF in pts with low CD4 cell counts who receive weekly or biweekly doses of INH, pts receive q24h (or minimally 3 times weekly) doses of RIF (or RFB) for initiation & continuation phase of rx (MMWR 51:214, 2002).
	INH + RIF (or RFB) q24h times 2 mos.		2. May treat up to 18 mos. in pts with delayed response.
	(Authors add **pyridoxine** 25-50 mg q24h to regimens that include INH)		3. Clinical and microbiologic response as in HIV-negative patient although there is considerable variability in outcomes among currently available studies (CID 32:623, 2001).
			4. Post-treatment suppression not necessary for drug-susceptible strains.
			5. Rate of INH resistance known to be <4% (↑ ↑ rates of resistance, see Section III.A).
			6. For more information, see MMWR 47(RR-20):1, 1998; CID 28:139, 1999; MMWR 52(RR-11):1, 2003
			7. INH resistant patient rx: daily or intermittent therapy: 1 dose per day for 2 weeks followed by 2-3 doses per week for 24 weeks (MMWR 47(RR-20), 1998].

Concomitant protease inhibitor (PI) therapy *(Modified from MMWR 49:185, 2000; AJRCCM 162:7, 2001)*

Initial & cont. therapy:		**Comments:** Rifamycins induce cytochrome CYP450 enzymes (RIF > RFB > RFP > RFB) & reduce serum levels of concomitantly administered PIs. Conversely, PIs (ritonavir > amprenavir > indinavir = nelfinavir > saquinavir) inhibit CYP450 & cause ↑ serum levels of RIF, RFP & RFB. If dose of RFB is not reduced, toxicity (ritonavir > amprenavir > indinavir = nelfinavir > saquinavir) inhibit CYP450 & cause ↑ serum levels of RIF, RFP & RFB. If dose of RFB is not reduced, toxicity
INH 300 mg + RFB (see below for dose) + PZA 25 mg per kg + ETB 15 mg per kg q24h times 2 mos., then INH + RFB times 4 mos. (up to 7 mos.)		

	RFB Dose		(↑ uveitis) may result. † RFB/PI combinations are therapeutically effective (CID 30:779, 2000). RFB has no effect on nelfinavir levels at dose of 1250 mg bid (Can J ID 12:69, 1999). **Although RFB is preferred, RIF can be used for rx of active TB in pts on regimens containing efavirenz or ritonavir. RIF should not be administered to pts on ritonavir + saquinavir because drug-induced hepatitis with marked transam elevations has been seen in healthy volunteers receiving this regimen (www.fda.gov).**
PI Regimen		
Nelfinavir 1200 mg q12h or indinavir 1000 mg q8h or amprenavir 1200 mg q12h:	150 mg q24h or 300 mg intermittently	
Lopinavir/ritonavir—standard dose	150 mg 2 times per wk.	

Alternative regimen:
INH + SM + PZA + ETB times 2 mos., then INH + SM + PZA 2-3 times per wk for 7 mos. May be used with any PI regimen. May be prolonged up to 18 mos. in pts with delayed response.

FOOTNOTES: * When DOT is used, drugs may be given 5 days per wk & the necessary number of doses adjusted accordingly. Although there are no studies that compare 5 with 7 q24h doses, extensive experience indicates this would be an effective practice. † Patients with cavitation on initial chest x-ray & positive cultures at completion of 2 months of rx should receive a 7-month (31 wk, either 217 doses [q24h] or 62 doses [2 times per wk] continuation phase. § 5-day a wk administration is always given by DOT. ¶ Not recommended for HIV-infected pts with CD4 cell counts <100 cells per mL. Options 1c & 2c should be used with caution in HIV-infected pts. # EMB can be d/c if drug sensitivities are known & strain is sensitive to INH & RIF. ◊ pts who do not have cavitation on initial chest x-ray. For pts started on this regimen & found to have a pos. culture from the 2-month specimen, rx should be extended an additional 3 months. ♣ Abbreviations: RIF, rifampin; RFB, rifabutin; RFP, rifapentine; INH, isoniazid; PZA, pyrazinamide; SM, streptomycin; EMB/ETB, ethambutol; PAS, para-aminosalicylic acid; AM-CL, linezolid. # Modified from MMWR 52(RR-11):1, 2003. See also JCP 11:329, 2002.

IV. Other Mycobacterial Disease ("Atypical") (See ATS Consensus: AJRCCM 152:51, 1997; IDC Rev, March 2002; CMR 15:716, 2002)

A. M. bovis

		INH + RIF + ETB		The M. tuberculosis complex includes M. bovis. All isolates resistant to PZA. 9-12 months of rx used by some authorities. Isolation not required.

B. Bacillus Calmette-Guerin (BCG) *(derived from M. bovis)*

Only fever (>38.5 C) for 12-24 hrs.	INH 300 mg q24h times 3 months		Intravesical BCG effective in superficial bladder tumors and carcinoma in situ. Adverse effects: fever (febrile reaction in 2.9%, granulomatous pneumonitis/hepatitis 0.7%, sepsis 0.4% (J Urol 147:596, 1992). With sepsis, consider INH + RIF + ETB
Systemic illness or sepsis	INH 300 mg q24h + (RIF 600 mg) + (ETB 1200 mg) q24h times 6 mos.		consider initial adjunctive prednisolone. Reports up to 40% BCG may cause regional adenitis or pulmonary disease in HIV-infected children (CID 37:1226, 2003).

C. M. avium-intra-cellulare complex (MAC, MAI, or Battey bacillus) ATS Consensus Statement: AJRCCM 156:51, 1997. Clin Chest Med 23:633, 2002

Immunocompetent patients with chronic pulmonary, disseminated disease (subcutaneous, bones)

Clarithro 500 mg bid or **azithro** 600 mg po q24h) + **ETB** 25 mg per kg po times 2 mos., then 15 mg per kg q24h) + **RIF** 600 mg po q24h (or **RFB** 300 mg po q24h). May add **AK** 15 mg per kg 3 times per wk for 2-6 mos. for severe disease. Alternative: **Clarithro** 500 mg bid (or **azithro** 600 mg po q24h until "ten", then 50 mg per kg 3 times per week), times 1 yr. Alternative: **Clarithro** 500 mg bid + **ETB** 15-25 mg per kg po + **RFB** 300 mg po q24h for up to 24 mos. (Curr Inf Dis Reps 2:163, 2000). Late in rx, consider intermittent dosing azithro 500 mg 3 times per week also effective (CID 32:1547, 2001).		**"Classic" pulmonary MAC:** (Men 50-70, smokers, COPD. May be associated with hot tub use (Clin Chest Med 23:675, 2002). **"New" pulmonary MAC:** Women 50-70, scoliosis, mitral valve prolapse, (bronchiectasis), pectus excavatum ("Lady Windermere syndrome"). May also be associated with hot tub use (Clin Chest Med 23:756, 2002). Susceptibility testing of MAC not recommended except clarithro testing of isolates from pts who have failed prior clarithro rx. **3 times per wk SM may be effective in immunocompetent patients (JID 178:1278, 1998; CID 30:288, 2000). Late "failures" (following completion of therapy) after treatment with clarithro or azithro in nodular bronchiectasis usually represent reinfection, not failure of rx (JID 186:266, 2002).**

See page 2 for abbreviations.   * *Dosages are for adults (unless otherwise indicated) and assume normal renal function*   † DOT = directly observed therapy

TABLE 12A (6)

CAUSATIVE AGENT/DISEASE; MODIFYING CIRCUMSTANCES	SUGGESTED REGIMENS		COMMENTS
	PRIMARY	**ALTERNATIVE**	

IV. Other Mycobacterial Disease ("Atypical") *(continued)*

CAUSATIVE AGENT/DISEASE; MODIFYING CIRCUMSTANCES	PRIMARY	ALTERNATIVE	COMMENTS
C. M. avium-intra-cellulare complex *(continued)* Immunocompromised pts: CD4 count <50–100 per mm³. Discontinue when CD4 count >100 per mm³ in response to HAART (NEJM 342:1085, 2000; CID 31:1245, 2000). Guideline: AnIM 137:435, 2002	**Azithro** 1200 mg po weekly OR **RFB** 300 mg po q24h OR **Azithro** 1200 mg po weekly + **RFB** 300 mg po q24h	**RFB** 300 mg po q24h OR **Azithro** 1200 mg po weekly + **RFB** 300 mg po q24h	RFB reduces MAC infection rate by 55% (no survival benefit); azithro by 68% (30% survival benefit); clarithro by 68% (69% survival benefit). RFB more effective than either alone but is not as well tolerated (NEJM 335:392, 1996). **Many drug-drug interactions, see Table 22, pages 148, 150.** Drug-resistant MAC disease seen in 29–58% of pts in whom disease develops while taking clarithro prophylaxis (J Inf 38:6, 1999). Clarithro resistance more likely in on azithro that has not been observed with RFB prophylaxis (CID 24:S; 1997, NEJM 335:384 & 428, 1996). RFB used for prophylaxis may be not to active M. tbc; RFB should be sure no active M. tbc. Poor selection of rifamycin-resistant M. tbc
Treatment Either presumptive dx or after positive culture of blood, bone marrow, or other usually sterile body fluids, e.g. liver	**Clarithro** 500 mg* po bid or **azithro** 600 mg po q24h) + **ETB** 15–25 mg per kg per day + **RFB** 300 mg po q24h *Higher doses of clari (1000 mg po bid) may be associated with ↑ mortality (CID 29:125, 1999)	**Clarithro** or **azithro** + **ETB** + one or more of: **CIP** 750 mg po bid or **Oflox** 400 mg po bid + **Amikacin** 7.5–15 mg per kg IV q24h In pts ketoconazole protease inhibitors can use clarithro 500 mg po bid (or **azithro** 600 mg) + **ETB** 15–25 mg per kg per day (if the pt has not had prior rifamycin therapy) (Johns Hopkins AIDS Report 9:2, 1997)	Median time to neg. blood culture: clarithro + ETB 4.4 wks vs azithro + ETB >16 wks. At 16 wks. clearance of bacteremia seen in 37.5% of azithro- & 85.7% of clarithro-treated pts (CID 27:1278, 1998). More recent study suggests similar clearance rates for azithro (46%) vs clarithro (56%) at 24 wks when combined with ETB (CID 27:1245, 2000). Azithro 250 mg po q24h not effective, but azithro 600 mg po q24h as effective as 1200 mg q24h & yields fewer adverse effects (AAC 43: 2869, 1999). Addition of RFB to clarithro + ETB ↑ emergence of resistance to clari, ↓ relapse rate & improves survival (CID 37:1234, 2003). Data on clofazimine difficult to assess. Earlier study suggested adding CLO of no value (CID 25:621, 1997). More recent study suggests it may be as effective as RFB in 3 drug regimens-containing clari, & ETB (CID 29:125, 1999) although it may not be as effective as RFB at present, early clari resistance (CID 28:136, 1999). Thus, pending more data, we still do not recommend CLO for MAI in HIV+ pts. Drug toxicity: With clarithro, 23% pts had to stop drug 2° to dose-limiting adverse reaction (AnIM 121: 905, 1994). Combination of clarithro, ETB and RFB led to uveitis and pseudojaundice (NEJM 343:1301, 1999). With low dose of RFB (300 mg)
Chronic post-treatment suppression—secondary prophylaxis	Always necessary. **Clarithro** (or **azithro**) 1-2 mg per kg per day (see dosage above)	**Clarithro** or **azithro** or **RFB** (dosage above)	Recommendations almost universal without chronic suppression. However, in patients on HAART with robust CD4 cell response, it may be possible to discontinue chronic suppression (JID 178:1446, 1998; NEJM 340:1301, 1999).
D. Mycobacterium celatum Treatment; optimal regimen not defined		May be susceptible to **clarithro**, **FQ** (Clin Micro Infect 3:582, 1997). Suggest rx "like MAI" but often resistant to RIF (J Inf 38:157, 1996). Most reported cases received 3 or 4 drugs.	Isolated from pulmonary disease and blood in AIDS patients (CID 24:144, 1997). Easily confused with M. xenopi (and MAC). Susceptibilities similar to MAC, but highly resistant to RIF (CID 24:140, 1997).
E. Mycobacterium chelonae ssp. abscessus ‐‐‐‐‐‐‐‐‐‐‐‐ **Mycobacterium chelonae ssp. chelonae**	Treatment; Surgical excision may facilitate clarithro rx in subcutaneous abscesses and is important adjunct to rx (CID 24:1147, 1997)	**Clarithro** 500 mg po bid times 6 mos. (AnIM 119:482, 1993) 2/3 of pts resistant to RIF, cefoxitin, & EMB (J Clin Micro 30: 2745, 2001). For serious disseminated infections add tobramycin + IMP for 1° 2 wks (Clin Micro Rev 15:716, 1997).	M. abscessus susceptible to AMK (70%), clarithro (95%), cefoxitin (70%), CLO, cefmetazole. Single isolates of M. abscessus often drug resistant associated with disease. Clarithro-resistant strains now described (J Clin Micro 39: 2745, 2001). M. chelonae susceptible to AMK (80%), clarithro, azithro, tobramycin (100%), IMP (60%), gatifloxacin (90%), moxifloxacin (AAC 46:3283, 2002). Resistant to cefoxitin, FQ (AJRCCM 156:51, 1997).
F. Mycobacterium fortuitum Treatment; optimal regimen not defined. Surgical exci-sion of infected areas.		**AMK** + **cefoxitin** + **probenecid** 2–6 wks, then po **TMP-SMX**, or **doxycycline** (usually responds to 6–12 mos. of rx with 2 drugs to which it is susceptible (AAC 46:3283, 2002). Clin Micro Rev 15:716, 2002). Nearly all strains respond to newer FQs & to macrolides.	**Resistant to all standard anti-TBc drugs.** Sensitive in vitro to doxycycline, minocycline, cefoxitin, IMP, AMK, TMP-SMX, CIP, ofloxacin, azithro, clarithro, gatifloxacin (80%) (AAC 46: 3283, 2002). Linezolid also active in vitro (JAC 45:764, 2002). M. fortuitum respond to rifabutin, rifabutin (JAC 39:567, 1997). May be resistant to azithromycin.

See page 2 for abbreviations.   * Dosages are for adults (unless otherwise indicated) and assume normal renal function   ¹ DOT = directly observed therapy

TABLE 12A (7)

CAUSATIVE AGENT/DISEASE; MODIFYING CIRCUMSTANCES	SUGGESTED REGIMENS		COMMENTS
	PRIMARY	**ALTERNATIVE**	
IV. Other Mycobacterial Disease ("Atypical") (continued)			
G. Mycobacterium haemophilum	Regimen(s) not defined. In animal model, **clarithro**, **rifabutin** effective (AAC 38:1987, 1994). **RIF + RFB + clarithro** shown effective though clinical experience limited (Clin Micro Inf 2:642, 1996). Surgical debridement may be necessary (CID 26:505, 1998).		Clinical: Ulcerating skin lesions, synovitis, osteomyelitis. Lab: Requires supplemented media to isolate. Sensitive in vitro to: CIP, cycloserine, rifabutin. Over ½ resistant to: INH, RIF, EMB, PZA (AVM 120:118, 1994).
H. Mycobacterium genavense	Regimens used include ≥2 drugs: **ETB, RIF, RFB, CLO, clarithro** in animal model, **clarithro** & **RFB** (& to lesser extent amikacin & **ETB**) shown effective in reducing bacterial counts (CID 26:505, 1998).		Clinical: CD4 <50. Symptoms of fever, weight loss, diarrhea. Lab: Growth in BACTEC vials slow (mean 42 days). Subcultures grow only on Middlebrook 7H11 agar containing 2 mcg per ml mycobactin J—growth still insignificant for in vitro testing (Ln 340:76, 1992; AnIM 117:586, 1992). Survival ↑ from 81 to 263 days in pts rx for at least 1 month with ≥2 drugs (AAC 46:3462, 2004).
I. Mycobacterium gordonae	Regimen(s) not defined, but consider **RIF + ETB + KM or CIP** (J Inf 38:157, 1999).		Susceptible in vitro to ETB, RIF, AMK, CIP, clarithro, linezolid (AAC 47:1736, 2003). Resistant to INH (CID 14:1229, 1992). Surgical excision.
J. Mycobacterium kansasii	[24q po: **INH** (300 mg) + **RIF** (600 mg) + **ETB** (25 mg per kg times 2 mos., then 15 mg per kg times 18 mos. (until culture-neg sputum times 12-15 mos. if HIV+ pt.) (See Comment)	If rifampin-resistant, po q24h: **INH** (900 mg) + **pyridoxine** (50 mg) + **ETB** (25 mg per kg) + **sulfamethoxazole** (1.0 gm tid) Rx until pt culture-neg sputum times 12-15 mos. (See Comment)	**All isolates are resistant to PZA**. Rifapentine, azithro, ETB effective alone or in combination in athymic mice (AAC 42:417, 2001). Highly susceptible to linezolid in vitro (AAC 47:1736, 2003). If HIV+ give rifabutin either clarithro (500 mg bid) or RFB (150 mg per day) for INH (AAC 156:S1, 1997). Because of variable susceptibility to INH, some substitute clarithro for INH. Resistance to clarithro reported (DMID 31:369, 1998), but most strains susceptible as well as moxifloxacin (AAC 55:S60, 2005) & levofloxacin (AAC 48:4562, 2004). Prognosis related to level of immunosuppression.
		Clari + **ETB** + **RIF** also effective in small study (CID 37:1178, 2003).	
K. Mycobacterium marinum	[**Clarithro** 500 mg (bid) **or** (**minocycline** 100-200 mg q24h) **or** (**TMP-SMX** 160/800 mg po bid), **or** (**RIF** + **ETB**) for 3 mos. (AJM 63:339, 1977). Rx 3 mos. after symptoms resolve, usually 3-4 mos. total (CID 31:439, 2000) **or** (**doxycycline** 100 mg po bid)		Resistant to INH & PZA (AJRCCM 156:S1, 1997). Also susceptible in vitro to linezolid (AAC 47:1736, 2003); CIP, gatifloxacin, moxifloxacin also show moderate in vitro activity (AAC 46:1114, 2002).
L. Mycobacterium scrofulaceum	Surgical excision. Chemotherapy seldom indicated. Although regimens not defined, start 4 drugs as for disseminated MAI.		In vitro resistant to INH, RIF, ETB, PZA, AMK, CIP (CID 20:549, 1995). Susceptible to clarithro, strep, erythromycin.
M. Mycobacterium simiae	Regimen(s) not defined. Start 4 drugs as for disseminated MAI.		Most isolates resistant to all 1st-line anti-tbc drugs. Isolates often not clinically significant (CID 26:625, 1998).
N. Mycobacterium ulcerans (Buruli ulcer)	**RIF + AMK** (7.5 mg per IM bid) **or** (**RIF** + **strep**) for 4-6 weeks. Surgical excision.	**ETB + TMP-SMX** (160/800 mg po tid) for 4-6 weeks. Surgical excision.	Susceptible in vitro to RIF, strep, CLO, ofloc, amikacin (AAC 42:2070, 1998; AAC 45: 231, 2000; AAC 46:3193, 2002). Monotherapy with RIF selects resistant mutants in mice (AAC 47:1228, 2003). RIF + strep effective in small study (AAC 49:3182, 2005). Treatment generally disappointing—see review, (Int J Inf Dis 6:80, 2002).
O. Mycobacterium xenopi	Regimen(s) not defined (CID 24:226 & 233, 1997). Some recommend a **macrolide** + (**RIF or rifabutin**) + **ETB ± SM** (AJRCCM 156:S1, 1997) or **RIF + INH ± ETB** (Resp Med 97:439, 2003) but recent study suggests no need to Rx HIV+ pts with MAI (CID 37:1250, 2003)		Susceptible in vitro to clarithro, strep, RIF, ofloc; resistant to ethionamide. Clarithro + RIF + EMB ± streptomycin improved survival in small study (Int J Tuberc Lung Dis 6:1203, 2002) and rifabutin (AAC 39:567, 1997) and many standard antimycobacterial drugs. Clarithro-containing regimens more effective than RIF/INH/ETB regimens in mice (AAC 45:3229, 2001). Also, linezolid active in vitro.
Mycobacterium leprae (leprosy) Paucibacillary (tuberculoid or indeterminate) Multibacillary (lepromatous or borderline) **See Comment for erythema nodosum leprosum** Rev. Lancet 363:1209, 2004	**Dapsone** 100 mg q24h unsupervised + **RIF** 600 mg once per month supervised for 6 months. **Ethionamide** (250 mg q24h) or **CLO** 50 mg q24h + (**CLO** 300 mg once per month supervised) + **RIF** 600 mg + month supervised) for 24 mg q24h unsupervised) for 24 mos. + (**CLO** 300 mg once per months; minimum of 2 yrs Rx. (CID 24:209 & 1994) Recent data suggest 12 mos. rx effective (Ln 353:655, 1999).	**Dapsone** + **(ofloc 400 mg + minocycline 100 mg) (Ln 353:655, 1999). Dapsone** + (**ofloc 400 mg** + **minocycline** 100 mg) q24h. For erythema nodosum leprosum, (prednisone 60-80 mg per day or thalidomide 100-300 mg per day) + **CLO** (See Comment) (Cin 26:S8, 1998). [Ofloc 400 mg po q24h, bactericidal and may be substituted for CLO [Ofloc 400 mg po q24h, bactericidal and clinically effective with 4 trials reference: Ln 345:4, 1995.] 1 recent study suggests dapsone monotherapy as effective as combination rx for multibacillary leprosy (AAC 38:2249, 1994). Regimens incorporating clarithro, minocycline, RIF. Ofloc showing promise as alternatives (AAC 44:2919, 2000). High relapse rate in pts treated with q24h RIF + ofloc for 4 wks (AAC 41:1953, 1997). Resistance to dapsone (Ln 349:103, 1997). Dapsone (or acedapsone^(a-3)) effective for prophylaxis (J Inf 41:137, 2000).	

See page 2 for abbreviations.   * Dosages are for adults (unless otherwise indicated) and assume normal/renal function   † **DOT** = directly observed therapy

TABLE 12B: DOSAGE, PRICE AND SELECTED ADVERSE EFFECTS OF ANTIMYCOBACTERIAL DRUGS[1]

AGENT (TRADE NAME)	USUAL DOSAGE*	ROUTE/[†] DRUG RESISTANCE (RES)†† US**/COST**	SIDE-EFFECTS, TOXICITY AND PRECAUTIONS	SURVEILLANCE
FIRST LINE DRUGS				
Ethambutol (Myambutol)	25 mg per kg per day for 2 months & then 15 mg per kg per day q24h as 1 dose [Bactericidal to both extracellular and intracellular organisms]	po RES: 0.3% (0–0.7%) 400 mg tab $1.80	**Optic neuritis** with decreased visual acuity, central scotomata, and loss of green and red perception; peripheral neuropathy and headache (~1%), rashes (rare). Anaphylactoid reaction (rare). **Comment:** Primarily used to inhibit resistance. Disrupts outer cell membrane in M. avium with ↑↑ activity to other drugs.	Monthly visual acuity & red/green with dose >15 mg per kg per day. ≥10% loss considered significant. Usually reversible if drug discontinued
Isoniazid (INH) (Nydrazid, Laniazid, Teebaconin)	Q24h dose: 5–10 mg per kg per day up to 300 mg per day as 1 dose. Twice weekly dose: 15 mg per kg per day. [Bactericidal to both extracellular and intracellular organisms] (< 10% protein binding) Add pyridoxine in alcoholic, pregnant, or malnourished pts.	po RES: 4.1% (2.6–6.8%) 300 mg tab $0.13 [IM (IV route not FDA-approved but has been used, esp. in AIDS)] 100 mg per ml in 10 ml vials (IM) $16.64	Overall ~1%. Liver: **Hepatitis** (children 10% mild ↑ SGOT, normalizes with continued rx, age <20 yrs rare, 20–34 yrs 1.2%, ≥50 yrs 2.3%) [also ↑ with q24h alcohol or for >2 months. Overall 0.1–2.3% (Ln ID 36:293, 2003)]. **Peripheral neuropathy** (17% on 6 mg per kg per day, less on 300 mg, increase in slow acetylators); **pyridoxine 10 mg q24h will ↓ incidence.** May be high. With prodromal sx, dark urine do LFTs; discontinue if SGOT >3–5 times normal. CNS toxicity, optic neuritis, convulsions, optic neuritis, toxic encephalopathy, psychosis, muscle twitching, dizziness, coma (all rare), allergic skin rashes, fever, minor disulfiram-like reaction, flushing after Swiss cheese, dark red blood dyscrasias (rare). **Drug-drug interactions common, see Table 22**	Pre-rx liver functions. Repeat if symptoms (fatigue, weakness, malaise, anorexia, nausea or vomiting >3 days (A/RCCM 152: 1705, 1995). Some recommend SGOT at 2, 4, 6 months esp. if age >50 years. Clinical evaluation every month.
Pyrazinamide	25 mg per kg per day (maximum 2.5 gm per day) q24h as 1 dose [Bactericidal for intracellular organisms]	po 500 mg tab $1.09	**Arthralgia; hyperuricemia** (with or without symptoms); hepatitis (high rx dose not exceeded); gastric irritation; photosensitivity (rare).	Pre-rx liver functions. Monthly SGOT, uric acid. Measure serum uric acid if symptomatic (gouty attack occurs).
Rifamate[*]—combination tablet	2 tablets single dose q24h	po (1 hr before meal) 1 tab $2.65	1 tablet contains 150 mg INH, 300 mg RIF	As with individual drugs
Rifampin (Rifadin, Rimactane, Rifocin)	10.0 mg per kg per day up to 600 mg per day q24h as 1 dose (60–90% protein binding)	po RES: 0.2% (0–0.3%) 300 mg cap $1.90 (IV available, Merrell Dow, Cost 600 mg $90.28)	INH/RIF dict in ~3% for toxicity, gastrointestinal irritation, antibiotic-associated colitis, drug fever (1%), pruritus with or without skin rash (1%), anaphylactoid reactions in HIV+ pts, mental confusion, transient abnormalities in liver function. **"Flu syndrome"** (fever, chills, headache, bone pain, shortness of breath) seen if RIF taken irregularly or if q24h dose given at an interval of more than 4x wk. **Discolors urine, tears, sweat, contact lens an orange–brownish color.** May cause drug-induced lupus erythematosus (LEJS 347: 1777).	Pre-rx liver function. Repeat if symptoms. **Multiple significant drug-drug interactions, see Table 22.**
Rifater[*] combination tablet (See Side-Effects)	Wt ≥55 kg, 6 tablets single dose q24h	po (1 hr before meal) 1 tab $1.96	1 tablet contains 50 mg INH, 120 mg RIF, 300 mg PZA. Used in 1st 2 months of rx. (PZA 25 mg per kg). Purpose is convenience ie, compliance (AnIM 122: 951, 1995). Swiss cost 1.58 more. Side-effects = individual drugs.	As with individual drugs. PZA 25 mg per kg
Streptomycin	15 mg per kg IM q24h; 0.75–1.0 gm per day initially then for 60–90 days, then 1.0 gm 2–3 times per week (15 mg per kg per day) q24h as 1 dose	IM (or IV) RES: 3.9% (2.7–7.6%) 1.0 gm $9.10	Overall 8%. **Ototoxicity**: vestibular dysfunction (vertigo); paresthesias (dizziness, nausea (all less in pts receiving 2–3 doses per week); tinnitus and high frequency loss (1%); nephrotoxicity (rare), peripheral neuropathy (rare), allergic skin rashes 4–5%, drug fever. Give deeply IM. (AMA Dept of Drugs, 607: 7441.) Ref: V—C/D 19:1150, 1994. Toxicity similar with rpt vs ltd dosing (CID 38:1538, 2004).	Monthly audiogram, (dizziness, serum creatinine or BUN at start of rx and weekly if pt stable

* Adult dosage only. ‡ Mean (range) (higher in Hispanics, Asians, and patients <10 years old); ** Average wholesale price according to 2005 Drug TOPICS Red BOOK, Medical Economics For review of adverse effects, see A/RCCM 167:1472, 2003.

* Adult dosage only • Dosages are for adults (unless otherwise indicated) and assume normal renal/renal function † **DOT** = directly observed therapy

[1] Note: Malabsorption of antimycobacterial drugs may occur in patients with AIDS enteropathy.
[2] **RES** = % resistance of M. tuberculosis

See page 2 for abbreviations • Dosages are for adults (unless otherwise indicated) and assume normal renal/renal function

94

TABLE 12B (2)

AGENT (TRADE NAME)	USUAL DOSAGE*	ROUTE/[1] DRUG RESISTANCE (RES) US[1]/COST**[1]	SIDE-EFFECTS, TOXICITY AND PRECAUTIONS	SURVEILLANCE
SECOND LINE DRUGS (more difficult to use and/or less effective than first line drugs)				
Amikacin (Amikin)	7.5–10.0 mg per kg per day (15 mg per kg per day) q24h[1]	IV or IM RES: (est. 0.1%) 500 mg $7.80	See Table 10, pages 64 & 74 Toxicity similar with gd vs tid dosing (CID 38:1538, 2004).	Monthly audiogram. Serum creatinine or BUN weekly if pt stable
Capreomycin sulfate (Capastat sulfate)	1 gm per day (15 mg per kg per day) q24h as 1 dose	IM RES: 0.1% (0–0.9%) 1 gm $25.54	Nephrotoxicity (36%), ototoxicity (auditory 11%), eosinophilia, leukopenia, skin rash, fever, hypokalemia, neuromuscular blockade.	Monthly audiogram, weekly serum creatinine or BUN
Ciprofloxacin (Cipro)	750 mg bid	po, IV 750 mg (po) $5.53	TB not an FDA-approved indication for CIP. Desired CIP serum levels 4-6 mcg per mL; requires median dose 800 mg (AJRCCM 151:2006, 1995). Discontinuation rates 6-7%. CIP well tolerated (AJRCCM 151:2006, 1995). FQ-resistant M. Tb identified in New York (Ln 345:1148, 1995) See Table 10, pages 64 & 71 for adverse effects.	None
Clofazimine (Lamprene)	50 mg per day (unsupervised) + 300 mg 1 time per month supervised or 100 mg per day	po (with meals) 50 mg $0.20	Skin pigmentation (pink-brown-black) 75–100%, dryness 20%, pruritus 5%. GI: abdominal pain 50% (rarely severe leading to exploratory laparoscopy), splenic infarction (VR), bowel obstruction (VR). Eye: conjunctival irritation, retinal crystal deposits.	None
Cycloserine (Seromycin)	750–1000 mg per day (15 mg per kg per day) 2–4 doses per day [Bacteriostatic for both extracellular & intracellular organisms]	po RES: 0.1% (0–0.3%) 250 mg cap $3.50	Convulsions, psychoses (5–10% of those receiving 1.0 gm per day), headache, somnolence, hyperreflexia, increased CSF protein and pressure, peripheral neuropathy. 100 mg pyridoxine per day concomitantly. Contraindicated in epileptics.	None
Dapsone	100 mg per day	po 100 mg $0.20	Blood ↓ hemoglobin (1–2 gm) & ↑ retics (2–12%) in most pts. Hemolysis in G6PD deficiency. Methemoglobinemia. CNS peripheral neuropathy (rare). GI: nausea, vomiting. Renal: albuminuria, nephrotic syndrome. Erythema nodosum leprosum in pts rx for leprosy (25% of pts).	None
Ethionamide (Trecator-SC)	500–1000 mg per day (15–20 mg per kg per day) 1–3 doses per day [Bacteriostatic for extracellular organisms only]	po RES: 0.8% (0–1.5%) 250 mg tab $3.09	Gastrointestinal irritation (up to 50% on large dose), goiter, peripheral neuropathy (rare), convulsions (rare), changes in affect (rare); difficulty in diabetes control, rashes, hepatitis, purpura, stomatitis; gynecomastia, menstrual irregularity. Give drug with meals or antacids; 50–100 mg pyridoxine per day concomitantly, SGOT thirony. Possibly teratogenic.	None
Ofloxacin (Floxin)	400 mg bid	po, IV 400 mg (po) $4.2	Not FDA-approved indication. Overall adverse effects 11%, 4% discontinued due to side-effects. GI: nausea 3%, diarrhea 1%. CNS: insomnia 3%, headache 1%, dizziness 1%.	None
Para-aminosalicylic acid (PAS, Paser) (Na+ or K+ salt)	4–6 gm bid (200 mg per kg per day) [Bacteriostatic for extracellular organisms only]	po RES: 0.8% (0–1.5%) 450 mg $0.08 (see Comment)	Gastrointestinal irritation (10–15%), goitrogenic action (rare); depressed prothrombin activity (rare); G6PD-mediated hemolytic anemia (rare), drug fever, rashes, hepatitis, myalgia, arthralgia. Retards hepatic enzyme induction; may ↓ INH hepatotoxicity. Available from CDC. (404) 639-3670, Jacobus Pharm. Co. (609) 921-7447	None
Rifabutin (Mycobutin)	300 mg per day (prophylaxis or treatment)	po 150 mg $7.19	Polymyalgia, polyarthralgia, leukopenia, granulocytopenia. Anterior uveitis when given with concomitant clarithromycin and used with rx per wk (MJM 330:438, 1994). Uveitis reported with 300 mg per day (AnIM 12:510, 1994). Reddish urine, orange skin (pseudojaundice).	None
Rifapentine (Priftin)	600 mg twice weekly for 1st 2 mos., then 600 mg q week	po 150 mg $3.00	Similar to other rifabutins. (See Rif, RFB.) Hyperuricemia seen in 2% on weekly rx (Ln 353:1843, 1999). Causes red-orange discoloration of body fluids.	None
Thalidomide (Thalomid)	100–300 mg po q24h (may use up to 400 mg q24h for severe erythema nodosum leprosum)	po 50 mg $42.36	Contraindicated in pregnancy. Causes severe life-threatening birth defects. Sedative, constipation. Available only through restricted distribution methods (Pregnancy Category X). Primarily causes drowsiness and somnolence. May cause peripheral neuropathy. (AJM 108:487, 2000.) For review, see Ln 363:1803, 2004	Available only through pharmacists participating in System for Thalidomide Education and Prescribing Safety (S.T.E.P.S.)

* Adult dosage only; † Mean (range) (higher in Hispanics, Asians, and patients <10 years old); ** Average wholesale price according to 2005 Drug Topics Red Book, Medical Economics

† **RES** = % resistance to drug. ‡ M. tuberculosis

See page 2 for abbreviations † Dosages are for adults (unless otherwise indicated) and assume normal renal function ‡ **DOT** = directly observed therapy

TABLE 13A: TREATMENT OF PARASITIC INFECTIONS*

Many of the drugs suggested are not licensed in the United States. The following are helpful resources available through the Center for Disease Control and Prevention (CDC) in Atlanta. Website is www.cdc.gov. General advice for parasitic diseases other than malaria: (770) 488-7760 or (770) 488-7775.
For CDC Drug Service: 8:00 a.m.–4:30 p.m. EST: (404) 639-3670 (or -2888); emergency after hours: (404) 639-2888; fax: (404) 639-3717.
For malaria: Prophylaxis advice (770) 488-7788 or (877) 394-3228 or (877) 394-8747, treatment (770) 488-7788; website: www.cdc.gov/travel, fax (888) 232-3299
NOTE: All dosage regimens are for adults with normal renal function unless otherwise stated.
For licensed drugs, suggest checking package inserts to verify dosage and side-effects. Occasionally, post-licensure data may alter dosage as compared to package inserts.
For abbreviations of journal titles, see page 3 **Reference with pediatric dosages:** Medical Letter on-line version: www.medletter.com **(August 2004)**

INFECTING ORGANISM	SUGGESTED REGIMENS		COMMENTS
	PRIMARY	**ALTERNATIVE**	
PROTOZOA—INTESTINAL (non-pathogenic: E. hartmanni, E. dispar, E. coli, Iodamoeba butschlii, Endolimax nana, Chilomastix mesnili)			
Balantidium coli	**Tetracycline** 500 mg po qid times 10 days	**Metronidazole** 750 mg po tid times 5 days	See Table 10C, for side-effects.
Blastocystis hominis: Role as pathogen controversial	**Nitazoxanide:** Adults 500 mg po bid times 3 days, children ages 1-3, 100 mg, ages 4-11 200 mg—both po bid times 3 days (TRSM 91:701, 1997)	**Metronidazole** 750 mg po tid times 10 days. Based on 1 placebo-controlled trial (J Travel Med 10:128, 2003). **Alternatives: Iodoquinol** 650 mg po tid times 20 days **or TMP-SMX-DS**, one bid times 7 days	
Cryptosporidium parvum and hominis Treatment is unsatisfactory Ref: CID 39:504, 2004	**HIV with immunodeficiency:** (1) Effective anti-retroviral therapy best therapy, (2) **Nitazoxanide** 500 mg po bid times 14 days in adults (60% response) in HIV+ children.		**Nitazoxanide:** Approved in liquid formulation for rx of children & 500 mg tabs for adults. Ref.: CID 40:1173, 2005. **C. hominis** assoc. with 1 in post-infection eye & joint pain, recurrent headache, & dizzy spells (CID 39:504, 2004).
	Immunocompetent—No HIV: Nitazoxanide 500 mg po bid times 3 days		
Cyclospora cayetanensis	Immunocompetent pts: **TMP-SMX-DS** tab 1 po bid times 10 days times 7-10 days	AIDS pts: **TMP-SMX-DS** tab 1 po qid times 10 days, then 1 tab 3 times per week times 2 wks.	If sulfa-allergic: **CIP** 500 mg po bid times 7 days & then 1 tab po 3 times per week times 2 wks.
Dientamoeba fragilis	**Iodoquinol** 650 mg po tid times 20 days	**Tetracycline** 500 mg po qid times 10 days OR **Metronidazole** 500-750 mg po tid times 10 days	Other alternatives: doxy 100 mg po bid times 10 days; paromomycin 500 mg tid times 7 days
Entamoeba histolytica; amebiasis Reviews: N Engl J 361:1025, 2003; NEJM 348:1563, 2003			
Asymptomatic cyst passer	**Paromomycin** (aminosidine in U.K.) 500 mg po tid times 7 days OR **Iodoquinol** 650 mg po tid times 20 days	**Diloxanide furoate**[NUS] (Furamide) 500 mg po tid times 10 days (Source: Panorama Compound Pharm., 800-247-9767)	Metronidazole not effective vs cysts.
Patient with diarrhea/dysentery; mild/moderate disease. Oral rx possible	**Metronidazole** 500-750 mg po tid times 10 days or **tinidazole** 2 gm once daily times 3 days followed by: Either [**paromomycin** 500 mg po tid times 7 days] or [**iodoquinol** 650 mg po tid times 20 days]	[**Tinidazole** 1 gm po q12h times 3 days] or [**ornidazole**[NUS] 500 mg po q12h times 5 days] followed by: **paromomycin** (was diiodohydroxyquin) 650 mg po tid times 20 days	**Dx:** antigen detection & PCR better than O&P (Clin Micro Ln 351:1672, 1998) Watch out for non-pathogenic E. dispar (Ln 351:1672, 1998)
Severe or extraintestinal infection, e.g., hepatic abscess	**Metronidazole** 750 mg **Iv** or **PO** tid times 10 days or **tinidazole** 2 gm once daily times 5 days followed by **paromomycin** 500 mg po tid times 7 days		**Serology positive (antibody present) with extraintestinal disease.**
Giardia lamblia; giardiasis	[**Tinidazole** 2 gm po times 1] OR [**nitazoxanide** 500 mg po bid times 3 days]	**Metronidazole** 500-750 mg po tid times 5 days (not approved in U.S.) See Comment. Rx if pregnant: **Paromomycin** 500 mg 4 times per day times 7 days	**Refractory pts** (metro 750 mg po + **quinacrine**[1] 100 mg po tid times 3 wks). Ref. CID 33:22, 2001; **Nitazoxanide** ref.: CID 40:1173, 2005.
Isospora belli	**TMP-SMX-DS** tab 1 po bid times 10 days; in AIDS pts: **TMP-SMX-DS** qid times 10 days & then bid times 3 wks.	[**Pyrimethamine** 75 mg per day po + **folinic acid** 10 mg per day po] times 14 days **OR CIP** 500 mg po bid times 7 days— 87% response (AnIM 132:885, 2000)	Chronic suppression in AIDS pts: either 1 TMP-SMX-DS tab 3 times per wk OR (pyrimethamine 25 mg per day po + folinic acid 5 mg per day po)

---

[1] **Drugs available from CDC Drug Service: 404-639-2888 or –3670 or www.cdc.gov/ncidod/srp/drugs/formulary.html: Bithionol, Bithionol, dehydroemetine, diethylcarbamazine (DEC), melarsoprol, nifurtimox, stibogluconate (Pentostam), suramin.**

[2] Quinacrine available from Panorama Compounding Pharmacy, (800) 247-9767, (818) 988-7979.

* See page 2 for abbreviations. All doses are for adults(unless otherwise indicated) and assume normal renal function.

TABLE 13A (2)

INFECTING ORGANISM	SUGGESTED REGIMENS		COMMENTS
	PRIMARY	ALTERNATIVE	
PROTOZOA—INTESTINAL (continued)			
Microsporidiosis			
Ocular: Encephalitozoon hellum or cuniculi, Vittaforma (Nosema) corneae, Nosema ocularum.	For HIV pts: antiretroviral therapy key	In HIV+ pts, reports of response of E. hellum to **Albendazole 400 mg po bid times 3 weeks**	To obtain fumagillin: 800-292-6773 or www.leiterrx.com. Neutropenia & thrombocytopenia serious adverse events. Dr. Molina labs use modified thromb/blue for corneal infection
	Albendazole 400 mg po bid times 3 weeks	For V. corneae, may need keratoplasty	
Intestinal (diarrhea): Enterocytozoon bieneusi, Encephalitozoon (Septata) intestinalis	**Albendazole 400 mg po bid times 3 weeks**; peds dose: 15 mg per kg per day div. into 2 daily doses times 7 days	Oral **fumagillin 20 mg po tid** reported effective for E. bieneusi (NEJM 346:1963, 2002)—see Comment	for micrographs for species identification. FA and PCR methods in development. Peds dose ref: PIDJ 23:915, 2004
Disseminated: E. hellum, cuniculi or intestinalis, Pleistophora sp., others in Comment	**Albendazole 400 mg po bid times 3 weeks**	No established rx for Pleistophora sp.	For Trachipleistophora sp., try itraconazole + albendazole (NEJM 351:42, 2004). Other pathogens: Brachiola vesicularum & algerae (NEJM 351:42, 2004)
PROTOZOA—EXTRAINTESTINAL			
Amebic meningoencephalitis			
Acanthamoeba sp.— no proven rx Rev: Clin Micro Rev 16:273, 2003	Success with IV **pentamidine**, topical **chlorhexidine** & 2% **ketoconazole** cream & then po **itra** (NEJM 331:85, 1994); 2 children responded to po TMP-SMX + rifampin + keto (CID 37:1304, 2003; Arch Path Lab Med 128:466, 2004)		For treatment of keratitis, see Table 1, page 11
Balamuthia mandrillaris	A cause of chronic granulomatous meningitis		
Naegleria fowleri. > 95% mortality.	**Pentamidine + clarithro + flucon + sulfadiazine + flucytosine**		
Sappinia diploidea	**Ampho B** 1.5 mg per kg per day in 2 div. doses & then 1 mg per kg per day IV times 6 days		
Babesia microti; babesiosis (CID 22:1117, 2001)	**Azithro** 500-600 mg po bid po times 7-10 days **+ atovaquone** 750 mg po q12h times 7-10 days (NEJM 343:1454, 2000)	**Clinda**mycin (600 mg po tid) + (**quinine** 650 mg po tid) times 7-10 days. For adults, can give **clinda** IV as 1.2 gm bid	Can cause overwhelming infection in asplenic patients. Reported in Washington State (EID 10:622, 2004).
Ehrlichiosis—See Table 1, page 42			
Leishmaniasis NOTE: Responses of various species differ—see references. U.S. military experience: CID 39:1674, 2004			
Visceral—Kala-azar L. donovani: India/Africa L. infantum: Mediterranean L. chagasi: New World **WARNING: Avoid combined antimony & ampho B** (Ln 351:1928, 1998)	**Miltefosine**[NUS] drug of choice—see Comment. **Adults:** 2.5 mg per kg per days po either as once or twice daily times 28 days **Children** (<12 yrs old): 2.5 mg per kg per day in 3 div. doses after meals times 28 days Refs: NEJM 347:1737, 1739, & 1794, 2002; PIDJ 22:434, 2003	**Lipid formulations** of ampho B effective in short-course regimens but impractical due to expense: **Children:** Liposomal ampho B >98% success (CID 38:560, 2003) in dose of 10 mg per kg per day times 2 days. **Adults:** Liposomal Ampho B 2 mg per kg per day times 5 days (CID 38:377, 2004).	**Antimony (stibogluconate or meglumine antimonate)** 20 mg per kg per day of antimony (Sb) (in 2 div. doses) IM or IV times 28 days. Not marketed in U.S. Contact CDC Drug Service: (404) 639-3670. **Miltefosine:** Available from Zentaris, Frankfurt, Germany: impavido@zentaris.de.
Mucosal—L. braziliensis	**Antimony,** as for Visceral	**Ampho B** 1 mg per kg IV every other day times 20-30 doses	Approx. cure rates: antimony 60%, AmB >75%
Cutaneous: **Most resolve spontaneously; Rx goal: ↓ time to cure & prevention of mucocutaneous spread** Old World: L. major New World: L. tropica & L. major Multiple species	**Fluconazole** 200 mg po once daily times 6 wks. Effective vs L. major (NEJM 346:891, 2002). New World—L.v. panamensis: **Miltefosine**[NUS] 2.5 mg per kg per day times 28 days 91% success (CID 38:1266, 2004).	Other options all IV: **Antimony,** as for visceral, or **Pentamidine** 2-4 mg per kg per day or qd times 4-7 doses	For **miltefosine**, contact Zentaris: impavido@zentaris.de. Treatment is species-specific. Good review (does not include miltefosine): JAC 53:158, 2004. **Other treatment options:** (1) Physical destruction by heat (CID 40:1148 & 1156, 2005; (2) Parenteral antimony + topical imiquimod (CID 40:1395, 2005); (3) Parenteral antimony + topical GM-CSF (JID 190:1793, 2004).

* See page 2 for abbreviations. All dosage recommendations are for adults (unless otherwise indicated) and assume normal renal function.

TABLE 13A (3)

INFECTING ORGANISM	SUGGESTED REGIMENS		COMMENTS
	PRIMARY	ALTERNATIVE	

PROTOZOA—EXTRAINTESTINAL (continued)

Malaria (Plasmodia species)—NOTE: CDC Malaria info—prophylaxis (877) 394-8747; treatment (770) 488-7788. After hours: 770-488-7100.
Websites: www.cdc.gov/ncidod/dpd/parasites/malaria.htm; www.who.int/health-topics/malaria.htm.

Prophylaxis—Drugs plus personal protection: screens, nets, 30–35% DEET skin repellent (Ultrathon), permethrin spray on clothing and nets *(AnIM 128:931, 1998)*

For areas **free of chloroquine-resistant** P. falciparum: Haiti, Dominican Republic, Central America west and north of the Panama Canal, and parts of the Middle East	**Chloroquine phosphate** (300 mg base) po per week, starting 1–2 wks before travel, during travel, & 4 wks post-travel (1 day prior to, during, & 7 days post-travel)	**CQ** may be taken. **CQ** safe during pregnancy. **The areas free of CQ-resistant falciparum malaria continue to shrink:** Central America west of Panama Canal, Haiti, and parts of Middle East. CQ-resistant falciparum malaria reported from Saudi Arabia, Yemen, Oman, & Iran.	
		CQ dose: 8.3 mg per kg (5 mg per kg base) per wk up to 300 mg (base) dose **or** **AP** by weight (peds tabs): 11–20 kg, 1 tab; 21–30 kg, 2 tabs; 31–40 kg, 3 tabs; >40 kg, 1 adult tab per day	
For areas with **CQ-resistant P. falciparum**	**Atovaquone-proguanil** 100 mg (**Malarone**) comb. tablet, 1 per day with food 1–2 days prior to, during, & 7 days post-travel. Peds dose in footnote¹ Cost per 2 wks.: $125. **Note:** May exacerbate psoriasis.	**Doxycycline** 100 mg po daily for adults & children >8 yrs of age¹ Cost per 2 wks.: $30 **OR** **Mefloquine (MQ)** 250 mg (228 mg base) po per week, 1 wk before, during, and for 4 wks after travel. Cost per 2 wks.: $80 [Peds dose in footnote]	**Pregnancy:** MQ current best option. Insufficient data with Malarone. **Avoid doxycycline and primaquine.** **Primaquine:** Used only if prolonged exposure to endemic area (e.g., Peace Corps). **Can cause hemolytic anemia if G6PD deficiency present.** MQ **not recommended** if cardiac conduction abnormalities, seizures, or psychiatric disorders, e.g., depression, psychosis. MQ outside U.S. 275 mg tab, contains 250 mg of base.
CDC voice info on prophylaxis in (888) 232-3228 or website: www.cdc.gov	Another option for adults: **primaquine (PQ)** 30 mg base po daily in non-pregnant G6PD-neg travelers 88% protective vs P. falciparum, > 92% vs P. vivax *(CID 33:1990, 2007)*.		Do not use halofantrine due to cardiac adverse events. Drug used for prophylaxis of P. vivax & P. ovale but presently not available in U.S. CDC Hotline: 770-488-7788.

Treatment—Based on CDC Guidelines (8/05) for drugs currently available in U.S. Artesunate drugs of major import in SE Asia & Africa but presently not available in U.S.

Clinical Severity/ Plasmodia sp.	Region Acquired	Suggested Treatment Regimens (Drug)		Comments
		Primary—Adults	Alternative & Peds	
Uncomplicated/ P. falciparum (or not identified)	Central America, west of Panama Canal, Haiti, Dominican Republic, & most of Middle East—**CQ-sensitive**	**CQ** 1 gm salt (600 mg base) po, then 0.5 gm in 6 hrs, then 0.5 gm daily times 2 days. Total: 2500 mg salt	**Peds CQ** 10 mg per kg of base po, then 5 mg per kg of base at 6, 24, & 48 hrs. Total: 25 mg per kg	Peds dose should never exceed adult dose.
Uncomplicated or unknown resistance	CQ-resistant or unknown resistance	**QS** 650 mg po tid + [(**Doxy** 100 mg po bid) or (**tetra** 250 mg po qid)] times 7 days **OR** **AP** 1 gm–400 mg (4 adult tabs) po once daily times 3 days with food	**MQ** 750 mg po, then 500 mg po in po div. tid times 7 days. **Peds:** (**QS** 10 mg per kg po tid + **clinda** 20 mg per kg per day div. tid)—both times 7 days	Can substitute clinda for doxycycline. **Doxy** 20 mg per kg per day MQ alternative due to neuropsych. reactions. Avoid if malaria acquired in SE Asia due to resistance.
Uncomplicated/ P. malariae	All regions	**CQ** as above for adults & peds		
Uncomplicated/ P. vivax or P. ovale	All except Papua, New Guinea & Indonesia (CQ-resistant)	**CQ** as above + **PQ** base 30 mg po once daily times 14 days	**Peds CQ** as above + **PQ** base 0.5 mg per kg po once daily times 14 days	PQ added to eradicate latent parasites in liver Screen for G6PD def. before starting PQ. (if G6PD positive, dose PQ as 45 mg po once weekly times 8 weeks. Avoid PQ in pregnancy.
Uncomplicated/ P. vivax	CQ-resistant: Papua, New Guinea & Indonesia	**QS** + (**doxy** or **tetra**) + **PQ** as above	**MQ** + **PQ** as above. **Peds** (<8 yrs old) **QS** alone times 7 days or **MQ** alone. If latter fail, add **doxy** or **tetra**	

¹ **Peds prophylaxis dosages** (Ref.: *CID 34:493, 2002*): **Mefloquine** weekly dose by **weight** in kg: <15 = 5 mg/kg; 15–19 = ¼ adult dose; 20–30 = ½ adult dose; 31–45 = ¾ adult dose; >45 = adult dose. **Atovaquone/proguanil** by weight in kg, single daily dose using peds tab (62.5 mg atovaquone & 25 mg proguanil): <11 kg not use; 11–20 kg, 1 tab; 21–30 kg, 2 tabs; 31–40 kg, 3 tabs; ≥41 kg, one adult tab. **Doxycycline** ages >8–12 yrs: 2 mg per kg per day up to 100 mg/day
* See page 2 for abbreviations. All dosage recommendations are for adults *(unless otherwise indicated) and assume normal renal function.*

TABLE 13A (4)

PROTOZOA—EXTRAINTESTINAL/Malaria/Treatment (continued)

Clinical Severity Plasmodia sp.	Region Acquired	Suggested Treatment Regimens (Drug) Primary—Adults	Alternative & Peds	Comments
Uncomplicated/ Pregnancy	CQ-sensitive areas CQ-resistant P. falciparum CQ-resistant P. vivax	**CQ** as above **QS + clinda** as above **QS** 650 mg tid times 7 days	If failing or intolerant, **QS → doxy**	Doxy or tetra used if benefits outweigh risks. No controlled studies of AP in pregnancy. Possible association of MQ & increased number of stillbirths. If P. vivax or P. ovale, after pregnancy check for G6PD & then primaquine.
Severe malaria, i.e. impaired consciousness, severe anemia, renal failure, pulmonary edema, ARDS, DIC, jaundice, acidosis, seizures, parasitemia >5%. One or more of latter. Almost always P. falciparum	All regions	**Quinidine gluconate** in normal saline: 10 mg per kg (salt) IV over 1 hr & then 0.02 mg per kg per min. by constant infusion OR 24 mg per kg IV over 4 hrs & then 12 mg per kg over 4 hrs q8h. Continue until parasite density <1% & can take po. QS as above times 7 days (SE Asia) or 3 days elsewhere **PLUS** **Doxy** 100 mg q12h times 7 days) OR (**clinda** 10 mg per kg IV load & then 5 mg per kg IV q8h times 7 days)	**Peds: Quinidine gluconate**—same IV mg per kg dose as for adults **PLUS** (**Doxy** [if >45 kg, 4 mg per kg IV; if <45 kg, 2 mg per kg IV q12h] times 7 days as for adults) OR **Clinda**, same mg per kg dose as for adults	Do aldosterone-sensitive QS monitor. BP, EKG (prolongation of QTc), & blood glucose (hypoglycemia). Consider exchange transfusion if parasitemia >10%. Switch to oral QS, doxy, & clinda when patient able. Steroids not recommended for cerebral malaria. **Outside U.S., the artemisinins (artemether, artesunate) are widely used in combination because of their efficacy vs resistant plasmodia, modest cost, & relative safety** e.g., artesunate 2 mg per kg po + clinda (CID 40:1777, 2005). For more info: NEJM 352:1565, 2005 & WHO website: www.rbm.WHO.int. Not available to date in U.S.

COMMENTS

Malaria—self-initiated treatment: Only for emergency situation where medical care not available

Atovaquone-proguanil (AP): 4 adult tabs (1 gm AP, 400 mg) po daily times 3 days

Microsporidia—systemic—see page 96, Intestinal Protozoa

INFECTING ORGANISM	SUGGESTED REGIMENS		COMMENTS
	PRIMARY	ALTERNATIVE	
Pneumocystis carinii Pneumonia (PCP). New name is **Pneumocystis jiroveci** (yee-row-vek-ee). Refs. NEJM 350:2487, 2004; CID 40(Suppl.3):S131, 2005			
Not acutely ill, able to take po meds: PaO₂ >70 mmHg	(**TMP-SMX-DS,** 2 tabs po q8h times 21 days) OR (**Dapsone** 100 mg po q24h + **trimethoprim** 5 mg per kg po q6h times 21 days) NOTE: Concomitant use of corticosteroids	[**Clindamycin** 300–450 mg po q6h + **primaquine** 15 mg base po q24h] times 21 days OR **Atovaquone** suspension 750 mg po bid with food times 21 days usually reserved for sicker pts with PaO₂ <70 (see below)	Mutations in the gene of the enzyme target (dihydropteroate synthetase) of sulfamethoxazole identified. Unclear whether mutations result in resistance to TMP-SMX or dapsone + TMP (EID 10:1721, 2004). Dapsone ref. CID 27:191, 1998. **After 21 days, chronic suppression in AIDS pts (see below).**
Acutely ill, po rx not possible: PaO₂ <70 mmHg	**Prednisone** (15–30 min. before TMP-SMX) (**TMP-SMX**): 40 mg q12h times 5 days, then 40 mg q24h times 5 days, then 20 mg q24h times 11 days. After 72 hrs, TMP component (po q24h) OR full IV component (per day) IV div. q6–8h times 21 days]	**Prednisone** as in primary rx **PLUS** (**Clinda** 600 mg IV q8h) + (**primaquine** 30 mg base po q24h) times 21 days OR **Pentamidine** 4 mg per kg per day IV times 21 days	**After 21 days, chronic suppression in AIDS pts (see below). PCP can occur in absence of HIV infection and steroids** (CID 23:215 & 219, 1997). Wait at least 4–8 days before declaring treatment failure & switching to clinda + primaquine or pentamidine. See above regarding gene mutations.
Primary prophylaxis and post-treatment suppression	Can substitute IV prednisone or **TMP-SMX-DS** or **SS**, 1 tab po q24h or 1 DS 3 times per wk) OR (**dapsone** 100 mg po q24h) [DC when CD4 >200 times 3 mos. (NEJM 344:159, 2001)].	[**Pentamidine** 300 mg q4 wks] OR (**dapsone** 200 mg po + **pyrimethamine** 75 mg po + **folinic acid** 25 mg, all once a week) or **atovaquone** 1500 mg once q24h with food.	TMP-SMX-DS regimen provides cross-protection vs toxo (reduce dose 25%), [or po] prednisone [aerosol q4 wks) OR (dapsone 200 mg po + pyrimethamine 1500 mg once q24h) protects vs toxo. Atovaquone suspension 1500 mg once daily as effective as daily dapsone (NEJM 1550:1889, 1998) or inhaled pentamidine (AID 7:60:369, 1999)

See page 2 for abbreviations. All dosage recommendations are for adults (unless otherwise indicated) and assume normal renal function.

TABLE 13A (5)

INFECTING ORGANISM	SUGGESTED REGIMENS		COMMENTS
	PRIMARY	ALTERNATIVE	
PROTOZOA—EXTRAINTESTINAL (continued)			
Toxoplasma gondii (Reference: Ln 363:1965, 2004)			
Immunologically normal patients (For pediatric doses, see reference)			
Acute illness with lymphadenopathy	No specific rx unless severe/persistent symptoms or evidence of vital organ damage		
Acquired via transfusion (lab accident) or in immunosuppressed pts	Treat as for acute illness or chorioretinitis		
Active toxo chorioretinitis in non-AIDS, lowered resistance due to steroids or cytotoxic drugs	**Pyrimethamine** (pyri) 200 mg po once on 1st day, then 50–75 mg po q24h] + **sulfadiazine** (see footnote[1]) 1–1.5 gm po qid] + **leucovorin** (folinic acid) 5–20 mg q8h while on pyri. Treat 1–2 wks beyond resolution of signs/symptoms; continue leucovorin 1 wk after stopping pyri.		For congenital toxo, toxo meningitis in adults, and chorioretinitis, **add prednisone 1 mg per kg per day in 2 div. doses** until CSF protein conc. falls or vision-threatening inflammation has subsided. Adjust folinic acid dose by following CBC results.
Acute in pregnant women	**Spiramycin** [From FDA, call (301) 827-2335] 1 gm po q8h (without food) until term or until fetal infection. NOTE: Use caution in interpretation of commercial tests for toxoplasma IgM antibody, for help, FDA Advisory (301) 594-3060 or Toxoplasma Serology Lab of Palo Alto Med. Found. (650) 853-4828.		IgG avidity test of help in 1st trimester (*J Clin Micro 42:941, 2004*).
Fetal/congenital	Management complex. Combination rx with pyrimethamine + sulfadiazine + leucovorin—see *Comment*		Details in *Ln 363:1965, 2004*). **Consultation advisable.**
Acquired immunodeficiency syndrome (AIDS)			
Cerebral toxoplasmosis Ref: *Ln 363:1965, 2004; CID 40(Suppl.3):S131, 2005*	[**Pyrimethamine** (pyri) 200 mg times 1 po, then (75 mg per day po)] + (**sulfadiazine** 1–1.5 gm po qid) + **folinic acid** 10–20 mg per day po) for 4–6 wks after resolution of signs/symptoms, and then suppressive rx (see below) OR **TMP-SMX** 10/50 mg per kg per day po or IV div. q12h times 30 days (*AAC 42:1346, 1998*)	[**Pyri + folinic acid** (as in primary regimen)] + 1 of the following: (1) **Clinda** 600 mg po/IV q6h or (2) **azithro** 1.2–1.5 gm po q24h or (3) **clarithro** 1 gm po bid or (4) **atovaquone** 1500 mg po q24h or (5) **atovaquone** 750 mg po q6h. then suppression.	Use alternative regimen for pts with severe sulfa allergy. If multiple ring-enhancing brain lesions (CT or MRI) >85% of pts respond to 7–10 days of empiric rx. If no response, suggest brain biopsy. Pyri penetrates brain even if no inflammation; folinic acid prevents pyrimethamine hematologic toxicity.
Primary prophylaxis: AIDS pts—IgG toxo antibody + CD4 count <100 per mcL	**TMP-SMX-DS**, 1 tab po q24h) or (**TMP-SMX-SS**, 1 tab po q24h)	**Dapsone** 50 mg po q24h) + (**pyri** 50 mg po q week) + **folinic acid** 25 mg po q week)] OR [**atovaquone** 1500 mg po q24h] OR [(**clinda** 300–450 mg po q6-8h) + (**pyri** 25–50 mg po q24h) + **folinic acid** 10–25 mg po q24h)] OR [**atovaquone** 750 mg po q6-12h]	Prophylaxis for pneumocystis also effective vs toxo. Refs: *MMWR 51(RR-8), 6/14/2002; AnIM 137:435, 2002*. (Pyri + sulfa) prevents PCP and toxo; (clinda + pyri) prevents toxo only.
Suppression after rx of cerebral toxo	[**Sulfadiazine** 500–1000 mg q6h + (**pyri** 25–50 mg po q24h) + **folinic acid** 10–25 mg po q24h)] DC if CD4 count >200 times 3 months.	[(**Clinda** 300–450 mg po q6-8h) + (**pyri** 25–50 mg po q24h)] OR **atovaquone** 750 mg po q6-12h	
Trichomonas vaginalis	See Vaginitis, Table 1, page 20		
Trypanosomiasis Ref: *Ln 362:1469, 2003*			
West African sleeping sickness (T. brucei gambiense)			
Early: Blood/lymphatic—CNS OK	**Pentamidine** 4 mg per kg IM daily times 10 days	**Suramin**[2] 100 mg IV (test dose), then 1 gm IV on days 1, 3, 7, 14, & 21	
Late: Encephalitis	**Melarsoprol**[2] 2.2 mg per kg per day IV times 10 days	**Eflornithine** 100 mg per kg per day IV times 14 days (*CID 41:748, 2005*)	Melarsoprol trial data: *JID 191:1793 & 1922, 2005*
Prophylaxis	**Pentamidine** 3 mg per kg IM q6 mos.		Not for casual visitor
East African sleeping sickness (T. brucei rhodesiense)			
Early: Blood/lymphatic	**Suramin**[2] 100 mg IV (test dose), then 1 gm IV on days 1, 3, 7, 14, & 21	None	

---

[1] Sulfonamides for toxo. Sulfadiazine now commercially available. Sulfisoxazole much less effective.
[2] Available from CDC Drug Service; see footnote 1 page 95
* See page 2 for abbreviations. All dosage recommendations are for adults (unless otherwise indicated) and assume normal renal function.

TABLE 13A (6)

INFECTING ORGANISM	SUGGESTED REGIMENS		COMMENTS
	PRIMARY	ALTERNATIVE	
PROTOZOA—EXTRAINTESTINAL/Trypanosomiasis/(East African sleeping sickness) *(continued)*			
Late: Encephalitis	**Melarsoprol**[1] 2–3.6 mg per kg per day IV times 3 days; repeat after 7 days & for 3rd time 7 days after 2nd course	**Prednisone** may prevent/alternate encephalopathy	
T. cruzi—**Chagas disease** or acute American trypanosomiasis Ref. *Ln 357;1777, 2001*	**Nifurtimox**[1] 8–10 mg per kg per day po div. 4 times per day after meals times 120 days Ages 11–16 yrs: 12.5–15 mg per kg per day po qid times 90 days Children 1–11 yrs: 15–20 mg per kg per day po div. qid po times 90 days	**Benznidazole**[1],[5] 5–7 mg per kg per day po div. 2 times per day times 30–90 days (*AJTMH 63;111, 2000*) NOTE: Avoid tetracycline and steroids.	Treatment of no benefit in chronic late disease. Nifurtimox reported 70–95% effective. Immunosuppression for heart transplant can reactivate chronic Chagas disease.
NEMATODES—INTESTINAL (Roundworms)			
Ascaris lumbricoides (**ascariasis**)	**Albendazole** 400 mg po times 1 dose or **mebendazole** 100 mg po bid times 3 days or 500 mg po bid times 1 dose	**Ivermectin** 150–200 mcg per kg times 1 dose or **Nitazoxanide: Adults**—500 mg po bid times 3 days; **children 4–11**—200 mg oral susp. po q12h	Can present with intestinal obstruction.
Capillaria philippinensis (**capillariasis**)	**Mebendazole** 200 mg po bid times 20 days	**Albendazole** 200 mg po bid times 10 days	
Enterobius vermicularis (**pinworm**)	**Albendazole** 400 mg po times 1 dose or **mebendazole** 100 mg po times 1, repeat in 2 wks	**Pyrantel pamoate** 11 mg per kg (to max. dose of 1 gm) po times 1 dose; repeat every 2 wks times 2.	*Side-effects in Table 13B, pages 103, 105*
Hookworm (Necator americanus and Ancylostoma duodenale)	**Albendazole** 400 mg po times 1 dose or **mebendazole** 500 mg po times 1 dose	**Pyrantel pamoate** 11 mg per kg po daily times 3 days	NOTE: Ivermectin not effective. Eosinophilia may be absent but eggs in stool (*NEJM 351;799, 2004*)
Strongyloides stercoralis (**strongyloidiasis**)	**Ivermectin** 200 mcg per kg per day po times 2 days	**Albendazole** 400 mg po bid times 2 days (7–10 days for hyperinfection syndrome)	Case report of ivermectin failure in pt with hypogammaglobulinemia (*Am J Med Sci 311;178, 1996*)
Trichostrongylus orientalis	**Albendazole** 400 mg po times 1 dose	**Pyrantel pamoate** 11 mg per kg (max. 1 gm) po times 1	**Mebendazole** 100 mg po bid times 3 days
Trichuris trichiura (**whipworm**)	**Albendazole** 400 mg po once daily times 3 days	**Mebendazole** 100 mg po bid times 3 days or 500 mg once	**Ivermectin** 200 mcg per kg daily po times 3 days
NEMATODES—EXTRAINTESTINAL (Roundworms)			
Angiostrongylus cantonensis—a cause of eosinophilic meningitis	Supportive care. Serial LPs to ↓ intracranial pressure	Antihelminth therapy may worsen meningitis (*NEJM 346;668, 2002*) Prednisone may help.	Mortality rate <1%. Ref.: *AJM 114;217, 2003*
Anisakis simplex (**anisakiasis**)	Physical removal: endoscope or surgery	Questionable response to albendazole (*Ln 354;54, 2002*)	Anisakiasis acquired by eating raw fish: herring, salmon, mackerel, cod, squid, snapper. Similar illness due to Pseudoterranova species acquired from cod, halibut, red
Ancylostoma braziliense & caninum; causes **cutaneous larva migrans**	**Ivermectin** 200 mcg per kg po times 1 dose per day times 1–2 days	**Albendazole** 200 mg po bid times 3 days	Also called "creeping eruption," dog and cat hookworm. Ivermectin cure rate 77% (1 dose) to 97% (2–3 doses) (*CID 31;493, 2000*)
Baylisascariasis (Raccoon ascaris)	No drug proven efficacious. Try po **albendazole**, 25 mg/kg po Both times 10 days	**Albendazole**, Peds: 25–50 per kg per day. Adults: 400	Some add steroids (*CID 39;1484, 2004*)
Dracunculus medinensis: **Guinea worm**	Slow extraction of pre-emergent worm		↓ inflammatory response and facilitate removal. Immersion in warm water promotes worm emergence. Mebendazole 400–800 mg per day times 6 days may kill worm.
Filariasis, Wolbachia bacteria needed for filarial development. Rx with doxy 100–200 mg ↓ number of microfilaria (*BMJ 326;207, 2003*)			
Lymphatic (**Elephantiasis**): Wuchereria bancrofti or Brugia malayi or B. timori	Prospective random DB trial shows efficacy of doxy vs both adult worms & microfilaria (200 mg po daily times 8 wks (*Ln 365; 2067 & 2116, 2005*)	**Diethylcarbamazine**[1],[2] (DEC) po over 14 days: Day 1, 50 mg, day 2, 50 mg tid, day 3, 100 mg tid; days 4–14, 2 mg per kg tid.	
		Metronidazole 250 mg po times 10 times used to ↓	
		Diethylcarbamazine[1],[2] (DEC) 6 mg per kg po once—similar effect as multiple doses	

[1] Available from CDC Drug Service, see footnote 1 page 95
[2] May need antihistamine or corticosteroid for allergic reaction from disintegrating organisms
* See pages 2 for abbreviations. All dosage recommendations are for adults (unless otherwise indicated) and assume normal renal function.

TABLE 13A (7)

INFECTING ORGANISM	SUGGESTED REGIMENS		COMMENTS
	PRIMARY	**ALTERNATIVE**	
NEMATODES—Extraintestinal (Roundworms)/Filariasis (continued)			
Cutaneous			
Loiasis: **Loa loa**, eyeworm disease Onchocerciasis (**onchocerciasis**)—river blindness (*Ln 360:203, 2002*)	**Diethylcarbamazine (DEC)**[1,2]—6 mg per kg po times 1 dose		DEC: 900 mg per wk po effective prophylaxis
	ivermectin 150 mcg per kg po times 1 dose; repeat q6 months to suppress dermal and ocular microfilariae. If eye involved, start **prednisone** 1 mg per kg per day po several days before ivermectin. NOTE: Worm survival requires symbiotic bacteria Wolbachia (*Science 296:1365, 2002*)		ivermectin ↓ number of microfilariae in skin and impairs female worm fertility, does not kill adult worms (nothing does). Ivermectin OK in pregnancy.
Body cavity			
Mansonella perstans (dipetalonemiasis)	**Mebendazole** 100 mg po bid times 30 days or **albendazole** 400 mg po bid times 10 days		Usually no or vague allergic symptoms + eosinophilia. Ivermectin has no activity against this species.
Mansonella streptocerca	**Diethylcarbamazine**[1,2] as above for Wuchereria OR **ivermectin** 150 mcg per kg times 1		Chronic pruritic hypopigmented lesions that may be confused with leprosy. Can be asymptomatic.
Mansonella ozzardi	**Ivermectin** 200 mcg per kg po times 1 dose may be effective		Usually asymptomatic. Articular pain, pruritus, lymphadenopathy reported. May have allergic reaction from dying organisms.
Dirofilarias: Heartworms			
D. immitis, dog heartworm	No effective drugs; surgical removal only option		Can lodge in pulmonary artery → coin lesion. Eosinophilia rare.
D. tenius (raccoon), D. ursi (bear), D. repens (dogs, cats)	No effective drugs		Worms migrate to conjunctiva, subcutaneous tissue, scrotum, breasts, extremities
Gnathostomiasis: eosinophilic myeloencephalitis	**Albendazole** 400 mg po q24h or bid times 21 days **ivermectin** 200 mcg per kg per day times 2 days		
Toxocariasis: *Clin Micro Rev 16:265, 2003*	**Rx directed at relief of symptoms as infection self-limited, e.g., steroids & antihistamines; use of anthelminthics controversial.**		
Visceral larval migrans	**Albendazole** 400 mg po bid times 5 days	**Mebendazole** 100–200 mg po bid	Severe lung, heart or CNS disease may warrant steroids. Differential dx of larval migrans syndromes: Toxocara canis and catis, Ancylostoma spp., Gnathostoma spp., Spirometra spp.
Ocular larval migrans	First 4 wks of illness: (Oral **prednisone** 30–60 mg po q24h) + subtenon **triamcinolone** 40 mg weekly/times 2 weeks.		No added benefit of anthelminthic drugs. Rx of little effect after 4 wks.
Trichinella spiralis (**trichinosis**)—muscle infection	**Albendazole** 400 mg po bid times 8–14	**Mebendazole** 200–400 mg po tid times 3 days, then 400–500 mg po tid times 10 days.	Use albendazole/mebendazole with caution during pregnancy.
	Concomitant **prednisone** 40–60 mg po q24h		
TREMATODES (Flukes)			
Clonorchis sinensis (liver fluke)	**Praziquantel** 25 mg per kg po tid times 1 day or **albendazole** 10 mg per kg per day po times 7 days		Same dose in children
Fasciola buski (intestinal fluke)	**Praziquantel** 25 mg per kg po tid times 1 day		Same dose in children
Fasciola hepatica (sheep liver fluke)	**Triclabendazole**[1,3] (Fasinex, Novartis Agribusiness) 10 mg per kg po times 1 dose. Ref.: *CID 32:1, 2001*		**Bithinol**: Adults and children: 30–50 mg per kg (max. dose 2 gm) per day every other day times 10–15 doses
Heterophyes heterophyes (intestinal fluke) Metagonimus yokogawai (intestinal fluke) Opisthorchis viverrini (liver fluke)	**Praziquantel** 25 mg per kg po tid times 1 day		Same dose in children. Same regimen for **Metorchis conjunctus** (North American liver fluke) **Nanophyetus salmincola**: Praziquantel 20 mg per kg po tid times 1 day
Paragonimus westermani (lung fluke)	**Praziquantel** 25 mg per kg po tid times 2 days or **bithionol**[1] 30–50 mg per kg po every other day times 10 days		Same dose in children

[1] Available from CDC Drug Service, see footnote 1 page 95

[2] May need antihistamine or corticosteroid for allergic reaction from disintegrating organisms

* See page 2 for abbreviations. *All dosage recommendations are for adults (unless otherwise indicated) and assume normal renal function.*

TABLE 13A (8)

INFECTING ORGANISM	SUGGESTED REGIMENS		COMMENTS
	PRIMARY	**ALTERNATIVE**	
TREMATODES (Flukes) (continued)			
Schistosoma haematobium; GU bilharziasis (NEJM 346:1212, 2002)	**Praziquantel** 20 mg per kg po bid times 1 day (2 doses)		Same dose in children. Alternative: metrifonate 10 mg per kg per dose po q2 wks for 3 doses.
Schistosoma intercalatum	**Praziquantel** 20 mg per kg po bid times 1 day (2 doses)		Same dose in children.
Schistosoma japonicum; Oriental schisto. (NEJM 346:1212, 2002)	**Praziquantel** 20 mg per kg po tid times 1 day (3 doses)		Same dose in children.
Schistosoma mansoni (intestinal bilharziasis) (JID 176:304, 1997) **Possible praziquantel resistance** (JID 176:304, 1997) (NEJM 346:1212, 2002)	**Praziquantel** 20 mg per kg po bid times 1 day (2 doses)	**Oxamniquine** single dose of 15 mg per kg po once; in North and East Africa 20 mg per kg po daily times 3 days Do not use during pregnancy	Same dose for children. Cures 60–90% pts. Report of success treating myeloradiculopathy with single dose of praziquantel. 50 mg per kg + prednisone for 6 months (CID 39:1618, 2004)
Schistosoma mekongi	**Praziquantel** 20 mg per kg po tid times 1 day (3 doses)		Same dose for children.
Toxemic schisto, Katayama fever	**Praziquantel** 25 mg per kg po q4h with food times 3 doses		Massive infection with either S. japonicum or S. mansoni
CESTODES (Tapeworms)			
Echinococcus granulosus (hydatid disease) (CID 37:1073, 2003; Ln 362:1295, 2003)	Meta-analysis supports percutaneous aspiration-injection-reaspiration (PAIR) + albendazole. Before **and** after drainage: **albendazole** ≥60 kg, 400 mg po bid or < 60 kg, 15 mg per kg per day div. bid, with meals. Then: Puncture (P) & needle aspirate (A) cyst content. Instill (I) hypertonic saline (15–30%) or absolute alcohol & wait 20–30 min., then re-aspirate (R) with final irrigation. **Continue albendazole times 28 days** Cure in 96% as compared to 90% pts with surgery.		
Echinococcus multilocularis (alveolar cyst disease) (CID 16:437, 2003)	**Albendazole** efficacy not clearly demonstrated, can try in dosages used for hydatid disease. Wide surgical resection only reliable rx, technique evolving (Radiology 198:259, 1996)		
Intestinal tapeworms			
Diphyllobothrium latum (fish), Dipylidium caninum (dog), Taenia saginata (beef), and Taenia solium (pork)	**Praziquantel** 5–10 mg per kg po times 1 dose for children and adults. **Alternative: Niclosamide** 2 gm po times 1. **NOTE:** Niclosamide preferred for Taenia solium because it is not absorbed; hence, avoid risk of CNS symptoms if pt has neurocysticercosis.		
Hymenolepis diminuta (rats) and H. nana (humans)	**Praziquantel** 25 mg per kg po times 1 dose for children and adults. **Alternative: Niclosamide** 500 mg po q24h times 3 days		
Neurocysticercosis (NCC): Larval form of T. solium Ref.: AJTMH 72:3, 2005	**NOTE: Treat T. solium intestinal tapeworms,** if present, with niclosamide		
Parenchymal NCC			
"Viable" cysts by CT/MRI	**Albendazole** ≥60 kg: 400 mg bid with meals or <60 kg: 15 mg per kg per day in 2 div. doses (max. 800 mg per day) + **Dexamethasone** 0.1 mg per kg per day ± Anti-seizure medication] — all times 8 days	(**Praziquantel** 50–100 mg per kg per day in 3 div. doses + **Dexamethasone** 0.1 mg per kg per day ± Anti-seizure medication) — all times 15 days	Albendazole assoc. with 46% ↓ in seizures (NEJM 350:249, 2004). Praziquantel less cysticidal activity. Steroids decrease serum levels of praziquantel.
"Degenerating" cysts	**Albendazole + dexamethasone** as above		Treatment improves prognosis of associated seizures.
Dead calcified cysts	No treatment indicated		
Subarachnoid NCC	**Albendazole + steroids** (as above) + shunting for hydrocephalus. Without shunt, 50% died within 9 yrs (J Neurosurg 66:686, 1987).		
Intraventricular NCC	**Albendazole + dexamethasone** + neuroendoscopic removal (if available)		
Sparganosis (Spirometra mansonoides) Larval cysts, source—frogs/snakes	Surgical resection or ethanol injection of subcutaneous masses (NEJM 330:1887, 1994).		

* See page 2 for abbreviations. All dosage recommendations are for adults (unless otherwise indicated) and assume normal renal function.

TABLE 13A (9)

DISEASE	INFECTING ORGANISM	SUGGESTED REGIMENS PRIMARY	ALTERNATIVE	COMMENTS
ECTOPARASITES Ref: *CID* 36:1355, 2003; *Ln* 363:889, 2004				
Head lice	Pediculus humanus, var. capitis *Med Lett* 47:68, 2005	**NOTE: Due to potential neurotoxicity, lindane not recommended.** **Permethrin** 1% generic lotion or cream rinse (Nix): Apply to shampooed dried hair for 10 min, repeat in 1 wk. **OR** **Malathion** 0.5% (Ovide): Apply to dry hair for 8-14 hrs, then shampoo	**Ivermectin** 200 mcg per kg po once; repeat in 7-10 days	**Permethrin** success in 78%. Extra combing of no benefit. Resistance increasing. No advantage to 5% **Malathion:** Report that 1-2 20-min. applications 98% effective *Ped Derm* 21:670, 2004). In alcohol—potentially flammable.
Pubic lice (crabs)	Phthirus pubis	Pubic hair: **Permethrin** OR **malathion** as for head lice	Eyelids: **Petroleum jelly** applied gid times 10 days OR **yellow oxide of mercury** 1% gid times 14 days	Costs: Permethrin 1% lotion/cream $8-9, Malathion 0.5% lotion $119, Ivermectin $20
Body lice	Pediculus humanus, var. corporis	No drugs for pt, treat the clothing. Organism lives in & deposits eggs in seams of clothing. Discard clothing; if not possible, treat clothing with 1% malathion powder or 10% DDT powder		
Scabies Immunocompetent patients	Sarcoptes scabiei	**Primary:** **Permethrin** 5% cream (ELIMITE): Apply entire skin from chin to toes. Leave on 8-10 hrs. Repeat in 1 week. Safe for children >2 mos. old. **Alternative:** **Ivermectin** 200 mcg per kg po times 1 (*NEJM* 333:26, 1995) **or** 10% **crotamiton** topically 1 time per day times 2 days		Trim fingernails. Reapply to hands after handwashing. Pruritus may persist times 2 wks after mites gone.
AIDS patients: $CD4 <150$ per mm^3 (Norwegian scabies—see Comments)		For Norwegian scabies: **Permethrin** 5% as above on day 1, then 6% sulfur in petrolatum daily on days 2-7, then repeat times seven weekly. **Ivermectin** 200 mcg per kg po times 1 reported effective.		Norwegian scabies in AIDS pts. Extensive, crusted. Can mimic psoriasis. Not pruritic. ELIMITE: 60 gm $18.60, ivermectin $19.62 Highly contagious—isolate!
Myiasis Due to larvae of flies		Usually cutaneous/subcutaneous nodule with central punctum. Treatment: Occlude punctum with petrolatum, fingernail polish, makeup cream or bacon. When larva migrates, manually remove.		Occlude punctum to prevent gas exchange with petrolatum, fingernail polish.

TABLE 13B: DOSAGE, PRICE, AND SELECTED ADVERSE EFFECTS OF ANTIPARASITIC DRUGS

NOTE: Drugs available from CDC Drug Service indicated by "CDC." Call (404) 639-3670 (or -2888)

Doses vary with indication. For convenience, drugs divided by type of parasite; some drugs used for multiple types of parasites, e.g., albendazole

COMMENT: Cost data represent average wholesale prices as listed in 2005 Drug Topics Red Book, Medical Economics.

CLASS, AGENT, GENERIC NAME (TRADE NAME)	USUAL ADULT DOSAGE (Cost)	ADVERSE REACTIONS/COMMENTS
Antiprotozoan Drugs **Intestinal Parasites**		
Albendazole (Albenza)*	Doses vary with indication, 200-400 mg po 200 mg tab $1.58	Teratogenic. Pregnancy Cat C; give after negative pregnancy test. Abdominal pain, nausea/vomiting, alopecia. ↑ serum transaminase. Rare leukopenia.
Dehydroemetine (CDC)*	1.5 mg per kg per day to max. of 90 mg IM	Local pain, ECG changes, cardiac dysrhythmias, precordial pain, paresthesias, weakness, peripheral neuropathy, GI: nausea/vomiting, diarrhea. Avoid strenuous exercise for 4 wks after rx.
Iodoquinol (Yodoxin) (650 mg $0.47)	Adults: 650 mg po tid; children: 40 mg per kg per day div. tid.	Rarely causes nausea, abdominal cramps, rash, acne. Contraindicated if iodine intolerance.
Metronidazole/Ornidazole^A,B (Tiberal)	Side-effects similar for all. *See metronidazole in Table 10A, page 66 & 10C, page 73*	
Paromomycin (Humatin) Aminosidine in U.K.	Up to 750 mg qid 250 mg caps $3.37	Drug is aminoglycoside similar to neomycin; if absorbed due to concomitant inflammatory bowel disease can result in oto/nephrotoxicity. Doses >3 gm assoc. with nausea, abdominal cramps, diarrhea.
Quinacrine (Atabrine, Mepacrine)^A,B	100 mg tid. No longer available in U.S.; 2 pharmacies will prepare as a service (1) Connecticut 203-785-6818; (2) California 800-247-9767	Contraindicated for pts with history of psychosis or psoriasis. Yellow staining of skin. Dizziness, headache, vomiting, toxic psychosis (1.5%), hemolytic anemia, leukopenia, thrombocytopenia, urticaria, rash, fever, minor disulfiram-like reactions.

* See page 2 for abbreviations. *All dosage recommendations are for adults (unless otherwise indicated) and assume normal renal function.*

TABLE 13B (2)

CLASS, AGENT, GENERIC NAME (TRADE NAME)	USUAL ADULT DOSAGE (Cost)	ADVERSE REACTIONS/COMMENTS
Antiprotozoan Drugs		
Tinidazole (Tindamax)	500 mg tabs, with food. Regimen varies with indication. Cost: 500 mg tab $4.56	Chemical structure similar to metronidazole but better tolerated. Seizures/peripheral neuropathy reported. **Adverse effects:** Metallic taste 4–6%, nausea 3–5%, anorexia 2–3%
Extraintestinal Parasites		
Antimony compounds[AUS] Stibogluconate sodium (Pentostam, Tricostam) (CDC) Meglumine antimoniate (Glucantime). Glucantim—French tradenames	Solution containing 30–34% pentavalent antimony	Cough/vomiting if IV infusion too fast. Arthralgia 50%. Others: myalgia, bradycardia, cramps/diarrhea, pruritus/rash, renal toxicity, ↑ amylase. **Abnormalities also occur. Combination rx with, or sequential rx with, ampho B may trigger fatal arrhythmias** (Ln 351:1928, 1998).
Atovaquone (Mepron) Ref: AAC 46:1163, 2002	Suspension: 1 tsp (750 mg) po bid 750 mg per 5 mL. Cost 210 mL: $744.00	No. pts stopping rx due to side-effects were 9%: rash 22%, GI 20%, headache 16%, insomnia 10%, fever 14%
Atovaquone and proguanil (Malarone) For prophylaxis of P. falciparum; little data on P. vivax	**Prophylaxis:** 1 tab po (250 mg + 100 mg) q24h with food **Treatment:** 4 tabs po (1000 mg + 400 mg) once daily with food times 3 days Adult tab: 250/100 mg. Peds tab 62.5/25 mg. Peds dosage: footnote 1 page 97. Cost: 250/100 mg adult tab $5.04	Adverse effects in rx trials: Adults—abd. pain 17%, N/V 12%, headache 10%, dizziness 5%. Rx stopped in 1%. Asymptomatic mild ↑ in ALT/AST. Children—cough, headache, anorexia, vomiting, abd. pain. See drug interactions, Table 22. Safe in G6PD-deficient pts. Can crush tabs for children and give with milk or other liquid nutrients. Renal insufficiency: contraindicated if CrCl <30 mL per min.
Benznidazole[AUS] (Rochagan, Roche, Brazil)	7.5 mg per kg per day po	Photosensitivity in 50% of pts. Rash 29%; abdominal pain, nausea/vomiting/anorexia, CNS: disorientation, insomnia, twitching/seizures, paresthesias, polyneuritis
Chloroquine phosphate (Aralen)	Dose varies—see Malaria prophylaxis and rx, pages 97-98. 500 mg tabs $6.04	Minor: anorexia/nausea/vomiting, headache, dizziness, blurred vision, pruritus in dark-skinned pts. Major: prolonged rx in rheumatoid arthritis doses can lead to retinopathy. Can exacerbate psoriasis. Can inhibit response to rabies vaccine. Contraindicated in pts with epilepsy.
Dapsone Ref: CID 27:191, 1998	100 mg po q24h 100 mg tab $0.20	Usually tolerated by pts with rash after TMP-SMX. Adverse effects: nausea/vomiting, rash, oral lesions (CID 18:630, 1994). Methemoglobinemia (usually asymptomatic); if >10–15%, stop drug. Hemolytic anemia if G6PD deficient. Sulfone syndrome: fever, rash, hemolytic anemia, atypical lymphocytes, and liver injury (West J Med 156:303, 1992).
Eflornithine[AUS] (Ornidyl)	Approved in U.S. for trypanosomiasis but not marketed. Contact Hoechst Marion Roussel, (800) 552-3188.	Diarrhea in ½ pts, vomiting, abdominal pain, anemia/leukopenia in ½ pts, seizures, alopecia, jaundice, ↓ hearing
Fumagillin	Eyedrops + po. 20 mg po tid. Call 800-547-1392.	Adverse events: Neutropenia & thrombocytopenia
Mefloquine (Lariam)	One 250 mg tab per week for malaria prophylaxis; for rx, 1250 mg times 1 or 750 mg & then 500 mg in 6–8 hrs. 250 mg tab $12.93. In U.S.: 250 mg tab = 228 mg base; outside U.S. 275 mg tab = 250 mg base	Side-effects in roughly 3%. Minor: headache, irritability, insomnia, weakness, diarrhea. Toxic psychosis, seizures can occur. Teratogenic—do not use in pregnancy. Do not use with quinine, quinidine, or halofantrine. Rare: Prolonged QT interval and toxic epidermal necrolysis (Ln 349:101, 1997). Not used for self-rx due to neuropsychiatric side-effects.
Melarsoprol (CDC) (Mel B, Arsobal) (Manufactured in France)	See Trypanosomiasis for adult dose. Peds dose: 0.36 mg per kg IV, then gradual ↑ to 3.6 mg per kg/d over 3–4 days to max 3.6 mg per kg po q24h times 3–4 doses.	Post-rx encephalopathy (10%) with 50% mortality overall; risk of death 2° to rx 4–8%. Prednisolone 1 mg per kg per day may ↓ encephalopathy. Other: Heart damage, albuminuria, abdominal pain, vomiting, peripheral neuropathy, Herxheimer-like reaction, pruritus.
Miltefosine[AUS] (Zentaris, Impavido)	100–150 mg (approx. 2.25 mg per kg per day) po times 28 days	Generally well-tolerated, q.v. Peds. Side-effects vary: kala-aza pts, Cutaneous leishmaniasis 2.25 mg per kg po q24h times 6 wks	Vomiting in up to 40%, diarrhea in 16%, rise in creatinine in moderate in severity—may resolve in <1 day
Nifurtimox (Lampit) (CDC) (Manufactured in Germany by Bayer)	8–10 mg per kg per day po div. 4 times per day	Side-effects in 40–70% of pts. GI: abdominal pain, nausea/vomiting. CNS: polyneuritis (1/3), disorientation, insomnia, twitching, seizures. Skin rash. Hemolysis with G6PD deficiency
Nitazoxanide (Alinia)	Adults: 500 mg po q12h. Children 4–11: 200 mg susp. po q12h. Take with food. 500 mg tab $13.02	Abdominal pain 7.8%, diarrhea 2.1%. Rev: CID 40:1173, 2005
Pentamidine (NebuPent)	300 mg via aerosol q month. Also used IM 300 mg $98.75 + admin. costs	Hypotension, hypocalcemia, hypoglycemia, pancreatitis. Neutropenia (15%), thrombocytopenia. Nephrotoxicity. Others: nausea/vomiting, ↑ liver tests, rash
Primaquine phosphate	26.3 mg[*] (=15 mg base) $0.77	In G6PD def. pts. can cause hemolytic anemia with hemoglobinuria, esp. African, Asian peoples. Methemoglobinemia. Nausea/abdominal pain if pt. fasting. (CID 39:1336, 2004)

* See page 2 for abbreviations. All dosage recommendations are for adults (unless otherwise indicated) and assume normal renal function.

TABLE 13B (3)

CLASS, AGENT, GENERIC NAME (TRADE NAME)	USUAL ADULT DOSAGE (Cost)	ADVERSE REACTIONS/COMMENTS
Antiprotozoan Drugs/Extraintestinal Parasites *(continued)*		
Pyrimethamine (Daraprim, Malocide) Also combined with sulfadoxine as **Fansidar** $4.13	100 mg, then 25 mg per day times 5 days $0.43 Cost of folinic acid (leucovorin) 5 mg $2.36	Major problem is hematologic: megaloblastic anemia, ↓ WBC, ↓ platelets. Can give 5 mg folinic acid per day to ↓ bone marrow depression and not interfere with antitoxoplasmosis effect. If high-dose pyrimethamine, ↑ folinic acid to 10–50 mg per day. Other: Rash, vomiting, diarrhea, xerostomia
Quinacrine[NUS]	For giardiasis: 100 mg po tid times 5 days Peds dose: 2 mg per kg po tid (max. 300 mg per day) times 5 days	Compounded by Med. Center Pharm., New Haven, CT. (203) 688–6816 or Panorama Compound. Pharm., Van Nuys, CA. (800) 247–9767
Quinidine gluconate	Loading dose of 10 mg (equivalent to 6.2 mg of quinidine base) per kg IV over 1–2 hrs, and then constant infusion of 0.02 mg of quinidine gluconate per kg per minute. 80 mg/10 ml $21.56	Adverse reactions of quinidine/quinine similar: (1) IV bolus injection can cause fatal hypotension, (2) hyperinsulinemic hypoglycemia, esp. in pregnancy, (3) ↑ rate of infusion of IV quinidine if QT interval ↑ >25% of baseline, (4) reduce dose 30–50% after day 3 due to ↓ renal clearance and ↓ vol. of distribution.
Quinine sulfate (300 mg salt = 250 mg base)	325 and 650 mg tabs. No IV prep. in U.S. Oral rx of chloroquine-resistant falciparum malaria: 650 mg po tid times 3 days, then tetracycline 250 mg po qid times 7 days 325 mg $0.16	Cinchonism: tinnitus, headache, nausea, abdominal pain, blurred vision. Rarely, blood dyscrasias, drug fever, asthma, hypoglycemia. Transient blindness in <1% of 500 pts (*AnIM* 136:339, 2002). Contraindicated if G6PD deficiency.
Spiramycin (Rovamycine) [*JAC 42:572, 1998*]	Up to 3–4 gm per day	GI and allergic reactions have occurred. Not available in U.S.
Sulfadiazine	1–1.5 gm po q6h. 500 mg $0.34	See *Table 10C, page 73*, for sulfonamide side-effects
Sulfadoxine and pyrimethamine combination (Fansidar)	Contains 500 mg of sulfadoxine and 25 mg of pyrimethamine One tab $4.13	Very long mean half-life of both drugs: Sulfadoxine 169 hrs, pyrimethamine 111 hrs allows weekly dosage. Do not use in pregnancy. Fatalities reported due to Stevens-Johnson syndrome and toxic epidermal necrolysis. Renal excretion—use with caution in pts with renal impairment
DRUGS USED TO TREAT NEMATODES, TREMATODES, AND CESTODES		
Bithionol (CDC)	Adults & children: 30–40 mg per kg (to max. of 2 gm per day) po every other day times 10–15 days	Photosensitivity, skin reactions, urticaria, GI upset
Diethylcarbamazine (Hetrazan) (CDC)	Used to treat filariasis. Licensed (Lederle) but not available in U.S	Headache, dizziness, nausea, fever. Host may experience inflammatory reaction to death of adult worms: fever, urticaria, asthma, GI upset (Mazzotti reaction).
Ivermectin (Stromectol, Mectizan)	Strongyloidiasis dose: 200 mcg per kg times 1 dose po Onchocerciasis: 150 mcg per kg po times 1 dose Scabies: 200 mcg per kg po times 1 3 mg tabs $4.35	Mild side-effects: fever, pruritus, rash, lnx of onchocerciasis, can cause tender lymphadenopathy, headache, bone/joint pain. Can cause Mazzotti reaction (see above).
Mebendazole (Vermox)	Doses vary with indication. 100 mg tab $5.91	Rarely causes abdominal pain, nausea, diarrhea. Contraindicated in pregnancy and children <2 yrs old
Oxamniquine (Vansil) [NUS]	For S. mansoni. Some experts suggest 40–60 mg per kg over 2–3 days in all of Africa.	Rarely, dizziness, drowsiness, neuropsychiatric symptoms, GI upset. Orange/red urine
Praziquantel (Biltricide)	Doses vary with parasite; see *Table 13A* 600 mg $11.90	Mild: dizziness/drowsiness, N/V, rash, fever. Only contraindication is ocular cysticercosis. Metab.-induced by anticonvulsants and steroids; can negate effect with cimetidine 400 mg po tid
Pyrantel pamoate (over-the-counter as Reese's Pinworm Medicine)	Oral suspension. Dose for all ages: 11 mg per kg (to max. of 1 gm) times 1 dose	Rare GI upset, headache, dizziness, rash
Suramin (Germanin) (CDC)	For early trypanosomiasis. Drug powder mixed to 10% solution with 5 mL water and used within 30 minutes.	Does not cross blood-brain barrier; no effect on CNS infection. Side-effects: vomiting, pruritus, urticaria, fever, paresthesias, albuminuria (discontinue drug if casts appear). Dies not well if renal/liver disease present. Deaths from vascular collapse reported
Thiabendazole (Mintezol)	Take after meals. Dose varies with parasite; see *Table 12A*. 500 mg $1.25	Nausea/vomiting, headache, dizziness. Rarely: liver damage, ↓ BP, angioneurotic edema, Stevens-Johnson syndrome. May ↓ mental alertness.

* See page 2 for abbreviations. All dosage recommendations are for adults (unless otherwise indicated) and assume normal renal/renal function.

TABLE 14A: ANTIVIRAL THERAPY (Non-HIV)*

VIRUS/DISEASE	DRUG/DOSAGE	SIDE EFFECTS/COMMENTS
Adenovirus—Cause of RTIs including fatal pneumonia in children & young adults. **Findings include:** fever, ↑ liver enzymes, leukopenia, thrombocytopenia, diarrhea, pneumonia, or hemorrhagic cystitis.	**No proven rx. Cidofovir** 5 mg per kg q wk times 2 wks, then q2 wks + **probenecid** 1.25 gm (see Comments). Cidofovir used successfully in 3/8 immunosuppressed children. Intravesical cidofovir (5 mg per kg in 100 ml saline instilled into bladder) successful in rx of adenovirus hemorrhagic cystitis (CID 40:199, 2005).	In virus load predicted responses to cidofovir (CID 38:45, 2004) successful (CID 40:1244, 2005). Value of rx controversial (CID 40:1244, 2005).
Coronavirus—SARS-CoV (Severe Acute Respiratory Distress Syn.) (see Comments) CID 36:1420, 2004. New coronavirus isolated in 2003 (NEJM 348:1953 & 1967, 2003). New coronavirus spread from Hong Kong to 30 countries. Effective infection control guidelines likely responsible for controlling the epidemic. Only 4 mini-outbreaks since 2004; 3/4 from research labs testing live virus (Science 304:1097, 2004); none reported so far to 2005 (7/05).	**Therapy remains predominantly supportive care.** Therapy tried or under evaluation (see Comments): **Ribavirin**—ineffective. Corticosteroids—small case series. Pegylated IFN-α effective in monkeys. Value of corticosteroids alone unclear. Inhaled nitric oxide improved oxygenation & improved chest x-ray (CID 39:1531, 2004).	Other coronaviruses (HCOV-229E, OC43, NL63, etc.) implicated as cause of croup, asthma exacerbations, & other RTIs in children (CID 40:1721, 2005; JID 191:492, 2005) may be associated with Kawasaki disease (JID 191:489, 2005).
Enterovirus—Meningitis: most common cause of aseptic meningitis. PCR on CSF valuable for early dx (Scand J Inf Dis 34:359, 2002) but ↓ sensitivity (CID >2 days of symptoms. PCR on feces pos. in 12/13 specimens, PCR in blood at clinical onset (CID 40:982, 2005).	**No rx currently recommended;** however, **pleconaril** (VP 63843) still under investigation. [For compassionate release use call Vinopharma (610) 458-7300, ext. 6287 (Donna Kobush, RN)].	No clinical benefit demonstrated in double-blind placebo-controlled trials in 21 infants with enteroviral aseptic meningitis (PID 22:335, 2003).
Hemorrhagic Fever Virus Infections: For excellent reviews, see Med Lab Observer, May 2005, p. 16, www.mlo-online.com and LnID 4:487, 2004		
Congo-Crimean Hemorrhagic Fever (HF) (CID 36:1254, 2004). Tick-borne. Symptoms include fever, headache, myalgia. Signs: conjunctival injection, hepatomegaly, petechiae (1/3). Lab: ↓ platelets, ↓ WBC, ↑ AST, LDH & CPK (100%)	**Oral ribavirin 30 mg per kg** as initial loading dose & then 15 mg per kg times 4 days & then 7.5 mg per kg times 6 days (WHO recommendation) (see Comment)	3/3 healthcare workers in Pakistan had complete recovery (Ln 346:472, 1995) & 61/69 (89%) with confirmed CCHF rx with ribavirin survived in Iran (CID 36:1613, 2003).
Ebola/Marburg HF (Central Africa). Severe outbreak in Angola 368 cases with 277 deaths by 5/3/05 (NEJM 352:2155, 2005; LnID 5:331, 2005)	**No effective antiviral rx** (J Virol 77:9733, 2003)	An intense inflammatory response within 4 days after infection may control virus proliferation & result in asymptomatic infection (Ln 355:2210, 2000). Can infect gorillas & chimps that come in contact with other dead animal carcasses (Science 303:387, 2004). Bats also suspected (LnID 5:331, 2005)
With pulmonary syndrome: Hantavirus	**No benefit from ribavirin has been demonstrated**	Acute onset of fever, headache, myalgias, non-productive cough, thrombocytopenia and non-cardiogenic pulmonary edema with respiratory insufficiency following exposure to rodents.
With renal syndrome: Lassa, Venezuelan, Korean, HF, Sabia, Argentinian HF, Bolivian HF, Junin, Machupo	**Ribavirin** IV 2 gm loading dose, then 1 gm q8h times 4 days then 0.5 gm q8h times 6 days (See Comment: Congo-Crimean HF)	Toxicity low, hemolysis reported but reversible. No significant changes in WBC, platelets, hepatic or renal function. Effective in Lassa and in 2 cases of Bolivian HF. No data on others. See CID 36:1254, 2003, for management of contacts (CID 24:718, 1997).
Dengue and dengue hemorrhagic fever (DHF) (see AnIM 104:545, 2004) www.cdc.gov/ncidod/dvbid/dengue/dengue-hcp.htm	**No data on antiviral rx.** Fluid replacement with careful hemodynamic monitoring. In DHF, use fluids. **DHF** with colloids may be preferred to crystalloids in children with low pulse pressures (J Ped 149:629, 2002)	Of 77 cases seen at CDC (2001-2004), recent (2-wk) travel to Caribbean island 30%, Asia 17%, Central America 15%, S. America 15% (MMWR 54:556, June 10, 2005). See www.clinicaltrials.gov/show/NCT0008055.
West Nile virus (see AnIM 104:545, 2004). A flavivirus transmitted by mosquitoes, blood transfusions, transplanted organs, & breast-feeding. IVIG (>200 species) are main host. Mosquito incidental host. Usually non-CNS disease but 1/150 cases develop meningitis or encephalitis, esp. elderly (CID 38:1257, 2004) & breast-feeding. Usually non-CNS disease but 1/150 cases develops meningitis or encephalitis (CID 38:1257, 2004; CID 41:1102, 2004). Long-term sequelae (neuromuscular weakness & psychiatric) common (IDCP 13:101, 2005)	**No proven rx to date.** 2 clinical trials in progress: (1) Interferon alfa-N3 (CID 40:764, 2005). See www.ny4.org/posting/nhal.html. (2) IVIG (Omr-IgG-am) with high titer antibody West Nile (JID 193:1), (Omrion (Israel)) 0.5 gm/kg IV q24h IV for 3-5 days; rapid ↑ in platelet counts (CID 36:1623, 2003). Contact NIH, 301-496-7453; see www.clinicaltrials.gov/show/NCT0008055.	Dx by ↑ IgM in serum & CSF or CSF PCR (contact State Health Dept / CDC). Blood supply now tested in U.S. ↑ serum lipase in some cases (NEJM 347:4161, 2003); cases (JAMA 276:1157, 1996)
Yellow fever		Reemergence in Africa & South America. Vaccination effective.
Hepatitis Viral Infections		
Hepatitis A (Ln 351:1643, 1998)	No therapy recommended. If within 2 wks of exposure, IMIG 0.02 mL per kg IM times 1 protective.	Vaccine recommendations in Table 20. Coverage of only 50% in states that recommend Hep A vaccination (MMWR 54:141, 2005); 40% of pts with chronic Hep C who developed superinfection with Hep A developed fulminant hepatic failure (NEJM 338:286, 1998).

* See page 2 for abbreviations. NOTE: All dosage recommendations are for adults (unless otherwise indicated) and assume normal renal function.
Costs from 2005 DRUG TOPICS RED BOOK, Medical Economics. Price is average wholesale price (AWP).

TABLE 14A (2)

VIRUS/DISEASE	DRUG/DOSAGE	SIDE EFFECTS/COMMENTS

Hepatitis Viral Infections *(continued)*

Hepatitis B

Acute — No therapy recommended | Most common cause of death from acute hepatitis in Italy *(Dig Liver Dis 35:404, 2003)*. Screen for HIV.

Chronic

HBeAg+:
Consider rx if:
(1) Persistent ↑ ALT/AST
(2) HBsAg positive
(3) HBV DNA plasma "viral load" > 10^5 copies/mL. If > 10^4 copies/mL, rx unless active inflammation/fibrosis on biopsy < 10^4: no rx.

HBeAg–: Rx indefinitely; consult specialist!
Refs: *NEJM 350:1118, 2004;*
Clin Gastro & Hep 2:87, 2004

Data on treatment changing rapidly; 4 approved options now approved & available—no cure available at all ages. **Goal of rx:** ↓ liver inflammation, stop progression of cirrhosis & prevent hepatocellular carcinoma (HCC) in all. If all cirrhosis, goals listed, desired response:
↓ plasma HB DNA to < 20,000 copies/ml;
Normal ALT/AST;
HBsAg to anti-HBs;
HBeAg to anti-HBe.

Lamivudine (LAV) 100 mg po q24h times 12 months or until HBsAg seroconversion. If hepatitis flare or persistent viral load elevation *(NEJM 351:1521, 2004)*, switch to ENT or ADF. Don't use for first-line rx in cirrhotics: ↑ clinical breakthrough with resistance & hepatitis flares.

Entecavir (ENT) 0.5 mg po fasting q24h: if previous LAV treatment or known YMDD mutation, use 1 mg q24h. Treat 1 year or min. 6 mos. after seroconversion.

Adefovir (ADF) 10 mg po q24h. For HBeAg+, 1 year or min. 6 mos. & recheck HBeAg; for HBeAg– (1 yr min) 6 mos. after seroconversion or indefinite).

Another option: **Tenofovir** 300 mg po q24h (also "Truvada" — combined as tab po q24h looks promising, but don't use alone in HIV co-infected patients.

• **PEG IFN alfa-2b** 180 mcg subcut. OR **PEG IFN alfa-2b** 1.5 mcg per kg once weekly times at least 1 year OR

Interferon alfa-2b 5 million units 3 times per week or 5 million units q24h subcut. for 16-24 weeks. Don't use IFNs in cirrhosis or decompensation, or post-transplant. Hepatitis flares common & associated with further decompensation.

Combination rx: PEG alfa-2a + LAV disappointing *(NEJM 352:26, 2005; AnIM 142:240, 2005)*

Specific drug comments *(side-effects & cost in Table 14B):*
LAV: Non-toxic. YMDD mutants less virulent than wild type. Sustained viral response (SVR) if initial ALT > 2x normal & is 65% at 3 yrs *(J Viral Hep 9:208, 2002)*. Active vs YMDD LAV mutants & ADV-resistant strains.

ENT: Min. toxicity. Active vs YMDD mutant strains.
Interferon PEG IFN alfa-2a 2 times more effective than standard IFN *(J Viral Hep 10:298, 2003)* & more effective than LAV or HBeAg(–) pts *(NEJM 351:1206, 2004)*. Genotypes A & B respond better (40–50%) than C & D (25–30%).
ADV: Effective vs YMDD mutant strains.
Headache & fatigue in 3–4%.

Based on limited studies: *Hpt 36:S225A, 1999; J Hpt 34:888 & 895, 2001*. Some add HBIG *(Hpt 28:585, 1998)*

Lamivudine 100 mg po q24h from 4 wks pre-transplant to 12 wks post-transplant.

Prevention of re-infection after liver transplant for Hepatitis B.

Hepatitis C (up to 3% of world infected, 4 million in U.S., 36,000 new cases annually). Co-infection with HIV common—see Sanford Guide to HIV/AIDS Therapy. See *AnIM 136:747, 2002;*
www.va.gov/hepatitis; www.hepnet.com/hepc.html

Acute
Usually asymptomatic (> 75%). Co-infection with HIV common—see text.
PCR within 13 days; antibody in 36 or more days *(JID 189:3, 2004; CID 40:951, 2005)*

Follow plasma HCV viral load by PCR
If clear within 3 mos., no treatment.
If persists: PEG IFN + ribavirin as below, albeit controversial *(NEJM 346:1091, 2002)*

Sustained viral response with IFN alfa-2b therapy 32% vs 4% with placebo. P 0.00007 *(Cochrane Database Sys & Rev CD000369, 2002)*

Chronic: www.va.gov/hepatitis; *Sem Liver Dis 23(Suppl 1):35, 2003; AASLD/IDSA Guidelines: Hpt 39:1147, 2004*

Treat it: persistent elevated ALT/AST, pos. HCV RNA plasma viral load, & inflammation on biopsy.

Genotypes 1 & 4
AnIM 140:346, 2004

PEG IFN: Either alfa-2a (Pegasys) 180 mcg subcut. once weekly OR alfa-2b (PEG-INTRON) 1.5 mcg per kg subcut. once weekly

Ribavirin

Weight	Ribavirin Dose
< 75 kg	400 mg a.m. & 600 mg p.m.
> 75 kg	600 mg a.m. & 600 mg p.m.

In U.S., 90% due to genotype 1. Sustained viral response (SVR) to 48-wk rx of genotype 1 42–51%; SVR to 24-wk rx of genotype 2 or 3 76-82%.
Avoid alcohol—accelerates HCV disease.
HIV accelerates HCV disease
See *Table 14B for drug adverse effects & cost*. Interferon alfa can cause serious depression.
Ribavirin is teratogenic & has dose-related hematologic toxicity.
For drugs in development, see *Hepatol Res, July 12, 2005.*

Monitor response by quantification:

HCV RNA	Result	Action
After 4 wks rx	Undetectable	Treat 48 wks
After 12 wks rx	< 2 log ↓ or undetectable	Discontinue therapy

Genotypes 2 or 3

PEG IFN alfa-2a or 2b—dose as for types 1 & 4 above

HCV RNA	Result	Action
After 4 wks rx	> 1 log ↓	Treat 24 wks

+ **Ribavirin** 400 mg po bid *(NEJM 352:2609, 2005)* — Treat 24 wks

For genotypes 2 & 3, some use standard IFN; results similar & ↓ cost.

For prevention of acute and chronic infection, see Table 15D, page 128

TABLE 14A (3)

VIRUS/DISEASE	DRUG/DOSAGE	SIDE EFFECTS/COMMENTS
Herpesvirus Infections (see review: CID 26:541, 1998)		
Cytomegalovirus (CMV)		
Normal host	No rx for acute mononucleosis-like syndrome and not established for congenital CMV (Sem Ped Int Dis 16:50, 2005)	
Immunocompromised host		
	Treatment of AIDS patients with highly active antiretroviral therapy (HAART) is effective in reducing mortality by 81% in pts with CMV infection in 44 immunocompetent pts with 1 month of viremia and elderly (Dig Dis Sci 50:609, 2005)	
Colitis/esophagitis	**Ganciclovir** as with retinitis except induction period extended for 3-6 wks. No agreement on use of maintenance rx. **Foscarnet** 90 mg per kg q12h effective in 9/10 pts (AAC 41:1226, 1997). **Valganciclovir also likely effective.** Switch to oral valganciclovir when po tolerated.	Consider in transplant & AIDS pts with dysphagia & retrosternal pain (Dig Dis Sci 50:609, 2005). CMV colitis: colitis reported in 44 immunocompetent pts with 1 yr of viremia in organ transplant pts. CMV DNA level >13 pg per mL correlated with active infection (JID 190:826, 2004). Ganciclovir (AIDS 19:S535-S538, 2005)
CMV of nervous system: Encephalitis & ventriculitis	**Ganciclovir** + **foscarnet** as in retinitis. Consider combination of ganciclovir and foscarnet if prior CMV rx used. Switch to valganciclovir when possible.	Treatment not defined, but disease develops while taking ganciclovir as suppressive therapy. (Neurology 48:1250, 1997)
Lumbosacral polyradiculopathy		(About 50% will respond (CID 20:747, 1995); survival ↑ (5.4 wks to 14.6 wks) (CID 27:345, 1998).
Mononeuritis multiplex	Not defined	
CMV pneumonia—predominantly transplants, rare in HIV	**Ganciclovir** 5 mg per kg IV q12h times 3 wks followed by maintenance. Valganciclovir 900 mg po q24h; or ganciclovir 5 mg per kg IV q24h.	Due to vasculitis and may not be responsive to antiviral rx (ArNeurol 29:139, 1991). In BMT recipients, serial measure of pp65 antigen was useful in early dx of CMV interstitial pneumonia; good results if GCV initiated within 6 days of antigen positivity (Bone Marrow Transplant 26:413, 2000). For preventive (see Table 15E, page 131
Retinitis (most common in AIDS) (most common in AIDS) 1996, 2004) Ophthalmology 111:1326, 2004). Marked reduction in CMV associated retinitis with HAART that was anti-CMV therapy (CID 37:1365, 2003). 33–63% with inactive CMV retinitis who responded to HAART (↑ of ≥50 CD4 cells per mL) developed immune recovery vitritis (vision ↓ & floaters — with posterior segment inflammation—vitreitis, papillitis & macular changes) an avg. of 43 wks after rx started (JID 179:697, 1999; AIDS 14:163, 2000; CID 38:1063, 2003). Continued ophthalmologic follow-up needed Corticosteroid for ↑ inflammatory reaction of immune recovery vitritis without reactivation of CMV retinitis (5th CROI, Abst 751).	**Induction therapy, primary: Valganciclovir** (GCV) 900 mg po bid with food (adjust for renal function) times 14–21 days **OR** ganciclovir (GCV) 5 mg per kg IV q12h (adjust for renal function) times 14–21 days **OR foscarnet** (FOS) 90 mg per kg IV q12h (adjust for renal function) at constant rate (requires infusion pump) times 14–21 days **OR** ganciclovir (GCV) 5 mg per kg IV q12h times 6–7 mos. + [either concomitant **intraocular ganciclovir implant** (delivers 1–2 mcg per hr] times 6–7 mos. + [either concomitant **IV GCV** 5 mg per kg IV q12h or oral valganciclovir 900 mg po q24h) when stabilized. **Induction therapy, alternative:** Cidofovir 5 mg per kg IV q week times 2 wks with **probenecid** (2 gm po 3 hrs before cidofovir dose, then 1 gm 2 hrs immediately after dose, and 1 gm 8 hrs after dose) and 1 liter of normal saline IV 1 hr before cidofovir infusion (J AIDS 8 HR 17:339, 1998; Blood 97:388, 2001) **OR** for pts who fail other rx regimens, consider combination rx with both: [**GCV** 5 mg per kg q12h or q24h IV and (2) **FOS** 90 mg per kg q12h up to total of 125 mg per kg q24h (CID 34:1337, 2002). **Suppression** (maintenance therapy): See CID 26:534, 1999. With immune reconstitution from HAART, maintenance may be dc if CD4 ≥100 mm³ after 6 mos of HAART (see www.aidsinfo.nih.gov for guidelines) and retinitis inactive.	**Alternative:** Combination of **GCV intraocular implant** q6 mos. + **valganciclovir** 900 mg po q24h **OR cidofovir** 5 mg per kg IV q2 wks + valganciclovir 900 mg po q24h were both above for induction and maintenance less predictable. Cannot use GCV ocular implant alone as approx. 50% risk of CMV retinitis in other eye at 6 mos. & 31% risk visceral disease. Risk ↓ with systemic rx (NEJM 337:83, 1997). Similarly, intraocular injections of fomivirsen will not prevent contralateral eye or systemic/visceral disease (Am J Ophth 133:467, 475, 494, 552, 2002). **Concurrent systemic rx recommended.** Intravitreal foscarnet used in Thailand in 193 AIDS pts with 66% eyes improved, but 35% developed vitreitis in the other eye (J Med Assoc Thai 88:170, 2005). Watch for retinal detachments. 50–60% within 1 yr of dx of retinitis. Equal efficacy of IV GCV & FOS. GCV avoids nephrotoxicity of FOS; FOS avoids bone marrow suppression of GCV & valganciclovir minimal even with prophylactic use (JID 189:1615, 2004; AAC 49:873, 2005). Reports indicate success of combination rx with GCV at 5 mg per kg q24h & FOS up to 125 mg per kg per day for 24 wks—resistant isolates in solid organ transplants (J Inf 337, 2002). Hypomagnesemia common complication. Valganciclovir 900 mg q24h has similar efficacy (17% progressed over 1 year) & toxicity profile as IV ganciclovir but with fewer V-related events (JAMS 30:392, 2002).
CMV in transplant patients: The prevention and management of CMV infections in transplant pts is beyond the scope of this Guide. Use of valganciclovir to prevent CMV infections in CMV seronegative recipients of an organ from a seropositive donor & in seropositive receivers has been highly effective (Ln 365:2105, 2005). Others suggest preemptive rx when pt develops CMV antigenemia post-transplant (Transplant 79:85, 2005)		
EBV—Mononucleosis (Ln ID 3:131, 2003)	**No treatment** complications. Corticosteroids for tonsillar obstruction or CNS	(See JAC 56:277, 2005 for current status of drugs in development).

TABLE 14A (4)

VIRUS/DISEASE	DRUG/DOSAGE	SIDE EFFECTS/COMMENTS
Herpesvirus Infections (continued)		
HHV-6—Implicated as cause of roseola (exanthem subitum) & other febrile diseases of childhood (NEJM 352:768, 2005). Reactivation in transplant pts documented in transplant pts (JID 179:311, 1999). Fever & rash documented in 47% of 110 U.S. HSCT pts treated with delayed monocytes & platelet engraftment (CID 40:932, 2005). Recognized in excellent rx with ganciclovir rx (CID 40:890 & 894, 2005). Foscarnet rx improved thrombotic microangiopathy (Am J Hematol 78:156, 2004).		
HHV-7—ubiquitous virus (>90% of the population is infected by age 4 yrs). No known human disease. Infects CD4 lymphocytes; transmitted via saliva		
HHV-8—The agent of Kaposi's sarcoma, Castleman's disease, & body cavity lymphoma	**No antiviral treatment.** Effective anti-HIV rx may help.	Systemic: chemotherapy. Localized lesions: radiotherapy, laser surgery or intralesional chemotherapy. Systemic: chemotherapy. Castleman's disease responsive to ganciclovir (Blood 103:1632, 2004). Valganciclovir reduced HHV8 replication in saliva by 79% vs placebo (IDSA 2005, Abst. 0066)
Herpes simplex virus (HSV) Types 1 & 2 (See also JID Suppl. 39:5237, 2004 or HSV in HIV-infected persons)	**Either** [Acyclovir (400 mg po 5 times per day for 10 days) or valacyclovir (400 mg po 5 times per day for 10 days) with without prednisone (60 mg/day for 5 days then taper by 10 mg per day) **or** prednisone (60 mg/day for 5 days then taper by 10 mg po q8h in children <12 yrs] **or no rx.**	HSV-1 is most common cause. Survival & recovery from neurological sequelae are related to mental status at time of initiation of rx. Early dx and rx imperative. Mortality has been reduced from >70% to 19% with acyclovir rx. With acyclovir in symptoms <3 days had better recovery and less neural degeneration when rx with acyclovir in symptoms <3 days. PCR of CSF for HSV-1 DNA is 100% specific & 75–98% sensitive. 8/31 (25%) CSF samples drawn before day 3 were neg, but another likely was positive. More data needed (Cochrane Database Syst Rev CD001849, 2004).
Bell's palsy (May also be caused by H. zoster, Lyme disease, HHV-6) (CID 50:529, 2000)	**Acyclovir** V 10 mg per kg IV (infuse over 1 hr) q8h times 14–21 days. Up to 20 mg per kg q8h in children <12 yrs	Surgical decompression within 14 days of symptoms controversial (NEJM 352:416, 2005). If saliva/CSF PCR pos, VZV acyclovir may help (PID 21:615, 2002)
Encephalitis Excellent reviews: CID 35: 254, 2002). UK experience (EID 9:234, 2003; Eur J Neurol 12:331, 2005)	**Acyclovir** V 10 mg per kg IV (infuse over 1 hr) q8h times 14–21 days. Up to 20 mg per kg q8h in children <12 yrs	PCR neg. Relapse after successful rx reported in 7/27 (27%) children. Relapse was associated with a lower total dose of initial acyclovir rx (285 ≥ 82 mg per kg in relapse group vs. 462 ± 149 mg per kg., p <0.03) (NEJM 30:185, 2000; Neuropediatrics 35:371, 2004).
Genital, immunocompetent Emerging problem in adolescents (Sem in Ped Inf Dis 16:24, 2005). ACOG guidelines for management (Herpes Management Forum, Herpes 12:15, 2005		
Primary (initial episode) See excellent reviews: NEJM 137:2571, 2004 & AnIM 137:2571, 2004 or CDC 2002 Guidelines	**Acyclovir** (Zovirax or generic) 400 mg po tid times 7–10 days (FDA-approved dosage is 200 mg po 5 times per day times 10 days). [NB $150 per course, OR $35 per course.] OR **Valacyclovir** (Valtrex) 1000 mg po bid times 10 days	CDC 2002 guidelines recommend treatment of international recommendations. By ↓ by 2 days time to resolution of signs & symptoms, ↓ by 7 days duration of viral shedding. Does not prevent recurrences. For severe cases only: 5 mg per kg IV q8h times 5–7 days.
	Famciclovir (Famvir) 250 mg po tid times 7–10 days (not FDA-approved for this indication). [$97–139 per course]	An ester of penciclovir, which is well absorbed, bioavailability 3–5 times greater than acyclovir. Found to be equal to acyclovir (Sex. Trans. Dis 24:481, 1997). Metabolized to penciclovir, which is active component. Side effects and activity similar to acyclovir.
Episodic recurrences	**Acyclovir** 400 mg po tid times 5 days OR **famciclovir** 125 mg po bid times 5 days OR **valacyclovir** 500 mg po bid times 3 days	Acyclovir 250 mg po tid found to be equal to acyclovir 200 mg 5 times per day. ↓ by 1 day, duration of lesions, ↓ by 4 days time to healing of lesions. ↓ by 7 day duration of rx. The 2-day course of valacyclovir 500 mg bid times 3 days was equivalent to 5 days, duration of episode & lesions 4.4 days (CID 34:958, 2002)
Chronic suppression (JAMA 280:928, 1998; JID 178:603, 1998) Decision to rx not arbitrary, but rx sig. improves quality of life for those with frequent recurrences (Clin Ther 17:1, 1995; Genitourin Med Infect 75:398, 1999).	Suppressive rx reduces the frequency of genital herpes recurrences by 70–80% among pts who have frequent recurrences (i.e., >6 recurrences per year) & many report no symptomatic outbreaks (MMWR 51:RR-6, 2002). **Acyclovir** 400 mg po bid (cost per yr $2983), **or valacyclovir** 1 gm po 250 mg po bid (cost per yr $562), **or famciclovir** 250 mg po bid (cost per yr $2983), **or valacyclovir** 1 gm po 500 mg po q24h ($1825 yr) in pts with <9 recurrences per yr. May use 1 gm po q24h if breakthrough of lower dose.	All suppress subclinical HSV-2 shedding between episodes of active disease. Vala = acyclovir in 69 immunocompetent pts & sig. better than placebo in double-blind crossover study (JID 190:1374, 2004). ↓ risk of transmission by 48% vs placebo (NEJM 350:11 & 67, 2004). Drug resistance unlikely in immunocompetent pts (HIV-1 & BMT) 6–7%. 3–5% develop resistance. However could also ↓ HIV transmission (JID 191:5107, 2005). Since 2/3 of pts demonstrate rx between any 1 & 5 days, daily suppressive rx should be reassessed periodically, and after 3–5 yrs, episodic rx may become more practical (AnIM 131:14, 1999). Rarely failure of suppression in immunocompetent pts (JID 150:156, 2005; CID 41:320, 2005)
Gingivostomatitis, primary (children)	**Acyclovir** 15 mg per kg po 5 times per day times 7 days	Efficacy demonstrated in randomized double-blind placebo-controlled trial (BMJ 314:1800, 1997).
Kerato-conjunctivitis and recurrent epithelial keratitis	**Trifluridine** (Viroptic), 1 drop 1% solution q2h (max. 9 drops per day for max. of 21 days (see Table I, page 11)	In controlled trials, response to suppressive rx with acyclovir (400 mg bid) reduced recurrences of ocular HSV from 32% to 19% over 18 mos (NEJM 339:300, 1998)
Mollaret's recurrent lymphocytic meningitis (HSV-2) (CID J 363:1772, 2004)	No controlled trials of antiviral rx. Resolves spontaneously in most cases. IV or po acyclovir or valacyclovir or famciclovir recommended.	Pos. PCR for HSV in CSF confirms dx (EJCMID 23:560, 2004). Daily suppression rx might ↓ frequency of recurrence but no clinical trials.

* See page 2 for abbreviations. NOTE: All dosage recommendations are for adults (unless otherwise indicated) and assume normal renal function.
Costs from 2005 DRUG TOPICS RED BOOK, Medical Economics. Price is average wholesale price (AWP).

TABLE 14A (5)

VIRUS/DISEASE	DRUG/DOSAGE	SIDE EFFECTS/COMMENTS
Herpesvirus Infections/Herpes Simplex Virus (HSV Types 1 & 2) (continued)		
Mucocutaneous		
Oral labial, "fever blisters":	Start rx with prodrome symptoms (tingling or burning) before lesions appear.	Penciclovir (J Derm Treat 13:67, 2002; JAMA 277:1374, 1997; AAC 46: 2848, 2002). Docosanol (J Am Acad Derm 45:222, 2001). Oral acyclovir 5% cream (AAC 46:2238, 2002). Oral famciclovir 1.77% topical available. Topical fluconazole (0.04% lidex gel) q8h times 5 days in combination with famciclovir. Lesion size and pain when compared to famciclovir alone (JID 181:1906, 2000).

Normal host See Ann Pharmacotherapy 38:705, 2004; JAC 53:703, 2004	**Drug** **Dose** **Duration Sx** **Cost**
	Oral: Valacyclovir 2 gm q12h times 1 day ↓ 1 day $36
	    Famciclovir 500 mg po bid times 7 days ↓ 2 days $123
	    Acyclovir[1][2] 400 mg 5 times per day
	                (q4h while awake) times 5 days ↓ ½ day $19 (generic)
	
	Topical:
	  Penciclovir 1% cream q2h during day times 4 days ↓ ½ day $25
	  Docosanol 10% cream[2] 5 times per day until healed ↓ ½ day $14
	  Acyclovir 5% cream[2] 6 times per day (q3h) times 7 days ↓ ½ day $37 per 2 gm
	                                     $86 per 5 gm
	
	[1] FDA approved only HIV. [2] Approved for immunocompromised	

	See Table 1, page 21	
Immunocompromised	**Acyclovir** 5 mg per kg IV (infused over 1 hr) q8h times 7 days (250 mg per M[2]) or 400 mg po 5 times per day times 14–21 days (see Comment if suspect acyclovir-resistant) **OR Famciclovir:** In HIV-infected, 500 mg po bid for 7 days for recurrent episodes of genital HSV. **OR Valacyclovir:** In HIV-infected, 500 mg po bid for 5–10 days for recurrent episodes of genital herpes or 500 mg po bid for chronic suppressive rx.	Acyclovir-resistant HSV occurs, esp. in large ulcers. Most will respond to **IV foscarnet,** but recur after drug discontinued (median 6 weeks (NEJM 325:551, 1991)). Suppressive rx with famciclovir (500 mg po bid) reduced viral shedding and clinical recurrences (total days with lesions 18% vs 5%) in HIV-infected pts (AnIM 128:21, 1998), similar to findings with acyclovir & valacyclovir (500 mg po bid) times 6 mos. 65% of valacyclovir were rx-free at 6 mos (JID 188:1009, 2003)]. Cidofovir (topical) has been used with moderate success (JID 176:892, 1997).
Perinatal (genital in pregnancy at delivery)	In 25% HSV reactivated in last month of pregnancy. Infant exposure to primary lesion 50% risk. If recurrent lesion 4%. 50% mortality in infected neonates. If visible genital lesion, deliver by **C-section,** regardless of duration of membrane rupture. If no lesions or symptoms, vaginal delivery. Routine HSV cultures no longer recommended. **Acyclovir** useful in those >36 weeks at 20 mg per kg if premature) times 10–21 days (J PIDJ 14:827, 1995; NEJM 337:509, 1997).	
Herpes Whitlow See Comment		
Oral labial or genital (includes pts with AIDS) and critically ill pts in ICU setting (See Comment)		
Herpes simiae—Monkey bite (Herpes B virus)	**Postexposure prophylaxis:** Valacyclovir 1 gm po q8h times 14 days or acyclovir 800 mg po 5 times per day times 14 days. **Treatment of disease:** (1) CNS symptoms absent. Acyclovir 12.5–15 mg per kg IV q8h or ganciclovir 5 mg per kg IV q12h (2) CNS symptoms present. Ganciclovir 5 mg per kg IV q12h	Fatal human cases of myelitis and hemorrhagic encephalitis have been reported following bites, scratches, or even inoculation of saliva from monkeys. Initial sx include fever, headache, myalgias and diffuse adenopathy. Incubation period of 2–14 days (EID 9:246, 2003).
CID 35:1191, 2002		
Herpes Varicella-Zoster Virus (VZV)		
Varicella: Vaccination has markedly ↓ incidence of varicella & morbidity (NEJM 352:450, 2005). Our understanding of the disease still undeveloped (COID 18:235, 2005).		
Normal host (2–12 years)		
Child	**Rx not recommended** by American Academy of Pediatrics. Oral acyclovir recommended for healthy persons at ↑ risk for moderate to severe varicella, i.e., >12 yrs of age; chronic cutaneous or pulmonary disorders. Oral rx of 2ª case in household (↑ risk of rash), use **acyclovir 20 mg per kg** po qid times 5 days. (start within 24 hrs of rash)	Acyclovir slowed development and ↓ number of new lesions; duration of disease ↓ in children receiving acyclovir (NEJM 325:1539, 1991; J PIDJ 21:739, 2002). Oral dosage of acyclovir in children should not exceed 80 mg per kg per day or 3200 mg per day.
Adolescents, young adults	**Acyclovir** 800 mg po 5 times per day times 5 days (start within 24 hrs of rash) or **valacyclovir**[EGA] 1000 mg po 3 times per day times 5 days) **Famciclovir**[EGA] 500 mg po 3 times per day also probably effective but data lacking (AnIM 130:922, 1999)	↓ duration of fever, time to healing, and symptoms (AnIM 117:358, 1962).
Pneumonia or chicken-pox in 3rd trimester of pregnancy	**Acyclovir** 800 mg po 5 times per day or 10 mg per kg IV q8h times 5 days. Risks and benefits to fetus and mother table unknown. Many experts recommend rx, especially in 3rd trimester. Some would add VZ/G (varicella-zoster immune globulin).	Varicella pneumonia severe in pregnancy (41% mortality) and acyclovir ↓ incidence and severity (AJO 185:422, 2002). If varicella-susceptible mother exposed and respiratory symptoms develop within 10 days after exposure, start acyclovir (CCTID 13:123, 1993). Acyclovir is pregnancy category B, no evidence for ↑ birth defects (MMWR 42:1, 1993). Dissemination with visceral involvement reported during puerperal rx of rheumatoid arthritis (J Rheum 31:2517, 2004).

111

TABLE 14A (6)

VIRUS/DISEASE	DRUG/DOSAGE	SIDE EFFECTS/COMMENTS
Herpesvirus Infections/Herpes Varicella-Zoster Virus (VZV) Varicella (continued)		
Immunocompromised host	Acyclovir 10–12 mg per kg IV (infused over 1 hr) q8h times 7 days (500 mg per M²)	Continuous infusion of high-dose acyclovir (2 mg per kg per hr) successful in 1 pt with severe hemorrhagic complications (Int J Inf Dis 6:6, 2002).
Prevention—Post-exposure prophylaxis Varicella was the leading cause of vaccine-preventable deaths in children in the U.S. before availability of vaccine, and has been reduced with vaccine, but still deaths in unvaccinated pts (MMWR 54:272, 2005).	**CDC Recommendations for Prevention:** Since <5% of cases of varicella (but >50% of varicella-related deaths occur in adults >20 yrs of age, the CDC recommends a more aggressive approach in this age group): **1st, varicella-zoster immune globulin** (VZIG) (125 units per 10 kg (22 lbs) body weight IM up to a max. of 625 units; minimum dose is 125 units) is recommended for post-exposure prophylaxis in susceptible persons at greater risk of complications (immunocompromised persons, pregnant women, and certain newborns). If given within 96 hrs of exposure and even up to 10 days after exposure, it will prevent or modify varicella if it develops. Initiate rx quickly (<24 hrs of rash) with **acyclovir** as below. Some would rx presumptively with acyclovir in high-risk pts. **2nd,** varicella develops, initiate rx quickly (<24 hrs of rash) with **acyclovir** as below. Some would rx presumptively with acyclovir in high-risk pts. **3rd,** susceptible adults should be vaccinated. Check antibody in adults with negative or uncertain hx of varicella (10–30% will be Ab-neg.) and vaccinate those who are Ab-neg. **3rd,** susceptible children should receive vaccination. Recommended routinely before age 12–18 mos. but OK at any age	
Herpes zoster (shingles) (See NEJM 342:635, 2000 & 347:340, 2002)	[NOTE: Trials showing benefit of rx only in pts treated within 3 days of onset of rash]	
Normal host Effective if most evident in pts >50 yrs.	Acyclovir 800 mg 5 times per day times 7–10 days. **OR** Valacyclovir 1000 mg po tid times 7 days (adjust dose for renal failure)	Valacyclovir ↓ post-herpetic neuralgia more rapidly than acyclovir in pts >50 yrs of age; median duration of zoster-associated pain was 38 days with valacyclovir and 51 days on acyclovir (AAC 39:1546, 1995).
(For rx of post-herpetic neuralgia, see CID 36:877, 2003)	**OR** Famciclovir 750 mg q24h or 500 mg po q8h times 7 days equal efficacy (J Clin Virol 29:248, 2004). Adjust for renal failure (see Table 17).	Toxicity of both drugs similar (Arch Fam Med 9:863, 2000). Time to healing rapid. Reduced post-herpetic neuralgia. Famciclovir similar to acyclovir in reduction of acute pain and PHN (J Microbiol Immunol Inf 37:75, 2004).
25-fold ↓ in zoster after immunization (MMWR 48:F1-6, 1999)	**OR** Acyclovir 800 mg po 5 times per day times 7–10 days	A meta-analysis of 4 placebo-controlled trials (691 pts) demonstrated that acyclovir accelerated by approx. 2-fold pain resolution by all measures. Post-herpetic neuralgia at 3 & 6 mos (CID 22:341, 1996); med. time to resolution of pain 41 days vs 101 days in those >50 yrs
New vaccine ↓ herpes zoster & post-herpetic neuralgia (NEJM 352:2271, 2005)	**Prednisone** 30 mg po bid days 1-7, 15 mg bid days 8-14 and 7.5 mg bid days 15-21 also recommended by some authorities in pts >50 yrs of age (NEJM 330:896, 1994) with moderate or severe pain at presentation (JID 178:9, 1999)	Prednisone added to acyclovir improved quality of life (↓ acute pain, sleep, and return to normal activity) (AnIM 125:376, 1996). In post-herpetic neuralgia, controlled trials demonstrated effectiveness of gabapentin, the lidocaine patch (5% & good analgesia in controlling pain (Drugs 64:937, 2004, J Clin Virol 29:248, 2004). Nortriptyline & amitriptyline are equally effective but nortriptyline is better tolerated (CID 36:877, 2003). Role of antiviral drugs in rx of PHN unproven (Neuro 64:21, 2005).
Immunocompromised host		
Not severe	Acyclovir 800 mg 5 times per day times 7 days. **OR** Valacyclovir 1000 mg po tid times 7 days (though both are not FDA-approved for this indication)	If progression, switch to IV
Severe: >1 dermatome, trigeminal nerve or disseminated	Acyclovir 10–12 mg per kg IV (infusion over 1 hr) q8h times 14 days. In older pts, or 7.5 mg per kg if nephrotoxicity and pt improving ↓ to 5 mg per kg q8h	A common manifestation of immune reconstitution in HIV-infected children (J All Clin Immun 113:742, 2004)
Influenza (A & B)		
Suspect or proven acute disease Rapid diagnostic tests available. Antiviral rx cost-effective without viral testing in febrile pt with typical symptoms during influenza season.	Rx must be begun within 72 hrs. Acyclovir-resistant VZV occurs in HIV+ pts. Foscarnet 40 mg per kg q8h for 14–26 days) successful in 4/5 pts (AnIM 115:19, 1991).	
Pathogenic avian influenza (H5N1) in poultry (mainly chickens & ducks) in East & Southeast Asia, 2004. 2 human cases reported with 57 deaths since Jan. 2004 (see www.cdc.gov/influenza) Human-to-human transmission reported (NEJM 352:333, 2005), most have had direct contact with poultry (NEJM 350:1179, 2004). Human isolates resistant to amantadine/rimantadine. Oseltamivir rx recommended (MMWR 53:97, 2004).	**If fever & cough; known symptoms A & B and last 48 hrs of illness, consider:** **For influenza A & B; also avian (H5N1)** Oseltamivir 75 mg po bid times 5 days (also approved for rx of children age 1–12 yrs, dose 2 mg per kg up to a total of 75 mg 5 days) or **Zanamivir** 2 inhalations (2 times 5 mg) bid times 5 days	Pts with COPD or asthma, **potential risk of bronchospasm with zanamivir** ↓ side effects (Cochrane Database Sys Rev:CD 001169, 2004). All ↓ duration of symptoms by approx. 50% (1–2 days) if given within 30–36 hrs after onset of symptoms. Benefit influenced by duration of sx before rx, initiation of oseltamivir within 12 hrs after fever onset associated with median illness duration by 74.6 hrs (JAC 51:123, 2003). ↓ risk of pneumonia & hospitalization (Curr Med Res Opin 21:761, 2005). **Disturbing report** of oseltamivir-resistant virus detected after 4 days of rx (Ln 364:733 & 759, 2004). In another study of 298 rx cases of adults (MMWR). Oseltamivir-resistant viruses found (AnIM 139:313, 2003).
Human infection possible (most recent report in returning travelers from Asia, Africa, Latin America, etc. esp. India (CID 40:1282, 2005).	For influenza A only: Rimantadine or amantadine.—Age: 1–9 yrs, 5 mg per kg per day (to max. of 150 mg) po bid; >65 yrs, 100 mg po qd (adjust for ↓ renal function) for 3–5 days or 1–2 days after disappearance of symptoms.	Higher incidence of CNS side effects (5–33%) with amantadine (e.g. dizziness, anxiety, insomnia) than rimantadine (6%); a danger in elderly and pts with renal disease. Oseltamivir & zanamivir effective for both influenza A & B (no resistance). Side effect of oseltamivir—nausea & vomiting (9% & 3% in pts on drug vs placebo respectively), esp. in community-acquired MRSA pneumonia (CID 40:1693, 2005).

* See page 2 for abbreviations. NOTE: All dosage recommendations are for adults (unless otherwise indicated) and assume normal renal function.
Costs from 2005 DRUGS TOPICS RED BOOK, Medical Economics. Price is average wholesale price (AWP).

TABLE 14A (7)

VIRUS/DISEASE	DRUG/DOSAGE	SIDE EFFECTS/COMMENTS
Influenza (A & B) (continued) Prevention: See *MMWR 54:RR-8;1, 2005*	**Prevention of influenza A & B,** give vaccine followed by **oseltamivir** 75 mg po q24h and if ≥13 yrs age, consider **zanamivir** for duration of peak influenza activity in community or for outbreak control in high-risk populations (*CID 39:459, 2004*). (Consider for similar populations as immunization recommendations)	**Prevention of influenza A:** give vaccine followed by **rimantadine** or **amantadine** (dosages as above) for duration of influenza A activity in community or for outbreak control in high-risk populations (*CID 39:459, 2004*). (Consider for similar populations as immunization recommendations)	Immunization contraindicated if hypersensitivity to hen's eggs. Both amantadine and rimantadine are about 60-90% effective against influenza A. Both oseltamivir and zanamivir reported efficacious (82 & 84% respectively) in clinical trials (*JAMA 285:748, 2001; JID 186:1582, 2002*). In families, rx of index case alone as well as contact cases was more effective than index case alone (p <0.01) (*JID 189:440, 2004*).
Measles Children	No therapy or **vitamin A** 200,000 units po times 2 days.		Vitamin A ↓ severity of measles in one study (*NEJM 323:160, 1990*), not in others.
Adults	No rx or **ribavirin** IV (!) 20-35 mg per kg per day times 7 days		↓ severity of illness in adults (*CID 20:454, 1994*).
Metapneumovirus (HMPV) A paramyxovirus isolated from pts of all ages, with bronchiolitis/bronchospasm to pneumonia (*PIDJ 23:S215, 2004*).	No proven antiviral therapy		Human metapneumovirus isolated from 6.2% of children with respiratory infections (*JID 190:20, 2004*), 12% of children with lower respiratory infections (*NEJM 350:443, 2004*) & 21% of hospitalized children with URI (*PIDJ 191:382, 2005*). Dual infection with RSV assoc. with severe bronchiolitis in healthcare setting rare (*JID 40:729, 2005*).
Monkey pox (orthopox virus) (see *LnID 4:17, 2004*) In 2003, 72 pts contracted monkeypox from contact with ill prairie dogs. Source likely imported Gambian giant rats (*MMWR 42:642, 2003*).	No proven antiviral therapy Cidofovir is active in vitro & in mouse model (*AAC 46:1329, 2002; Antivir Res 57:13, 2003*)		Incubation period of 12 days, then fever, headache, cough, adenopathy, & a vesicular papular rash that pustulates, umbilicates, & crusts on the head, trunk, & extremities. Transmission in healthcare setting rare (*JID 40:729, 2005*).
Norovirus (Norwalk-like virus, or NLV) Caused 93% of outbreaks of non-bacterial gastroenteritis reported to CDC between 1997 & 2000. Transmission is by contaminated food, fecal-oral contact, or fomites.	No antiviral therapy. Replete volume.		Sudden onset of nausea, vomiting, & watery diarrhea lasting 12-60 hours. Ethanol-based hand rubs ineffective against norovirus (*J Hosp Inf 60:144, 2005*)
Papillomaviruses. 81.7% of 60 adolescent females infected over 2.2 yrs (*JID 191:182, 2005*). Therapies unsatisfactory with limited efficacy, high recurrence rates (*JAC 53:137, 2004*). **Anogenital Warts.** Condyloma acuminatum (HPV types 6 & 11 most common; HPV types 16 & 18 most likely premalignant) [See *CID 28(Suppl.1):S37, 1999*] [NOTE: Results of Pap smear should be available prior to rx; avoid rx in pregnant women] NOTE: Recurrences common after all treatments.	**Podofilox:** Apply 0.5% soln twice daily application with cotton swab for 3 days followed by 4 days of no rx; repeat cycle 4-6 times as necessary (max 4 cycles) **OR** [25% **podophyllin** in tincture of benzoin (Podocon-25): apply once weekly for up to 6 wks; wash after 1-4 hrs.] If no		Podofilox: Local reactions—pain, burning, inflammation in 50%. No systemic effects. Efficacy in penile warts: 74% vs placebo 0%. Recurrences 36% vs 100% with placebo (Podocon-25 15 mL $32.40, Condylox 3.5 mL $56.64). Warts recur in 1/3 with either agent within 1st month after rx.
	interferon alfa-2b (intron A), **alfa-n3** (Alferon N): 1 million units (0.1 mL) into lesion 3 times per week times 3 weeks		Painful; dilute to 10 million units per 1 mL. Other concentrations are hypertonic (*CID 28:S37, 1999*). Use when other rx fails, esp. in AIDS
Warts occurred within 36 mos. after infection with HPV-16/18 in 64% (*JID 119:731, 2005*).	intralesional injection of skin test antigens (mumps, candida or trichophyton) w/o or without interferon alfa-2b		More effective than placebo in ↓ warts. IFN alfa-2b did not ↑ response rate & given alone, not better than placebo in one 235-pt randomized single-blind placebo-controlled trial (*ArDerm 141:589, 2005*). An in vitro positive delayed hypersensitivity to antigen predicted resolution of wart.
	imiquimod (5% cream). Apply 3 times per wk prior to sleep; remove 6-10 hrs later when awake. Continue until cleared or 16 wks.		Clearance rates of 62% vs 14% for controls if applied 3 times per wk for up to 16 wks or until warts completely cured (*AAC 42:789, 1998*). Less effective in immunosuppressed pts. Benefit in 5/12 pts who completed 24-month course (*J Derm 152:122, 2005*). Cost of 1-4 wks = $108-432. Local reactions—mild erythema 60%, erosion 30%
Skin papillomas	Topical α-lactalbumin, Oleic acid (from human milk) applied daily for 3 wks		↓ Lesion size & recurrence vs placebo (p <0.0001) (*NEJM 350:2663, 2004*).
Parvo B19 Virus (Erythrovirus B19) Uncomplicated or self-limited acute arthritis. May be chronic in children.	No treatment recommended		Bone marrow shows selective erythrocyte maturation arrest with giant pronormoblasts. IgM antibody for diagnosis. Parvo B19 also associated with respiratory distress syndrome (*OID 27:40, 1998*) and myocardial/hydrops fetalis (*OID 220:1343, 1998*). Parvo found in a 5-year-old boy with chronic infection (likely multifocal) (*PIDJ 24:272, 2005*)
Acute profound anemia: in children, in hemolytic anemia, in HIV	**IVIG** 0.4 gm per kg IV q24h times 5 days in immune def states with severe anemia has been reported successful.		IVIG contains anti-parvo B19 antibody. Longterm remission reported (*Transpl Inf Dis 7:30, 2005*). In pts with pre-existing hemolytic anemia, parvo B19-induced bone marrow arrest can result in sudden severe anemia.

TABLE 14A (8)

VIRUS/DISEASE	DRUG/DOSAGE	SIDE EFFECTS/COMMENTS
Papovavirus/Polyomavirus		
Progressive multifocal leukoencephalopathy (PML)/JC virus	See SANFORD GUIDE TO HIV/AIDS THERAPY	Cytarabine of no value in controlled trial (NEJM 338:1345, 1998). Camptothecin, a human topoisomerase I inhibitor, was administered to a single pt with slowing of progression (Ln 349:1366, 1997). Use of cidofovir controversial (Clin Micro Rev 16:569, 2003; J Child Neurol 19:35, 2004; Transpl Inf 17:658, 2005)
Pts with advanced HIV disease or organ transplant. Reported in 3 pts receiving natalizumab, a monoclonal antibody against alpha 4 integrins for Crohn's disease (1) & multiple sclerosis (2) (NEJM 353:353, 362, & 369, 2005).	**HAART** ↑ survival (545 days vs 60 days, p 0.001) and either improved (50%) or stabilized (50%) neurological deficits in 12 pts (AIDS 12:2467, 1999). Others less optimistic (CID 28:1152, 1999)	DC immunosuppression in transplant pts resulted in successful outcome (Am J Transpl 5:1151, 2005)
Polyomavirus-associated nephropathy	**Due to BK virus post renal transplant**	Possible role for cidofovir (LnID 3:611, 2003)
Rabies (see Table 20C, pages 144–146; see Mayo Clin Proc 79:671, 2004; MMWR 54:RR-3:1, 2005)		
Rabid dogs account for 50,000 cases per year worldwide. Most cases in the U.S. are cryptic, i.e., no documented evidence of bite or contact with a rabid animal (CID 35:738, 2003). 70% assoc. with 2 rare bat species (EID 9:151, 2003). An organ donor infected 4 recipients (2 kidneys, liver & artery) who all died of rabies avg. 13 days after transplant (NEJM 352:1103, 2005).		**Mortality 100% with only survivors those who receive rabies vaccine before the onset of illness/symptoms** (CID 36:61, 2003). A 15-year-old female who developed rabies 1 month post-exposure but survived after drug induction of coma (+ other rx) for 7 days; did not receive immunoprophylaxis (NEJM 352:2508, 2005). Corticosteroids: ↑ mortality rate and ↓ incubation time in mice. Therapies that have failed after symptoms develop include rabies vaccine, rabies immunoglobulin, rabies virus neutralizing antibody, ribavirin, alfa interferon, & ketamine
Respiratory Syncytial Virus		
Major cause of pneumonia in neonates/infants. In adults, RSV accounted for 10.6% of hospitalizations for pneumonia, 11.4% for COPD, 7.2% for asthma & 5.4% for CHF in pts >65 yrs of age (NEJM 352:1749, 2005). RSV caused 11% of clinically important respiratory illnesses in infants (JID 191:1093, 2005).	Rapid dx by antigen detection on nasopharyngeal wash. **No rx proven to ↑ survival.** Various combinations of ribavirin, RSV-IVIG & palivizumab have been used, see Comments (PIDJ 23:707, 2004; Pharmacother 24:932, 2004; Ped Drugs 6:1, 2004)	Ribavirin reported to ↓ fever and other symptoms and signs. However, in controlled studies, **ribavirin had no beneficial effect** (J Ped 128: 422, 1996; AJRCCM 160:829, 1999). Still recommended by some authorities for immunocompromised children (PIDJ 19:253, 2000) & still controversial (PIDJ 22:588, 2003).
(1) Children <24 mos. old with bronchopulmonary dysplasia (BPD) requiring supplemental O₂	**RSV immune globulin intravenous** (RSV-IVIG) 100 mg per kg IV once monthly Nov. through April (for northern hemisphere) 1st year of life for prematures. Perhaps up to 60 months of age for pts with BPD. **OR**	RSV-IVIG very expensive—estimated cost per infusion $1175. See consensus opinion for details: Ped Inf Dis J 15:1059, 1996. See Ln 354:847, 1999 for updated review.
(2) Perhaps premature infants (<26 wks gestation) and <6 mos. old at start of RSV season	**Palivizumab** 15 mg per kg IM q month Nov.–April as above (Scand J Inf Dis 33:323, 2001). Cost: $3000–5000(AWP).	Palivizumab reduced hospitalization rates for RSV in 1500 premature infants & BPD children with chronic lung disease from 10.6% to 4.8% (Pediatrics 102:531, 1998). Expense argues against its use, but in 2004 approx. 100,000 infants received drug annually in U.S. (PIDJ 23:1051, 2004).
Rhinovirus (Colds) See Ln 361:51, 2003	No antiviral rx indicated (Ped Ann 34:53, 2005)	Rx sniffl: ipratropium nasal spray ↓ rhinorrhea and sneezing vs placebo (AnIM 125:89, 1996). Clemastine (an antihistamine) ↓ sneezing, rhinorrhea, mouth & throat in 6–19% (CID 22:656, 1996). Zinc lozenges were ineffective (CID 31:1202, 2000). Oral **pleconaril** given within 24 hrs of onset reduced duration of symptoms in DBPCT (p < .001) (CID 38:1523, 2003). A combination of intranasal interferon alfa-2b, oral chlorpheniramine & ibuprofen ↓ symptom score by 33–73% vs placebo when started 24 hrs after exptl rhinovirus (JID 186:147, 2002). Echinacea didn't work (CID 38:1387, 2004 & 40:807, 2005)—put it to rest
Found in ⅓ of children with community-acquired pneumonia, role in pathogenesis unclear (CID 39:681, 2004). Antiviral Kleenex may reduce spread (Med Lett 47:3, 2005)	Symptomatic rx: • **ipratropium bromide nasal** (2 sprays per nostril tid) • **clemastine** 1.34 mg 1–2 tab po bid-tid (OTC)	
SARS-CoV See page 106		
Smallpox vaccine (NEJM 346:1300, 2002)	Smallpox vaccine (if within 4 days of exposure) + cidofovir (dosage uncertain; contact CDC: 770-488-7100)	
Contact vaccinia (JAMA 288:1901, 2002)	From vaccination: Progressive vaccinia—vaccinia immune globulin may be of benefit. To obtain immune globulin, contact CDC: 770-488-7100 (CID 39:759, 776 & 819, 2004)	
West Nile virus See page 106		

* See page 2 for abbreviations. NOTE: All dosage recommendations are for adults (unless otherwise indicated) and assume normal renal function. Costs from 2005 DRUG TOPICS RED BOOK, Medical Economics. Price is average wholesale price (AWP).

TABLE 14B: ANTIVIRAL DRUGS (Other Than Retroviral)

DRUG NAME(S) GENERIC (TRADE)	DOSAGE/ROUTE/COST*	COMMENTS/ADVERSE EFFECTS
CMV (See Sanford Guide to HIV/AIDS Therapy)		
Cidofovir (Vistide)	5 mg per kg IV q week times 2, then q2 weeks. (375 mg) ($888) Properly timed IV prehydration with normal saline and oral probenecid **must be used with each cidofovir infusion** (see pkg insert for details). Renal function (serum creatinine and urine protein) must be monitored prior to each dose (see pkg insert for details).	**Adverse effects: Nephrotoxicity:** dose-dependent proximal tubular injury (Fanconi-like syndrome): proteinuria, glycosuria, bicarbonaturia, phosphaturia, polyuria (nephrogenic diabetic insipidus, Ln 350:413, 1997), ↑ creatinine. Concomitant saline prehydration, probenecid, extended dosing intervals allowed use. 25% of pts do IV cidofovir due to nephrotoxicity. Other toxicities: nausea 48%, fever 31%, alopecia 16%, myalgia 16%, proboscipod hypersensitivity 16%, neutropenia 29%. No effect on hematocrit, platelets, LFTs. **Comment:** Recommended strict dosage, frequency, or infusion rate must not be exceeded. Dose must be reduced or discontinued if changes in renal function occur during rx. For ↑ of 0.3–0.4 mg per dL in serum creatinine, cidofovir dose must be ↓ from 5 to 3 mg per kg; discontinue cidofovir if ↑ of 0.5 mg per dL above baseline or 3+ proteinuria develops (for 2+ proteinuria, observe pts carefully and consider discontinuation).
Foscarnet (Foscavir)	90 mg per kg IV q12h (induction) 90 mg per kg IV q24h (maintenance) Dosage adjust. with renal dysfunction (see Table 17) (6 gm) ($83)	**Adverse effects: Major clinical toxicity is renal impairment (1/3 of patients)**—↑ creatinine, proteinuria, nephrogenic diabetes insipidus. ↓ K⁺, ↓ Ca⁺⁺, ↓ Mg⁺⁺. Toxicity ↑ with other nephrotoxic drugs (ampho B, aminoglycosides or pentamidine (especially severe ↓ Ca⁺⁺)). CNS: seizures. Hematol.: ↓ WBC, ↓ Hgb. Hepatic: liver function tests ↑. Neuropathy. Penile ulcers.
Ganciclovir (Cytovene)	5 mg per kg IV q12h times 14 days (induction) 5 mg per kg IV q24h or 6 mg per kg 5 times per wk (maintenance) Dosage adjust. with renal dysfunction (see Table 17) (500 mg IV) ($45) Oral: 1.0 gm tid with food (fatty meal) (Oral 1 gm cap $9.60)	**Adverse effects:** Absolute neutrophil count dropped below 500 per mm³ in 15%, thrombocytopenia 21%, anemia 6%. Fever 48%, GI 50%: nausea, vomiting, diarrhea, abdominal pain 19%, rash 10%. Retinal detachment 11% (relationship to ganciclovir ?). Confusion, headache, psychiatric disturbances and seizures. Neutropenia may respond to granulocyte colony stimulating factor (G-CSF or GM-CSF). Severe myelosuppression may be ↑ with coadministration of zidovudine or azathioprine. 32% dc/interrupted rx, principally for neutropenia. Hematologic: less than with IV. Granulocytopenia 18%, anemia 12%, thrombocytopenia 6%. GI, skin same as with IV. Retinal detachment 8%.
Valganciclovir (Valcyte)	900 mg (two 450 mg tabs) po bid times 21 days for induction, followed by 900 mg po q24h. Take with food. (450 mg cap $31.70, ~$1.90/60 cap)	**Adverse effects:** late retinal detachment (7/30 eyes). Does not prevent CMV retinitis in good eye or visceral dissemination. **Comment:** Replacement every 6 months recommended. A prodrug of ganciclovir with better bioavailability. ~60% with food. **Adverse effects:** Similar to ganciclovir.
Herpesvirus (non-CMV)		
Acyclovir (Zovirax or generic)	Doses: see Table 14A 400 mg tab G $0.30–0.70 (or $110–200/yr for chronic suppression) IV $90 per g Suspension 200 mg per 5 mL $137 Ointment 5% 15 gm $90	**po:** Generally well-tolerated with occ. diarrhea, vertigo, arthralgia. Less frequent rash, fatigue, insomnia, fever, menstrual abnormalities, acne, sore throat, muscle cramps, lymphadenopathy. **IV:** Phlebitis, caustic with vesicular lesions with IV infiltration, CNS (1%): tremors, confusion, hallucinations, delirium, seizures, coma (CID 21:435, 1995). Improve 1–2 weeks after rx stopped. Renal (5%): ↑ creatinine, hematuria. With high doses may crystallize in renal tubules → obstructive uropathy (rapid infusion, dehydration, renal insufficiency and ↑ dose ↑ risk). Adequate pre-hydration may prevent such nephrotoxicity. Hepatic: ↑ ALT, AST. Uncommon: neutropenia (CID 20:1557, 1995), rash, diaphoresis, hypotension, headache, nausea.
Famciclovir (Famvir)	250 mg cap $4.70 500 mg cap $9.93	Metabolized to penciclovir. **Adverse effects:** similar to acyclovir, included headache, nausea, diarrhea, and dizziness but incidence did not differ from placebo (JAMA 276:47, 1996). May be taken without regard to meals. Dose should be reduced if CrCl <60 mL per min (see package insert & Table 14A, page 109 & Table 17, page 138).
Penciclovir (Denavir) Trifluridine (Viroptic)	Topical 1% cream 1.5 gm $26 1 drop 1% solution q2h (max. 9 drops per day) for max. of 21 days (7.5 mL, 1% solution) $105	Apply to area of recurrence of herpes labialis with start of sx, then q2h while awake times 4 days. Well tolerated. Mild burning (5%), palpebral edema (3%), punctate keratopathy, stromal edema
Valacyclovir (Valtrex)	500 mg cap $5	An ester pro-drug of acyclovir that is well-absorbed. Bioavailability 3–5 times greater than acyclovir. **Adverse effects** similar to acyclovir (see JID 186:340, 2002). Thrombotic thrombocytopenic purpura/hemolytic uremic syndrome reported in pts with advanced HIV disease and transplant recipients participating in clinical trials at doses of 8 gm per day.

* See page 2 for abbreviations. NOTE: All dosage recommendations are for adults (unless otherwise indicated) and assume normal renal function. Costs from 2005 Drug Topics Red Book, Medical Economics. Price is average wholesale price (AWP).

TABLE 14B (2)

DRUG NAME(S) GENERIC (TRADE)	DOSAGE/ROUTE/COST*	COMMENTS/ADVERSE EFFECTS
Hepatitis		
Adefovir dipivoxil (Hepsera)	10 mg po q24h (with normal CrCl); see Table 17A for renal impairment. Intron \$18 ea. = \$546 per month	Adefovir dipivoxil is a prodrug of adefovir. It is an acyclic nucleotide analog with activity against hepatitis B (HBV) at 0.2–2.5 mM (IC₅₀). See Table 9 for Cmax & T½. Primarily renal excretion—adjust dose. No food interactions. Remarkably few side effects. No nephrotoxicity at 10 mg per day. Monitor renal function, esp. with pts with pre-existing or other risks for renal impairment. Exacerbations, even acute hepatic decompensation, have occurred with discontinuation. Pregnancy (category C): minimal; limited, but hepatic decompensation has occurred.
Entecavir (Baraclude)	0.5 mg q24h; if refractory to lamivudine: 1 mg per day (\$714.60 per month)	A nucleoside analog active against HBV including lamivudine-resistant mutants. Minimal adverse effects reported: headache, fatigue, dizziness, & nausea reported in 22% of pts. Potential for lactic acidosis but not reported to date. Adjust dosage in renal impairment (see Table 17, page 197).
Interferon alfa is available as alfa-2a (Roferon-A), alfa-2b (Intron-A)	3 million units (Roferon: \$40; Intron \$39; Intergen 9 mcg \$52)	**Adverse effects:** Flu-like syndrome (headache, fever, myalgia, arthralgias, esp. during 1st week of rx: fever 98%, fatigue 89%, myalgia 73%; headache 71%. GI: anorexia 46%, diarrhea 29%. CNS: dizziness 21%. Rash 18%, later profound fatigue & psychiatric symptoms in up to ⅓ of pts (J Clin Psych 64:708, 2003) (depression, anxiety, emotional lability and agitation), alopecia. ↑ TSH, autoimmune thyroid disorders with hypo- or hyperthyroidism. Graves disease reported (J Inv Med 53:26, 2005). Hematol.: ↓ WBC 49%, ↓ Hgb 27%, ↓ platelets 35%. Consider prophylactic antidepressant in pts with history. Acute reversible hearing loss and/or tinnitus in up to 1/3 (Arch IM 343:1134, 1994). Non-neuropathy (retinal hemorrhage, cotton wool spots, ↓ in color vision) reported (AJO 18:1365, 2004). Cryoglobulinemia assoc. with HCV usually responds to IFN but exacerbations with vasculitis also reported with rx (Clin Rheum, e30, June 2005). Side-effects ↑ with ↑ doses and dose reduction may be needed.
PEG interferon alfa-2b (PEG-Intron)	0.5–1.5 mcg per kg subcut. q wk (120 mcg \$591)	
Pegylated-40k interferon alfa-2a (Pegasys)	180 mcg subcut. q wk times 48 wks (180 mcg \$404)	Attachment of IFN to polyethylene glycol (PEG) prolongs half-life and allows weekly dosing. Better efficacy data with similar adverse effects profile compared to standard IFN.
Lamivudine (3TC) (Epivir-HBV)	100 mg po q24h (\$100.14 for 1 yr for hepatitis B. [100 mg] tab \$7 or \$205 per month)	
Ribavirin/interferon alfa-2b combination pack (Rebetron)	**Adverse effects:** See Table 14D, page 122. NOTE: 100 mg po q24h times 1 yr for hepatitis B. (100 mg) tab \$7 or \$205 per month) Combination kit contains 3 wk supply of IFN and 42, 70, or 84 caps of 200 mg ribavirin. **Dose:** ≤75 kg give Rebetron 3 million units IFN alfa-2b 3 x per week AND ribavirin 1000 mg po q.a.m. (<75 kg) or 600 mg po bid (>75 kg). Rebetron (1000 mg per day ribavirin dose pack). (\$9652 per 24 wk course)	**Ribavirin.** Hemolytic anemia common but usually responds to ↓ ribavirin dosage. ARDS reported (Chest 124:406, 2003). Erythropoietin (Epoetin alfa) effective in ↑ Hgb levels & quality of life while allowing adequate dosage of ribavirin to be maintained (Pharmacotherap 25:662, 2005); does not apply to anemia due to antiretrovirals (Gastro 100:1415, 2005). **Since ribavirin is teratogenic, drug must not be used during pregnancy or within 6 months of pregnancy.** Also should not be used in pts with endstage renal failure, severe heart disease, or hemoglobinopathies. Ribavirin efficacy against HBV (but not with other degree of anemia (but 5 wk efficacy against HBV (but with only degree of anemia). A pilot study suggests levels between 3000 to 3500 ng per mL 8 wks after initiating rx is optimal (Intervirol 48:138, 2005).
PEG IFN + ribavirin in combination		**Interferon alfa.** Severe psychiatric effects, esp. depression, most common reason for discontinuation of rx. **Suicidal behavior reported.** Preemptive rx with antidepressants effective in 1 open-label study (J Hpt 42:793, 2005). Hyper- & hypothyroidism. Alopecia (30%) including reversible alopecia universalis (J Chemother 17:212, 2005) & other thyroid dysfunction. Uncommon side-effects include exacerbation of psoriasis, lichen planus, Behçet's syndrome, sarcoidosis, pulmonary disease (Medscape Gen Med 7:6, 2005), and sudden sensory neural hearing loss (Anticancer Res 23:1151, 2003) & other hematological conditions. Sexual dysfunction with ↓ testosterone levels (J Endo 185:345, 2004), & risk of lipoatrophy 2° to mitochondrial toxicity when administered with nucleoside analogs to HIV-HCV co-infected pts (Antivir Ther 10:557, 2005), & sarcoidosis (AbDerm 141:865, 2005).

	Ribavirin	Interferon
Dose changes	Hgb: <10	↓ to 200 mg q a.m.	No change
	<8.5	DC	DC
	WBC <1500		↓ to 1.5 million units subcut. 3 times per wk
	<1000		DC
	Abs. PMNs <750		↓ to 1.5 million units subcut. 3 times per wk
	<500	No change	DC
	Platelets <50,000	No change	↓ to 1.5 million units subcut. 3 times per wk
	<25,000	DC	DC

* See page 2 for abbreviations. NOTE: All dosage recommendations are for adults (unless otherwise indicated) and assume normal renal function.
Costs from 2005 Drug Topics Red Book, Medical Economics. Price is average wholesale price (AWP).

TABLE 14B (3)

DRUG NAME(S) GENERIC (TRADE)	DOSAGE/ROUTE/COST*	COMMENTS/ADVERSE EFFECTS
Hepatitis *(continued)* Ribavirin (Rebetol)	Use with pegylated interferons (alfa-2a & 2b) for treatment of hepatitis C. Available as: 200 mg caps (rebetol). Dose: <75 kg BW – 2 caps in a.m. & 3 caps in p.m.; >75 kg BW 3 caps in a.m. & 3 caps in p.m. Cost: 200 mg $10.60	Side-effects as above, esp. hemolytic anemia (during 1st 1–2 wks of rx) with hemoglobin ↓ 1 or 2 gm. Should not be used with CrCl <50 mL per min & cautiously with cardiac disease.
Influenza A Amantadine (Symmetrel) or Rimantadine (Flumadine)	Amantadine and rimantadine doses are the same (rimantadine approved only for prophylaxis in children, not treatment). Amantadine 100 mg po bid; >65 y.o., 100 mg po or 100 mg per 10 mL soln. G: 100 mg cap $0.50, 100 mg tab/syrup $2 Rimantadine 100 mg tab/syrup $2	Side-effects/toxicity: CNS (nervousness, anxiety, difficulty concentrating, and lightheadedness). Symptoms occurred in 6% on rimantadine vs 14% on amantadine. They usually ↓ after 1st week and disappear when drug dc. GI (nausea, anorexia). Some serious side-effects—delirium, hallucinations, and seizures—are associated with high plasma drug levels resulting from renal insufficiency, esp. in older pts, those with prior seizure disorders, or psychiatric disorders. Dosages of both drugs should be reduced (amantadine: creatinine clearance <50 mL per min; rimantadine CrCl <10 mL per min); see package inserts and Table 17, pages 137 & 138. Both drugs teratogenic in animals and contraindicated during pregnancy [Med Lett 39:72, 1997].
Influenza A and B—For therapy, initiate within 48 hrs of symptom onset		
Zanamivir (Relenza) For pts ≥12 yrs of age	2 inhalations (2 times 5 mg) bid times 5 days. Powder is inhaled using a specially designed breath-activated device. Each inhalation containing blister contains 5 mg of zanamivir. $60/course	Active by inhalation against neuraminidase of both influenza A and B and inhibits release of virus from epithelial cells of respiratory tract. Approx. 4–17% of inhaled dose absorbed by kidney but with low absorption, dose reduction not necessary in renal failure. Minimal side-effects: <3% cough, sinusitis, diarrhea, nausea and vomiting. **Reports of respiratory adverse events in pts with or without h/o airways disease, should be avoided in pts with respiratory disease.**
Oseltamivir (Tamiflu)	75 mg po bid for treatment (pediatric suspension (12 mg per mL)) approved for treatment, not prevention, in children age 1–12 at dose of 2 mg per kg (up to 75 mg) bid times 5 days. For prevention 75 mg po q24h for duration of peak of flu. $73 per 5 day course	Well absorbed (80% bioavailable) from GI tract as ethyl ester of active compound GS 4071. T½ 6–10 hrs; excreted unchanged by kidney. Adverse effects in 15% include diarrhea 1.6%, nausea 0.5%, vomiting. Nausea ↓ with food. Also available as 12 mg per mL oral suspension. headache [J Am Geri Soc 50:608, 2002].
Respiratory Syncytial Virus (RSV) and other		
Palivizumab (Synagis) (See Med Lett 41:1, 1999) Used only for prevention of RSV infection in high-risk children Pediatrics 102:1211, 1998)	15 mg per kg IM q month 100 mg vial (1 injection) $1560	A monoclonal antibody directed against the F glycoprotein on surface of virus; side-effects are nominal. occ. ↑ ALT [JID 176:1215, 1997].
Ribavirin (Virazole)	1.1 gm per day (6 gm vial for inhalation $1574)	**Ribavirin side-effects:** Anemia, rash, conjunctivitis. Read package insert. Avoid procedures that lead to drug precipitation in ventilator tubing with subsequent dysfunction. Significant teratogenicity in animals. **Contraindicated in pregnant women and partners.** Pregnant health care workers should avoid direct care of pts receiving aerosolized ribavirin.
RSV-iV immunoglobulin (iG) (RespiGam)	100 mg per kg IV q month (50 mL, $1487)	RespiGam side-effects rare but include fatal anaphylaxis, pruritus, rash, wheezing, fever, joint pain.
Warts (See CID 28:S37, 1999)		
Interferon alfa-2b or alfa-n3	Apply 1 million units into lesion. Cost: $10	Interferon alfa-2b 3 million units per 0.5 mL, interferon alfa-n3 5 million units per 1 mL. Cost: $10.
Podofilox (Condylox)	3.5 mL, for topical application; $130	Side-effects: Local reactions—pain, burning, inflammation in 50%. No systemic effects.
Imiquimod (Aldara)	Cream applied 3 times per week to maximum of 16 wks. 250 mg packets $15	Mild erythema, erosions, itching and burning

* See page 2 for abbreviations. NOTE: All dosage recommendations are for adults (unless otherwise indicated) and assume normal renal function.
Costs from 2005 Drug Topics Red Book, Medical Economics. Price is average wholesale price (AWP).

TABLE 14C: ANTIRETROVIRAL THERAPY IN TREATMENT-NAIVE ADULTS

(See the 2005 SANFORD GUIDE TO HIV/AIDS THERAPY, Table 6, for additional information regarding treatment and complications of antiretroviral agents)

In 2005, guidelines and recommendations for the treatment of individuals infected with HIV-1 were updated: DHHS guidelines for the use of antiretroviral therapy (ART) in pediatrics, and recommendations for ART in pregnant women. All documents are available online at www.aidsinfo.nih.gov. New treatment recommendations by the International AIDS Society-USA Panel were also released (JAMA 292:251, 2004), as were guidelines for primary care management of HIV-infected persons provided by the HIV Medicine Association of the IDSA (CID 39:609, 2004). For additional explanation and alternatives, see www.aidsinfo.nih.gov.

A. When to start therapy?

HIV Symptoms	CD4 cells per mcL	Start Treatment	Comment
Yes	Any	Yes	
No	<200	Yes	
No	>200–350	Offer (see Comment)	Risk for progression to AIDS also depends on viral load; consider on individual basis
No	>350	No (see Comment)	Maybe if CD4 decreasing rapidly and/or viral load >100,000 copies per mL

* Acute retroviral syndrome—*See page 118, section C.*

B. Suggested Initial Therapy Regimens for Untreated Chronic HIV Infection *(For pregnancy, see below and Table 8 of the SANFORD GUIDE TO HIV/AIDS THERAPY, 2005)*

1. Preferred Regimens

Regimen	Pill strength (mg)	Usual Daily Regimen (oral)	No. pills per day	Cost per month (Avg. Wholesale Price)	Comment (See also individual agents)
a. (Zidovudine + Lamivudine)+ Efavirenz	(300 + 150) + 600	(Combination—Combivir 1 tab bid) + 1 tab q24h at bedtime, empty stomach (see Comment)	3	$1135	Good efficacy, low pill burden; low AE profile. If rx stopped, dc efavirenz 1–2 wks before other agents (for explanation, see page 120). Avoid efavirenz in pregnancy or in women who might become pregnant (Pregnancy Category D). Food may ↑ serum efavirenz concentration, which can lead to ↑ adverse events.
b. (Tenofovir + Emtricitabine)+ Efavirenz	(300 + 200) + 600	(Combination—Truvada 1 tab q24h) + 1 tab q24h at bedtime, empty stomach. Food may ↑ serum efavirenz concentration, which can lead to ↑ adverse events.	2	$1258	Good efficacy, low pill burden. Tenofovir: emerging reports of renal toxicity. Avoid efavirenz in pregnancy or in women might become pregnant (Pregnancy Category D). Interim analysis of ongoing trial suggests superiority of emtricitabine/tenofovir/ efavirenz over 3TC/ZDV/efavirenz in rx-naive pts (27 IAS, 2005)
c. (Zidovudine + Lamivudine)+ Lopinavir/Ritonavir	(300 + 150) + 200/50	(Combination—Combivir 1 tab bid) + 2 tabs bid without regard to food	6	$1394	Good virologic efficacy and durable effect. Tolerable AEs. ↓ accumulation of resistance mutations than nelfinavir regimen (NEJM 346:2039, 2002). Lopinavir/ ritonavir can be given as 4 tabs once daily in rx-naive pts.

2. Alternative Regimens

Regimen	Pill strength (mg)	Usual Daily Regimen (oral)	No. pills per day	Cost per month (Avg. Wholesale Price)	Comment (See also individual agents)
a. Didanosine EC + Lamivudine + Efavirenz	400 + 300 + 600	1 cap q24h at bedtime, fasting + 1 tab q24h + 1 tab q24h at bedtime, empty stomach. Didanosine dosage shown for ≥60 kg	3	$1071	Low pill burden. Efficacy and durability under study. Potential didanosine AEs (pancreatitis, peripheral neuritis). Avoid efavirenz in pregnancy or in women who might become pregnant (Pregnancy Category D). Food may ↑ serum efavirenz concentration, which can lead to adverse events. Can substitute emtricitabine 200 mg (po) q24h for lamivudine 300 mg (po) q24h.
b. (Zidovudine + Lamivudine)+ Fosamprenavir + Ritonavir	(300 + 150) + 700 + 100	(Combination—Combivir 1 tab bid) + 1 tab bid fed or fasting + 1 tab bid fed or fasting	6	$1892	Take without regard to meals. Skin rash. GI symptoms. Contains sulfa moiety. Alternative fosamprenavir regimen available for rx-naive pts: fosamprenavir without ritonavir (see label for doses).
c. (Zidovudine + Lamivudine)+ Nelfinavir	(300 + 150) + 625	(Combination—Combivir 1 tab bid) + 2 tabs bid, with food	6	$1490	For peds: oral solution of amprenavir available. Nelfinavir-associated diarrhea in 20%. Nelfinavir contraindicated with drugs highly dependent on CYP3A4 elimination where ↑ levels may cause life-threatening toxicity.
d. (Zidovudine + Lamivudine)+ Atazanavir	(300 + 150) + 200	(Combination—Combivir 1 tab bid) + 2 caps q24h, with food	4	$1485	Lower potential for lipid derangement by atazanavir than other PIs. May ↑ PR interval & bilirubin.

TABLE 14C (2)

Regimen	Pill strength (mg)	Usual Daily Regimen (oral)	No. pills per day	Cost per month (Avg. Wholesale Price)	Comment (See also individual agents)
2. Alternative Regimens *(continued)*					
e. **Zidovudine + Lamivudine) + Indinavir + Ritonavir**	(300 + 150) + 400 + 100	(**Combination—Combivir** 1 tab bid) + 2 caps q12h + 1 cap q12h	8	$1672	Nephrolithiasis—hydrate! May ↑ bilirubin. Metabolic effects of PI.
3. Triple nucleoside or nucleoside/nucleotide regimen: Due to inferior virologic activity, use only when preferred or alternative regimen not possible.					
Zidovudine + Lamivudine + Abacavir	(300 + 150 + 300)	(**Combination—Trizivir** 1 tab bid)	2	$1110	Reduced efficacy as compared to preferred & alternative regimens. Potential serious abacavir AEs. *(See comments for individual agents)*
4. During pregnancy: Expert consultation mandatory. Timing of rx initiation & drug choice must be individualized. Viral resistance testing should be strongly considered. Longterm effects of agents unknown. Certain drugs hazardous or contraindicated *(see SANFORD GUIDE TO HIV/AIDS THERAPY, Table 17)*. See www.aidsinfo.nih.gov for additional information & alternative rx options, and *(see SANFORD GUIDE TO HIV/AIDS THERAPY, Table 8A)* for regimens to prevent mother-child transmission.					
a. **Zidovudine + Lamivudine + Nevirapine**	(300 + 150 + 200)	(**Combination—Combivir** 1 tab bid) 1 tab bid fed or fasting [after 14-day lead-in period of 1 tab q24h)]	4	$1097	See nevirapine **Black Box warnings** *(page 120)*—among others, ↑ risk of **potentially fatal hepatotoxicity** in women with CD4 >250. Avoid in this group unless benefits clearly > risks; monitor intensively if drug must be used.
b. **Zidovudine + Lamivudine+ Nelfinavir**	(300 + 150) + 625	(**Combination—Combivir** 1 tab bid) 2 tabs bid with food	6	$1490	*(See section 2.c above)*
c. **Zidovudine + Lamivudine+ Saquinavir + Ritonavir**	(300 + 150) + 500 + 100	(**Combination—Combivir** 1 tab bid) 2 tabs bid + 1 cap bid	8	NA	Use saquinavir tabs only in combination with ritonavir. Certain drugs metabolized by CYP3A4 are contraindicated with saquinavir/ritonavir. (LHHS recommendations based on saquinavir softgel caps, which are no longer available, plus ritonavir. www.aidsinfo.nih.gov).

C. Suggested Regimen for Acute Primary HIV Infection *(see Comment)*

Regimen	Pill Strength (mg)	Usual Daily Regimen (oral)	No. pills per day	Cost per month (Avg. Wholesale Price)	Comment (See also individual agents)
Zidovudine + Lamivudine)+ Efavirenz	(300 + 150) + 600	(**Combination—Combivir** 1 tab bid) 1 tab q24h at bedtime, empty stomach. Food may ↑ serum efavirenz concentration, which can lead to ↑ adverse events.	3	$1135	Benefits of rx acute HIV infection uncertain; treatment is considered optional and best undertaken in research setting. Perform resistance testing. Optimal duration of rx unknown. (See www.aidsinfo.nih.gov). Avoid efavirenz in pregnancy or in women who might become pregnant **(Pregnancy Category D).**

D. Some Antiretroviral Therapies Should NOT Be Offered. see *Comment)*

E. Selected Characteristics of Antiretroviral Drugs
1. **Selected Characteristics of Nucleoside/Nucleotide Reverse Transcriptase Inhibitors (NRTIs)**
   All agents have Black Box warning: Risk of lactic acidosis/hepatic steatosis. Also, labels note risk of fat redistribution/accumulation with ARV rx. For combinations, see warnings for component agents.

Generic/Trade Name	Pharmaceutical Prep. (Avg. Wholesale Price)	Usual Adult Dosage & Food Effect	Absorbed, %, po	Serum T½, hrs	Intracellular T½, hrs	Elimination	Major Adverse Events/Comments (See Table 14D)
Abacavir (ABC; Ziagen)	300 mg tabs or 20 mg per mL oral solution ($448 per month)	300 mg bid or 600 mg po q24h. Food OK	83	1.5	20	Liver metab., renal excretion of metabolites, 82%. Alcohol ↑ AUC	**Hypersensitivity reaction:** fever, rash, N/V, malaise, diarrhea, abdominal pain, respiratory symptoms. (Severe reactions may be ↑ with 600 mg dose.) **Do not rechallenge!** Report to 800-270-0425.

TABLE 14C (3) (continued)

1. **Selected Characteristics of Nucleoside or Nucleotide Reverse Transcriptase Inhibitors (NRTIs) (3)**
   All agents have **Black Box warning**: Risk of lactic acidosis/hepatic steatosis. Also, labels note risk of fat redistribution/accumulation with ARV rx. For combinations, see warnings for component agents.

Generic/Trade Name	Pharmaceutical Prep. (Avg. Wholesale Price)	Usual Adult Dosage & Food Effect	Absorbed, %, po	Serum T½s, hrs	Intracellular T½s, hrs	Elimination	Major Adverse Events/Comments (See Table 14D)
Abacavir/lamivudine/ zidovudine (Trizivir)	Film-coated tabs: ABC 300 mg + 3TC 150 mg + ZDV 300 mg ($1170 per month)	1 tab po bid (not recommended for wt. <40 kg or CrCl <50 mL per min or impaired hepatic function)	(See individual components)			(See Comments for individual components) **Note: Black Box warnings** for ABC hypersensitivity reaction & others. Should only be used for regimens intended to include these 3 agents. **Black Box warning**—limited data for VL >100,000 copies per mL.	
Didanosine (ddI, Videx or Videx EC) Comment: Potential ↑ toxicity & ↓ efficacy if used with tenofovir (see AIDS Reader 15:4/3, 2005).	25, 50, 100, 150, 200 mg chewable tabs; 100, 167, 250 mg powder for oral solution; 125, 200, 250, 400 enteric-coated caps ($332 per month Videx EC)	260 kg: Usually 400 mg enteric-coated tabs q24h ½ hr before or 2 hrs after meal **Do not crush** <60 kg: 250 mg EC po q24h Food ↓ levels *See Comment*	30–40	1.6	25–40	Renal excretion, 50%	**Pancreatitis**, peripheral neuropathy; lactic acidosis & hepatic steatosis (rare but life-threatening), esp. combined with stavudine in pregnancy. Retinal, optic nerve changes reported. **If ddI + TDF is used, reduce dose from 400 mg to 250 mg EC q24h (or from 250 mg EC to 200 mg EC for adults <60 kg).**
Emtricitabine (FTC, Emtriva) Exacerbation of Hep B reported after stopping FTC	200 mg caps; 10 mg per mL solution ($318 per month)	200 mg po q24h. Food OK.	93	Approx. 10	39	Renal excretion 86%, minor biotransformation; 14% excretion in feces	Well tolerated; headache, nausea, vomiting & diarrhea occasionally, skin rash rarely. Skin hyperpigmentation. Differs only slightly in structure from lamivudine (5-fluoro substitution)
Emtricitabine/tenofovir disoproxil fumarate (Truvada)	Film-coated tabs: FTC 200 mg + TDF 300 mg ($770 per month)	1 tab q24h for CrCl ≥50 mL per min Food OK	92/25	10/17	—	Primarily renal/renal	See Comments for individual agents **Black Box warning**—not indicated for rx of Hep B. Exacerbation after stopping.
Lamivudine (3TC, Epivir)	150, 300 mg tabs; 10 mg per mL oral solution ($331 per month)	150 mg po bid or 300 mg po q24h. Food OK.	86	5–7	18	Renal excretion, minimal metabolism	**Use HIV dose, not Hep B dose.** Usually well-tolerated. Risk of exacerbation of Hep B after stopping 3TC.
Lamivudine/abacavir (Epzicom)	Film-coated tabs: 3TC 300 mg + abacavir 600 mg ($781 per month)	1 tab po q24h. Food OK.	86/86	5–7/1.5	—	Primarily renal metabolism	See Comments for individual agents. **Note abacavir hypersensitivity Black Box warnings** (severe reactions may be ↑ with 600 mg dose)
Lamivudine/zidovudine (Combivir)	Film-coated tabs: 3TC 150 mg + ZDV 300 mg ($722 per month)	1 tab po bid. Not recommended for CrCl <50 mL per min or impaired renal/hepatic function Food OK.	86/64	5–7/0.5–3	—	Primarily renal metabolism with renal excretion of glucuronide	See Comments for individual agents **See Black Box warning**—exacerbation of Hep B in pts stopping 3TC
Stavudine (d4T, Zerit)	15, 20, 30, 40 mg capsules; 1 mg per mL oral solution ($330 per month 40 mg caps)	260 kg: 40 mg po bid <60 kg: 30 mg po bid Food OK; high-fat meal ↑ absorption	86	1.2–1.6	3.5	Renal excretion, 40%	**Highest incidence of lactic acidosis of all NRTIs.** (See Comments for didanosine.) Pancreatitis. Peripheral neuropathy. High incidence of lipoatrophy, hyperlipidemia.
Tenofovir disoproxil fumarate (TDF; Viread)—a nucleotide **Black Box warning**—Not indicated for treatment of Hep B. exacerbations of Hep B reported after stopping tenofovir.	300 mg tabs ($478 per month)	CrCl ≥50 mL per min: 300 mg po q24h. Food OK; high-fat meal ↑ absorption	39 (with food); 25 (fasted)	17	>60	Renal excretion 70–80%	Headache, N/V. Cases of renal dysfunction reported; avoid concomitant nephrotoxic agents. Must adjust dose of ddI if used concomitantly (see ddI Comments above). Atazanavir & lopinavir/ritonavir ↑ tenofovir concentrations; monitor for adverse effects.

TABLE 14C (4) *(continued)*

1. Selected Characteristics of Nucleoside or Nucleotide Reverse Transcriptase Inhibitors (NRTIs)

All agents have Black Box warning: Risk of lactic acidosis/hepatic steatosis. Also, labels note risk of fat redistribution/accumulation with ARV rx. For combinations, see warnings for component agents.

Generic/Trade Name	Pharmaceutical Prep. (Avg. Wholesale Price)	Usual Adult Dosage & Food Effect	Absorbed, % po	Serum T½, hrs	Intracellular T½, hrs	Elimination	Major Adverse Events/Comments (See Table 14D)
Zalcitabine (ddC; Hivid)	0.375, 0.75 mg (0.375, 0.75 tabs [$623 per month)	0.75 mg po q8h. Food OK	85	2	3	Renal excretion, 70%.	**Peripheral neuropathy.** Rarely life-threatening: lactic acidosis, pancreatitis.
Zidovudine (ZDV, AZT; Retrovir)	100, 300 mg (100 mg caps; 300 mg tabs; 10 mg per mL IV solution; 10 mg per mL oral syrup [$389 per month)	300 mg po q12h. Food OK	60	1.1	11	Metabolized to glucuronide & excreted in urine	Bone marrow suppression, GI intolerance, headache, insomnia, malaise, myopathy

2. Selected Characteristics of Non-Nucleoside Reverse Transcriptase Inhibitors (NNRTIs)

Generic/Trade Name	Pharmaceutical Prep. (Avg. Wholesale Price)	Usual Adult Dosage & Food Effect	Absorbed, % po	Serum T½, hrs	Intracellular T½, hrs	Elimination	Major Adverse Events/Comments (See Table 14D)
Delavirdine (Rescriptor)	100, 200 mg tablets ($253 per month)	400 mg po q8h.	85	5.8		Cytochrome P450 (3A inhibitor) 51% excreted in urine (<5% unchanged), 44% in feces.	Rash severe enough to stop drug in 4.3%.
Efavirenz (Sustiva) **Pregnancy Category D—may cause fetal harm—avoid in pregnant women or those who might become pregnant** (Note: No single method of contraception is 100% reliable)	50, 100, 200 mg capsules, 600 mg tablet ($479 per month)	600 mg po q24h at bedtime. ↑ serum food. Food may ↑ serum conc., which can lead to ↑ in risk of adverse events.	42	40–55 See Comment		Cytochrome P450 (3A mixed inducer/inhibitor) 14–34% of dose excreted in urine as glucuronidated metabolites, 16–61% in feces.	Rash severe enough to dc use of drug in 1.7%. High frequency of diverse CNS AEs: somnolence, dreams, confusion, agitation. Serious psychiatric symptoms. False-pos. cannabinoid screen. Very long tissue T½. If efavirenz to be discontinued, stop efavirenz & continue other two drugs in regimen for 1-2 weeks before stopping companion agents. Otherwise, risk of developing efavirenz resistance, as after 1–2 days only efavirenz in blood and/or tissue (11th CROI 2004, Abst. 131).
Nevirapine (Viramune) **Black Box warning—fatal hepatotoxicity.** Women with CD4 >250 esp. vulnerable, including pregnant women. Avoid in this group unless benefit clearly > risks (www.fda.gov/cder/drug/advisory/nevirapine.htm)	200 mg tabs, 50 mg per 5 mL oral suspension ($424 per month)	200 mg po q24h for 14 days & then 200 mg po bid (see Comments & Black Box warning) Food OK	> 90	25–30		Cytochrome P450 (3A4, 2B6) inducer, 80% of dose excreted in urine as glucuronidated metabolites, 10% in feces.	Rash severe enough to stop drug in 7%, severe or life-threatening skin reactions in 2%. Do not restart if any discontinuation for severe skin rxn. Rash escalation period may ↓ skin reactions. As with efavirenz, because of long T½, consider continuing companion agents for several days if nevirapine is discontinued. Men with CD4 >400 also at ↑ risk. Rash severe enough to stop drug in 7%, severe reactions in 2%. If serious, intensive monitoring required.

3. Selected Characteristics of Protease Inhibitors (PIs).

All PIs: Glucose metabolism: new diabetes mellitus or deterioration of glucose control; fat redistribution; possible hemophilia bleeding; hypertriglyceridemia or hypercholesterolemia. Exercise caution re: potential drug interactions.

Generic/Trade Name	Pharmaceutical Prep. (Avg. Wholesale Price)	Usual Adult Dosage & Food Effect	Absorbed, % po	Serum T½, hrs	Elimination	Major Adverse Events/Comments (See Table 14D)
Atazanavir (Reyataz)	100, 150, 200 mg capsules ($857 per month)	400 mg po q24h with food (exception is atazanavir 300 mg po q24h + ritonavir 100 mg po q24h when used with efavirenz (atazanavir 400 mg q24h) or with TDF 300 mg po q24h). Take with food 2 hrs pre or 1 hr post buffered ddI. Ritonavir-boosted dose also recommended for ARV rx-experienced pts.	Good oral bioavailability; food enhances bioavailability & ↓ pharmacokinetic variability. Absorption ↓ by antacids, H₂-blockers, proton pump inhibitors.	Approx. 7	Cytochrome P450 (3A4, 1A2 & 2C9 inhibitor), & UGT1A1 inhibitor. 7% excreted in urine (13% unchanged), 79% excreted in feces (20% unchanged)	No ↑ lipids in available studies. Asymptomatic unconjugated hyperbilirubinemia common. Headache, rash, GI symptoms. **Prolongation of PR interval (1st degree AV block) with ↑ interval with ritonavir. Avoid/adjust/monitor. Caution in pre-existing conduction system disease. Efavirenz & tenofovir ↓ atazanavir exposure: use atazanavir/ritonavir regimen; also, atazanavir ↑ tenofovir concentrations—watch for adverse events.**

3. **Selected Characteristics of Protease Inhibitors (PIs)** *(continued)*

TABLE 14C (5)

Glucose metabolism: new diabetes mellitus or deterioration of glucose control, fat redistribution, possible hemophilia bleeding, hypertriglyceridemia or hypercholesterolemia. Exercise caution re. potential drug interactions.

Generic/Trade Name	Pharmaceutical Prep. (Avg. Wholesale Price)	Usual Adult Dosage & Food Effect	Absorbed, %, po	Serum T½, hrs	Elimination	Major Adverse Events/Comments (See Table 14D)
Fosamprenavir (Lexiva)	700 mg tablet ($632 per month if with ritonavir)	1400 mg (two 700 mg tabs) po bid OR With ritonavir: [1400 mg fosam-prenavir (2 tabs) + ritonavir 200 mg] po q24h OR [700 mg fosamprenavir (1 tab) + ritonavir 100 mg] po bid	Bioavailability not established. Food OK	7.7	Hydrolyzed to amprenavir, then Cytochrome P450 (3A4 substrate, inhibitor, inducer)	Amprenavir prodrug. (See major adverse events, Table 14D(2).) Once-daily regimen (1) not recommended for PI-experienced pts, (2) additional ritonavir needed if given with efavirenz (see label). Boosted twice-daily regimen is recommended for PI-experienced pts.
Indinavir (Crixivan)	100, 200, 333, 400 mg capsules Store in original container with desiccant	Two 400 mg caps (800 mg) po q8h. Without food or with light meal. Can take with ritonavir (e.g., 800 mg indinavir + 100 mg ritonavir q12h), no food restriction	65	1.2-2	Cytochrome P450 (3A4 inhibitor)	**Maintain hydration. Nephrolithiasis,** nausea, inconsequential ↑ of indirect bilirubin, ↑ AST/ALT, headache, asthenia, blurred vision, metallic taste, hemolysis. ↑ urine WBC (>100 per hpf) has been assoc. with nephrolithiasis/medullary calcification, cortical atrophy.
Lopinavir + ritonavir (Kaletra)	(200 mg lopinavir + 50 mg ritonavir) tablets. Tabs do not need refrigeration. Oral solution: (80 mg lopinavir + 20 mg ritonavir) per mL. (NOTE: drug content of tabs is not equal to that of previous 133.3/33.3 mg capsules.)	(400 mg lopinavir + 100 mg ritonavir)—2 tabs po bid. Higher dose may be needed in non-rx-naive pts when used with efavirenz, nevirapine, amprenavir (caps), or unboosted fosamprenavir (tabs). (See Table 22B & C & pkg labeling for specific agents.)	No food effect (Earlier capsule formulation required food.)	5-6	Cytochrome P450 (3A4 inhibitor)	Nausea, vomiting, diarrhea, ↑ AST/ALT, pancreatitis. Oral solution 42% alcohol. Lopinavir + ritonavir can be taken as single daily dose of 4 tabs (total 800 mg lopinavir + 200 mg ritonavir), except in rx-experienced pts or those taking concomitant efavirenz, nevirapine, amprenavir, or nelfinavir.
Nelfinavir (Viracept)	625, 250 mg tabs; 50 mg per gm oral powder ($726 per month)	2 625 mg tabs (1250 mg) po bid, with food	20-80 Food ↑ exposure & variability	3.5-5	Cytochrome P450 (3A4 inhibitor)	Diarrhea. Coadministration of drugs with life-threatening toxicities & which are cleared by CYP3A4 is contraindicated.
Ritonavir (Norvir)	100 mg capsules; 600 mg per 7.5 mL solution. Refrigerate caps but not solution. Room temperature times 1 mo. OK ($10.29 per capsule)	Full dose: 6 caps (600 mg) po Escalate to full dose: 300 mg po times 2 days; 400 mg bid times 3 days; 500 mg bid times 7 days; then 600 mg bid. Booster drug —see Comment	Food ↑ absorption	3-5	Cytochrome P450. Potent 3A4 & 2D6 inhibitor	Nausea/vomiting/diarrhea, extremity & circumoral paresthesias, hepatitis, taste perversion. ↑ CPK & uric acid. **Used to enhance pharmacokinetics of other PIs, using lower ritonavir doses. Black Box warning**—potentially fatal drug interactions—see Table 22A–C, pages 149 & 152
Saquinavir (Invirase—hard gel caps or tabs) + ritonavir	Saquinavir 200 mg caps, 500 mg film-coated tabs; ritonavir 100 mg caps ($718 per month)	(2 tabs saquinavir (1000 mg) OR 5 caps saquinavir (1000 mg)) + 1 cap ritonavir (100 mg) po bid, with food	Erratic, 4 (saquinavir alone)	1-2	Cytochrome P450 (3A4 inhibitor)	Nausea, diarrhea, headache. ↑ AST/ALT. Avoid rifampin with saquinavir + ritonavir—hepatitis (see http://www.fda.gov/cder/drug/InfoSheets/HCP/saquinavirHCP.htm, accessed 2/26/05). **Black Box warning**—Invirase to be used only with ritonavir.
Tipranavir (Aptivus) For rx-experienced pts or PI-resistant strains	250 mg capsules. Refrigerate unopened bottles. Use opened bottles within 2 months.	[500 mg (two 250 mg caps) + ritonavir 200 mg] po bid, with food	Absorption low, ↑ with high fat meal, ↓ with Al+++ & Mg++ antacids	5.5-6	Cytochrome 3A4. But with ritonavir most of drug is eliminated in feces	Contains sulfa moiety. **Black Box warning**—hepatitis, fatal hepatic failure. Use cautiously in pts with liver disease, esp. Hep B or C; contraindicated in Child-Pugh class B-C. Monitor LFTs. Coadministration of certain drugs contra-indicated (see Drug-Drug Interactions, Table 22).

4. Selected Characteristics of Fusion Inhibitors

TABLE 14C (6)

Generic/Trade Name	Pharmaceutical Prep. (Avg. Wholesale Price)	Usual Adult Dosage & Food Effect	Absorbed, %	Serum $T^{1/2}$, hrs	Elimination	Major Adverse Events/Comments (See Table 14D)
Enfuvirtide (T20, Fuzeon) Hypersensitivity reactions reported (fever, rash, chills, N/V, ↓ BP, ↓ or ↑ AST, ALT—do not restart if occur	Single-use vials of 90 mg (set ml when reconstituted). Inject in deltoid, ant. thigh, or abdomen. Rotate injection sites, avoiding those currently inflamed.	90 mg (1 mL) subcut. bid. Reconstituted with sterile water for injection. Reconstituted vials can be refrigerated for 24 hrs only. ($23,980 per year)	84	3.8	Catabolism to its constituent amino acids with subsequent recycling of the amino acids in the body pool. Specific metabolic pathway(s) have not been performed in humans. Does not alter the metabolism of CYP3A4, CYP2D6, CYP1A2, CYP2C19 or CYP2E1 substrates.	Local reaction site reactions 98%, 4% discontinue; erythema/induration ~80-90%, nodules/cysts ~80%, pruritus 65%, ecchymosis ~50%; neuropathy 8.9%, insomnia 11.3%, ↓ appetite 6.3%, myalgia 5%, lymphadenopathy 2.3%, eosinophilia ~10%. ↑ incidence of bacterial pneumonias. Alone offers little benefit to a failing regimen (NEJM 348:2249, 2003)

TABLE 14D: ANTIRETROVIRAL DRUGS AND ADVERSE EFFECTS (www.aidsinfo.nih.gov—accessed February 2005)

DRUG NAME(S): GENERIC (TRADE)	ADVERSE EFFECTS
Nucleoside Reverse Transcriptase Inhibitors (NRTI) (Black Box warning for all nucleoside/nucleotide RTIs: lactic acidosis/hepatic steatosis, potentially fatal. Also carry Warnings that fat redistribution has been observed)	
Abacavir (Ziagen)	**Most common:** Headache 7-13%, nausea 7-19%, diarrhea 7-19%, malaise 7-12% **Most significant: Hypersensitivity reaction** in 8% with malaise, fever, GI upset, rash, lethargy, & respiratory symptoms most commonly reported, myalgia, arthralgia, edema, paresthesia less commonly reported. Severe hypersensitivity reaction may be more common with once-daily dosing. **Rechallenge contraindicated; may be life-threatening.**
Didanosine (ddI) (Videx)	**Most common:** Diarrhea 28%, nausea 6%, rash 9%, headache 7%, fever 12%, hyperuricemia 2% **Most significant: Pancreatitis 1-9%. Black Box warning—Cases of fatal and nonfatal pancreatitis** have occurred in pts receiving ddI, especially when used in combination with d4T or d4T + hydroxyurea. Fatal lactic acidosis in pregnancy with ddI + d4T. Peripheral neuropathy in 20%, 12% required dose reduction. Rarely retinal changes.
Emtricitabine (FTC, Emtriva)	**Most common:** Headache 20%, diarrhea, nausea, rash, skin hyperpigmentation **Most significant:** Potential for lactic acidosis (as with other NRTIs), **exacerbation of hepatitis B on stopping drug**
Lamivudine (3TC) (Epivir)	**Most common:** Headache 35%, nausea 33%, malaise 27%, nasal Sx 20%, cough 18%, diarrhea 18%, insomnia 11% (all in combination with ZDV. Pancreatitis more common in pediatrics (15%). **Black Box warning.** Make sure to use HIV dosage, not Hep B dosage. **Exacerbation of hepatitis B on stopping drug.**
Stavudine (d4T) (Zerit)	**Most common:** Diarrhea, nausea, vomiting, headache **Most significant: Peripheral neuropathy** 15-20%. Pancreatitis 1%. Appears to produce lactic acidosis more commonly than other NRTIs. **Black Box warning— Fatal & nonfatal pancreatitis with d4T + ddI + hydroxyurea. Fatal lactic acidosis/steatosis in pregnant women receiving d4T + ddI.** Motor weakness in the setting of lactic acidosis mimicking the clinical presentation of Guillain-Barré syndrome (including respiratory failure) (rare)
Zalcitabine (ddC) (Hivid)	**Most common:** Oral ulcers 13%, rash 8% **Most significant: Black Box warning—Pancreatitis** <1%, **peripheral neuropathy** 22-35%. Severe continuous pain, slowly reversible when ddC is discontinued, ↑ risk in diabetes mellitus and heart failure in pts with Hep B.
Zidovudine (ZDV, AZT) (Retrovir)	**Most common:** Nausea 50%, anorexia 20%, vomiting 17%, **headache 62%.** Also reported: asthenia, myalgias, myopathy. **Anemia** (<8 gm, 1%) **granulocytopenia** (<750, 1.8%). Anemia may respond to epoetin alfa if endogenous serum erythropoietin levels are ≤500 million units per mL.
Nucleotide Reverse Transcriptase Inhibitor (NtRTI) (Black Box warning for all nucleoside/nucleotide RTIs: lactic acidosis/hepatic steatosis, potentially fatal. Also carry Warnings that fat redistribution has been observed)	
Tenofovir (TDF) (Viread)	**Most common:** Diarrhea 11%, nausea 8%, vomiting 5%, headache **Most significant: Severe exacerbations of hepatitis B reported in pts who stop tenofovir.** Not indicated to treat Hep B. Monitor carefully if drug is stopped; anti-HBV rx may be warranted if TDF stopped. Possible ↑ bone demineralization. Reports of Fanconi syndrome & renal injury induced by tenofovir alfa. (CID 37:e174, 2003; JAIDS 35:269, 2004). Modest decline in Ccr with TDF vs other NRTIs (CID 40:1194, 2005).
Non-Nucleoside Reverse Transcriptase Inhibitors (NNRTI)	
Delavirdine (Rescriptor)	**Most common:** Nausea, diarrhea, vomiting, headache **Most significant: Skin rash** has occurred in 18%, can continue or restart drug in most cases. Stevens-Johnson syndrome and erythema multiforme have been reported rarely. ↑ in liver enzymes in 5% of patients.

TABLE 14D (2)

DRUG NAME(S): GENERIC (TRADE)	ADVERSE EFFECTS
Non-Nucleoside Reverse Transcriptase Inhibitors (NNRTI) *(continued)*	
Efavirenz (Sustiva)	**Most common:** CNS **side-effects 52%,** symptoms include dizziness, insomnia, somnolence, impaired concentration, psychiatric sx, and abnormal dreams; symptoms are worse during first 2–4 weeks; discontinuation rate 2.6%. Rash 26%, improves with continued rx; discontinuation with antihistamines; discontinuation rate 1.7%. Can cause false-positive urine test results for cannabinoid with CEDIA DAU multi-level THC assay. **Most significant:** Serious neuropsychiatric symptoms, including severe depression 2.4% & suicidal ideation 0.7%. Elevation in liver enzymes. **Teratogenicity reported in primates; pregnancy category D—may cause fetal harm, avoid in pregnant women or those who might become pregnant** (see *2005 SANFORD GUIDE TO HIV/AIDS THERAPY, Table 9*). NOTE: No single method of contraception is 100% reliable. Contraindicated with certain drugs metabolized by CYP3A4.
Nevirapine (Viramune)	**Most common:** Rash 37%; occurs during 1st 6 wks of therapy. Follow recommendations for 14-day lead-in period to ↓ risk of rash *(see Table 14D).* Women experience 7-fold ↑ in rate of rash as compared to men. Rx & drug may need to be stopped if severe. Severe life-threatening rash in 6.6–7% of pts. About 50% will resolve w/o discontinuation of drug. **Most significant: Black Box warning—Severe life-threatening skin reactions reported:** Stevens-Johnson syndrome, toxic epidermal necrolysis, and hypersensitivity reaction or drug rash with eosinophilia and systemic symptoms (DRESS) *(AIM 145:2501, 2001)*. For severe rashes, dc drug immediately and do not restart. In a clinical trial, the use of prednisone ↑ the risk of rash *(see Table 14D).* **Life-threatening hepatotoxicity reported:** 2/3 during the first 12 wks of rx. Overall 1% develop hepatitis. Pts with pre-existing ↑ in ALT or AST and/or hepatitis of chronic Hep B or C ↑ susceptible *(Hpt 35:182, 2002)*. Women with CD4 >250, including pregnant women, at ↑ risk. Avoid in this group unless no other option. Men with CD4 >400 also at ↑ risk. Monitor pts intensively (clinical and LFTs), esp. during the first 12 wks of rx. If clinical hepatotoxicity, severe skin or hypersensitivity reactions occur, dc drug and never rechallenge.
Protease Inhibitors (PI)	Abnormalities in glucose metabolism, dyslipidemias, fat redistribution syndromes (fat redistribution). Pts taking PI may be at increased risk for developing osteopenia/osteoporosis. Spontaneous bleeding episodes have been reported in HIV+ pts with hemophilia being treated with PI. Rheumatoid complications have been reported with use of PIs *(Ann Rheum Dis 61:82, 2002)*. **Caution for all PIs**—Coadministration with certain drugs dependent on CYP3A for elimination & for which ↑ levels can cause serious toxicity may be contraindicated.
Amprenavir (Agenerase)	**Most common:** Nausea 43–74%, vomiting 24–34%, diarrhea 39–60%, paresthesia 26–31%. ↑ ALT/AST. Contains sulfa moiety. **Most significant:** Skin rash 28%. Most maculopapular of mild-moderate intensity, some with pruritus. Severe or life-threatening rash, including Stevens-Johnson syndrome, in 1% of pts. Severe rash seen 7–73 days after start. Can resolve w/o discontinuation 11 days. **Black Box warning**—potential propylene glycol toxicity with oral solution. Do not use in pregnancy, children <4 yrs old, renal/hepatic failure, with metronidazole.
Atazanavir (Reyataz)	**Most common:** Asymptomatic unconjugated hyperbilirubinemia in up to 60% of pts, jaundice in 7–9%. Moderate to severe events: Diarrhea 1–3%, nausea 6–14%, abdominal pain 4%, headache 6%, rash 5–7%. **Most significant:** Prolongation of PR interval (1° degree AV block) reported, rarely 2° AV block. One case acute interstitial nephritis *(Am J Kidney Dis 44:E81, 2004)*.
Fosamprenavir (Lexiva)	**Most common:** Skin rash 20–30% (moderate or worse in 3–8%), nausea, headache, diarrhea. **Most significant:** Rarely Stevens-Johnson syndrome, hemolytic anemia.
Indinavir (Crixivan)	**Most common:** ↑ in indirect bilirubin 10–15% (≥2.5 mg per dL), due to a drug-induced Gilbert's syndrome (of no clinical significance). Nausea 12%, vomiting 4%, diarrhea 5%. Pyuria reported in ~35% of children *(CID 32:E43, 2001)*. **Most significant: Kidney stones.** Due to indinavir crystals in collecting system. Nephrolithiasis in 12% of adults, higher in pediatrics. Prevent (minimize) by good hydration (at least 48 oz. water per day) *(AAC 42:332, 1998)*. Tubulointerstitial nephritis/renal colic reported in association with asymptomatic ↑ urine WBC. Severe hepatitis reported in 3 cases *(Ln 349:924, 1997)*. Hemolytic anemia reported.
Lopinavir/Ritonavir (Kaletra)	**Most common:** GI: diarrhea 14–24%, nausea 2–16%, ↑ lipid abnormalities in up to 20–40%. More diarrhea with q24h dosing. **Most significant:** Pancreatitis, inflammatory edema of the face *(AIDS 16:673, 2002)*.
Nelfinavir (Viracept)	**Most common:** Mild–moderate **diarrhea** 20%. For diarrhea: Oat bran tabs, calcium, or oral anti-diarrheal agents (e.g. loperamide, diphenoxylate/atropine sulfate).
Ritonavir (Norvir)	**Most common:** GI: better absorbed if taking with chocolate milk, Ensure, or Advera; nausea 23%, ↓ by initial dose escalation (titration) regimen; vomiting 13%, diarrhea 15%. Circumoral & peripheral paresthesias 6%, ↓ over time. Many drug-drug interactions & ↑ in lipid abnormalities. **Most significant:** Hepatic failure *(AnIM 129:670, 1998)*. **Black Box warning** relates to many important drug-drug interactions—inhibits P450 CYP3A & CYP2D6 system—may be life-threatening. *(see Table 22).* Rarely Stevens-Johnson syndrome, anaphylaxis.
Saquinavir (Invirase hard cap, tablet)	**Most common: Diarrhea,** abdominal discomfort, nausea, headache. **Black Box Warning**—Invirase & Fortovase are not bioequivalent. (NOTE: Fortovase discontinued in 2006.) **Use Invirase only with ritonavir.**
Tipranavir (Aptivus)	**Most common:** Nausea & vomiting, diarrhea, abdominal pain. Rash in 8–14%, more common in women, & 33% in women taking ethinyl estradiol. Major lipid effects. **Most serious: Black Box warning**—associated with hepatitis & fatal hepatic failure. Risk of hepatotoxicity ↑ in Hep B or Hep C co-infection. Potential for major drug interactions.
Fusion Inhibitor: Enfuvirtide (T20, Fuzeon)	**Most common:** Local injection site reactions (98% at least 1 local ISR), 4% dc because of ISR (pain & discomfort, induration, erythema, nodules & cysts, pruritus, & ecchymosis). **Most significant:** ↑ rate of bacterial pneumonia (6.7 pneumonia events per 100 pt yrs), hypersensitivity reactions ≤1% (rash, fever, nausea & vomiting, chills, rigors, hypotension, & ↑ serum liver transaminases).

TABLE 15A: ANTIMICROBIAL PROPHYLAXIS FOR SELECTED BACTERIAL INFECTIONS*

CLASS OF ETIOLOGIC AGENT/DISEASE/CONDITION	PROPHYLAXIS: AGENT/DOSE/ROUTE/DURATION	COMMENTS
Group B streptococcal disease (GBS), neonatal: Approaches to management [CDC Guidelines, *MMWR 51(RR-11):1, 2002*]:		
Pregnant women—intrapartum antimicrobial prophylaxis procedures: 1. Screen all pregnant women with vaginal & rectal swab for GBS at 35–37 wks gestation (unless other indications for prophylaxis exist. GBS bacteriuria during this pregnancy or previously delivered infant with invasive GBS disease, even then cultures may be useful for susceptibility testing). Use vaginal-rectal swab specimen, enriched broth culture (Lim broth), subculture to blood agar; hold 18–24 hrs. **Rx during labor if swab culture positive.** 2. Rx during labor if previously delivered infant with invasive GBS infection, or if any GBS bacteriuria during this pregnancy (*MMWR 53:506, 2004*). 3. Rx if GBS status unknown but if any of the following are present: (a) delivery at <37 wks gestation [see *MMWR 51(RR-11):1, 2002* algorithm for threatened preterm delivery]; or (b) duration of ruptured membranes ≥18 hrs; or (c) intrapartum temp. ≥100.4°F [≥38.0°C].	**Prophylactic regimens during labor:** **Pen G** 5 million units IV q4h (load then 2.5 million units IV q4h) **Alternative: Ampicillin** 2 gm IV (load) then q4h (1 gm IV) q8h **Pen-allergic: Pts not at high risk for anaphylaxis: Cefazolin** 2 gm IV initial dose, then 1 gm IV q8h. **Pts at high risk for anaphylaxis:** GBS susceptible to clinda & erythro. **Clindamycin** 900 mg IV q8h or **erythromycin** 500 mg IV q6h. **Vancomycin** 1 gm IV q12h for pts at high risk for anaphylaxis when alternative to clindamycin or erythromycin needed (e.g., GBS-resistant or unknown susceptibility). Continue treatment until delivery	Careful observation of signs & symptoms. 95% of infants will show clinical signs of infection during the 1st 24 hrs whether mother received intrapartum antibiotics or not (*Pediatrics 106:244, 2000*). For gestational age < 35 wks of observation see algorithm: *MMWR 51(RR-11):1, 2002.*
Neonate of mother given prophylaxis	Careful observation of signs & symptoms. See algorithm. *MMWR 51(RR-11):1, 2002.*	
Preterm, premature rupture of the membranes in Group B strep-negative women	IV **ampicillin** 2 gm q6h + IV **erythromycin** 250 mg q6h) for 48 hrs followed by po **amoxicillin** 250 mg q8h + po **erythromycin** base 333 mg q8h times 5 days. Decreases infant morbidity. (*JAMA 278:989, 1997*)	Antibiotic rx reduced infant respiratory distress syndrome (50.6% vs 40.8%, p = 0.03), necrotizing enterocolitis (5.8% to 2.3%, p = 0.03) and prolonged pregnancy (2.9 to 6.1 days, p = 0.0001) vs placebo. Rx in labor, po erythromycin did not improve neonatal outcomes vs placebo (11% vs 14.4% poor outcomes; p=0.02 for single births) but not on AM-CL or both drugs in combination (both assoc. with ↑ necrotizing enterocolitis) (*Ln 357:979, 2001*). (*See ACOG discussion, Ob Gyn 102:875, 2003*)
Post-splenectomy bacteremia Likely agents: Pneumococcus (90%), meningococcal, H. influenzae type b (also at ↑ risk of fatal malaria, severe babesiosis). Ref. *2003 Red Book, 26th Ed. Amer Acad Pediatrics*	**Immunizations:** Ensure admin. of pneumococcal vaccine, H. influenzae B, & quadrivalent meningococcal vaccines at recommended times. In addition, asplenic children with sickle cell anemia, thalassemia, & perhaps others, daily antimicrobial prophylaxis until at least age 5—See **Comments.**	Antimicrobial prophylaxis until age 5. Amox 20 mg/kg po once per day or Pen V-K 125 mg bid. Consider Pen V-K 250 mg bid for at least 1 yr in children after splenectomy. Maintain immunizations plus self-administer AM-CL with any febrile illness while seeking physician assistance. Pen allergy: TMP-SMX or clarithro. May need to consider other alternatives re: pen-resistant S. pneumoniae prevalence increases.
Sexual Exposure		
Sexual assault survivor [likely agents and risks, see *NEJM 332:234, 1995; MMWR 51(RR-6):1, 2002*]	(**Ceftriaxone** 125 mg IM) + (**metronidazole** 2 gm po single dose) + (**azithromycin** 1 gm po single dose) or (**doxycycline** 100 mg po bid times 7 days) *MMWR 51(RR-6):1, 2002*	Obtain expert advice re: forensic exam & specimens, pregnancy, physical trauma, psychological issues. At initial exam. Culture for gonococci & chlamydia (if available), wet mount for T. vaginalis & culture (vaginal swab). Serologic evaluation for syphilis, Hep B, HIV, others as appropriate. Initiate post-exposure prophylaxis for HIV & hepatitis B as appropriate (see Table 15D.) Follow-up exam for STD at 1–2 wks. Retest syphilis & HIV serology at 6, 12, 24 wks if negative earlier.
Sexual contacts, likely agents: N. gonorrhoeae, C. trachomatis	(**Ceftriaxone** 125 mg IM once) + (**doxycycline** 100 mg po bid, po times 7 days) or (**cefixime** 400 mg po) + (**azithromycin** 1 gm po), each as single dose)	Be sure to check for syphilis since all regimens may not eradicate incubating syphilis. Identify & rx chlamydia as appropriate to suspected STD [see *MMWR 51(RR-6):1, 2002* for other etiologies & rx options].
Syphilis exposure		Presumptive rx for exposure within 3 mos., as tests may be negative. Make effort to do syphilis
Sickle-cell disease Likely agent: S. pneumoniae (see post-splenectomy, above) Ref. *2003 Red Book, 26th Ed. Amer Acad Pediatrics*	Children <5 yrs: **Penicillin V** 125 mg po bid ≥5 yrs: **Penicillin V** 250 mg po bid (Alternative in children: Amoxicillin 20 mg/kg per day)	Start prophylaxis by 2 mos. (*Pediatrics 106:367, 2000; http://aappublications.org*). Age-appropriate vaccines, including pneumococcal (Hib, influenza ± meningococcal. Treating infections, consider possibility of penicillin non-susceptible pneumococcal.

* See page 2 for abbreviations

TABLE 15B: SURGICAL ANTIBIOTIC PROPHYLAXIS* (EID 7:220, 2001; CID 38:1706, 2004; Am J Surg 189:395, 2005)

Surgical Procedures: To be optimally effective, antibiotics must be started within the last hr (2 hrs before the surgical incision (NEJM 326:281, 1992). For most procedures the number of doses needed for optimal coverage is not defined. Most applications employ a single dose (Med Lett 43:92, 2001) although some FDA-approved and other regimens call for 3 or more doses. If the surgical procedure lasts > 3 hrs, additional intraoperative doses should be given at approx. 3-hr intervals. A recent consensus statement from the National Surgical Infection Prevention Project (CID 38:1706, 2004) advises antibiotic prophylaxis be started within 1 hr before incision and prophylaxis lasts no more than 2 half-lives of the prophylactic agent, and in most cases not be extended beyond 24 hrs. (Note: The dose/route/durations listed below for adults with normal renal function & not intolerant of these agents are for the most part those approved in FDA product labeling. For single dose regimens, the dosage & route are the same.) See Table 15C for regimens to reduce risk of endocarditis.

General Comments: In some centers, ↑ resistance has render certain regimens (e.g., quinolones) unsuitable for prophylaxis. Pharmacologic considerations suggest that typical prophylaxis dosing may yield suboptimal serum/tissue levels in pts with high BMI (see Surgery 136:738, 2004 for cefazolin; Eur J Clin Pharm 54:632, 1998 for vancomycin), although clinical implications uncertain.

TYPE OF SURGERY	PROPHYLAXIS	COMMENTS
Cardiovascular Surgery Antibiotic prophylaxis in cardiovascular surgery has been proven beneficial only in the following procedures. • Reconstruction of abdominal aorta • Procedures on the leg that involve a groin incision • Any vascular procedure that inserts prosthesis/foreign body • Lower extremity amputation for ischemia • Cardiac surgery • Perhaps permanent pacemakers (see Comment)	**Cefazolin** 1–2 gm IV as a single dose or q8h for 1–2 days or **cefuroxime** 1.5 gm IV as a single dose or q12h for total of 6 gm or **vancomycin** 1 gm IV as single dose or q12h for 1–2 days. Consider **intranasal mupirocin** evening before, day of surgery & bid for 5 days post-op in pts with pos. nasal culture for S. aureus.	Single injection just before surgery probably as effective as multiple doses. Not recommended for cardiac catheterization. For prosthetic heart valves, customary to stop prophylaxis either after removal of retrosternal drainage catheters or just a 2nd dose after coming off bypass. Vancomycin may be preferable in hospitals with ↑ frequency of MRSA or in high-risk pts (CID 38:1555, 2004), or those colonized with MRSA (CID 38:1706, 2004); however, does not cover Gm-neg. bacilli, therefore would add cefazolin for groin incisions. Meta-analysis failed to demonstrate overall superiority of vancomycin over β-lactam prophylaxis for cardiac surgery (CID 38:1357, 2004). A meta-analysis of 7 placebo-controlled randomized studies of antimicrobial prophylaxis for implantation of permanent pacemakers: sig. ↓ in incidence of infection (Circulation 97: 1796, 1998). Intranasal mupirocin ↓ sternal wound infections from S. aureus in 1850 pts; used historical controls (An Thor Surg 54:632, 1998) in another trial, it reduced nosocomial S. aureus infections only in nasal carriers (NEJM 346:1871, 2002).
Gastric, Biliary and Colonic Surgery **Gastroduodenal/Biliary** Gastroduodenal, includes percutaneous endoscopic gastrostomy (high-risk only, see Comments)	**Cefazolin or cefoxitin or cefotetan or ceftizoxime or cefuroxime** 1.5 gm IV as a single dose (some give additional doses q12h for 2–3 days).	Gastroduodenal: High-risk is marked obesity, obstruction, ↓ gastric acid or ↓ GI motility. Biliary: Cephalosporins not active vs enterococci yet clinically effective as prophylaxis in biliary surgery. With cholangitis, treat as infection, not prophylaxis: TC-CL 3.1 gm q4–6h IV or PIP-TZ 3.375 gm q6h or 4.5 gm q8h IV; AM-SB 3.0 gm q6h IV. Biliary high-risk: age >70; acute cholecystitis, non-functioning gallbladder, obstructive jaundice or common duct stones. Meta-analysis supports use in percutaneous endoscopic gastrostomy (Am J Gastro 95:3133, 2000).
Biliary, includes laparoscopic cholecystectomy (high-risk only, see Comments)	In biliary surgery, cefazolin 1 gm & ceftizoxime 1 gm (± repeat dosing at 12 & 24 hrs) were equivalent (AAC 40:70, 1996).	
Endoscopic retrograde cholangiopancreatography	No iv without obstruction. If obstruction: **Ciprofloxacin** 500–750 mg po 2 hrs prior to procedure	Most studies show that achieving adequate drainage will prevent postprocedural cholangitis or sepsis and no further benefit from prophylactic antibiotics. With inadequate drainage antibiotics may be of value. American Society for GI Endoscopy recommends use for known or
Biliary—controversial. No benefit from single dose piperacillin in randomized placebo-controlled trial, AnIM 125:442, 1996 (see Comment)	**Ceftizoxime** 1.5 gm IV 1 hr prior to procedure or **Piperacillin** 4 gm IV 1 hr prior to procedure	suspected biliary obstruction. Oral CIP as effective as cephalosporins in 2 studies & less expensive (CID 23:380, 1996).
Colorectal, includes appendectomy Elective surgery	**Neomycin ± erythromycin** po (see Comment for dose) or **[Cefazolin** 1–2 gm IV + **metronidazole** 0.5 gm IV (single dose)] or **cefoxitin or cefotetan** 1–2 gm IV	Elective colorectal prep: Pre-op day: (1) 10 am 4 L polyethylene glycol electrolyte solution (Colyte, GoLYTELY) po over 2 hr. (2) Clear liquid diet only. (3) 1 pm, 2 pm and 11 pm, neomycin 1 gm + erythro base 1 gm po. (4) NPO after midnight. There are alternative regimens which have been less well studied. GoLYTELY 1–6 pm, then neomycin 2 gm po + metronidazole 2 gm po at 7 pm and 11 pm. Oral regimen as effective as parenteral; parenteral in addition to oral not required. For emergency colorectal surgery, use parenteral. (CID 15 Suppl. 1:S313, 1992).
Emergency surgery		
Ruptured viscus: See Peritoneum/Peritonitis, Secondary, Table 1, page 34		

* See page 2 for abbreviations

TABLE 15B (2)

TYPE OF SURGERY	PROPHYLAXIS	COMMENTS
Head and Neck Surgery (Am Otol Rhinol Laryngol 101 Suppl 16, 1992) Antimicrobial prophylaxis in head & neck surgery appears efficacious only for procedures involving oral/pharyngeal mucosa (e.g., laryngeal or pharyngeal tumor) but even with prophylaxis, wound infection rate high (41% in 1 center) (Head Neck 23:447, 2001). Uncontaminated-head and neck surgery does not require prophylaxis.		
Clean, non-implant; e.g., craniotomy	**Cefazolin** 1 gm IV once. Alternative: **vanco** 1 gm IV once	**Cefazolin** 2 gm IV (single dose) or **clindamycin** 600–900 mg IV (single dose) + **gentamicin** 1.5 mg per kg IV (single dose)
Neurosurgical Procedures [Prophylaxis most effective in ↓ infection rate with intracranial pressure monitors in retrospective analysis of 215 pts (J Neurol Neurosurg Psych 69:381, 2000)]		Reference: Ln 344:1547, 1994
Clean, contaminated (cross sinuses, or naso/oropharynx)	**Clindamycin** 900 mg IV (single dose)	British recommend amoxicillin-clavulanate 1.2 gm IV[a,b] or (cefuroxime 1.5 gm IV + metronidazole 0.5 gm IV).
CSF shunt surgery; controversial (Meta-analysis CID 17:98, 1993)	**Vancomycin** 10 mg into cerebral ventricles + **gentamicin** 3 mg into cerebral ventricles (Ln 344:1547, 1994)	Efficacy when infection rate >15%. Alternative: TMP (160 mg) + SMX (800 mg) IV pre-op and q12h times 3 doses
Obstetric/Gynecologic Surgery		
Vaginal or abdominal hysterectomy	**Cefazolin** 1–2 gm or **cefoxitin** 1–2 gm or **cefotetan** 1–2 gm or **cefuroxime** 1.5 gm all IV 30 min. before surgery.	1 study found cefotetan superior to cefazolin (CID 20:677, 1995) For prolonged procedures, doses can be repeated q4-8h for duration of procedure.
Cesarean section for premature rupture of membranes or active labor	**Cefazolin** once, administer IV as soon as umbilical cord clamped.	Prophylaxis decreases risk of endometritis/wound infection in elective as well as non-elective C-section; single dose equivalent to multiple dose regimens (Cochrane Database System Rev 2002, Issue 3, & 1999, Issue 1).
Abortion	1st trimester: aqueous **pen G** 2 mU IV or **doxycycline** 300 mg po. 2nd trimester: **Cefazolin** 1 gm IV	Meta-analysis showed benefit of antibiotic prophylaxis in all risk groups. One regimen was doxy 100 mg orally 1 hr before procedure, then 200 mg after procedure (Ob Gyn 87:884, 1996).
Orthopedic Surgery [Most pts with prosthetic joints do not require prophylaxis for routine dental procedures, but individual considerations prevail for high-risk procedures & prostheses (J Am Dental Assn 134:895, 2003; Med Lett 47:59, 2005)].		
Hip arthroplasty,[1] spinal fusion	Same as cardiac	Customarily stopped after "Hemovac" removed. NSIPP workgroup recommends stopping prophylaxis within 24 hrs of surgery (CID 38:1706, 2004).
Total joint replacement (other than hip)	**Cefazolin** 1–2 gm IV pre-op (& 2nd dose) or **vancomycin** 1 gm IV on call to OR	Post-op: some would give no further rx (Med Lett 39:98, 1997). NSIPP workgroup recommends stopping prophylaxis within 24 hrs of surgery (CID 38:1706, 2004).
Open reduction of closed fracture with internal fixation	**Ceftriaxone** 2 gm IV once	3.6% vs 8.3% (for placebo) infection found in Dutch trauma trial (Ln 347:1133, 1996)
Peritoneal Dialysis Catheter Placement	**Vancomycin** single 1000 mg dose 12 hrs prior to procedure	Effectively reduced peritonitis during 14 days post-placement in 221 pts: vanco 1%, cefazolin 7%, placebo 12% (p=0.02) (Am J Kidney Dis 36:1014, 2000).
Urologic Surgery/Procedures Antimicrobials not recommended in pts with sterile urine. Pts with pre-operative bacteriuria should be treated.	Recommended antibiotic to pts with pre-operative bacteriuria: **Cefazolin** 1 gm IV q8h times 1–3 doses perioperatively, followed by oral antibiotics (**nitrofurantoin** or TMP-SMX) until catheter is removed or for 10 days. Modify based on susceptibility test results.	
Transrectal prostate biopsy	**Ciprofloxacin** 500 mg po 12 hrs prior to biopsy and repeated 12 hrs after 1st dose	Bacteremia 7% with CIP vs 37% (gentamicin) (Urology 38:84, 1991; review in JAC 39:115, 1997). Levo 500 mg 30–60 min. before procedure was effective in low-risk pts; additional doses were given for ↑ risk (J Urol 168:1021, 2002).
Other		
Breast surgery, herniorrhaphy	**P Ceph 1,2**, dosage as Gynecologic Surgery, above	Meta-analysis did not show clear evidence of benefit from prophylaxis in elective inguinal hernia repair (Cochrane Database System Rev 2004, Issue 4).

[1] Gentamicin (12.5 mg per gm of acrylic bone cement) is released for at least 3 weeks. Usefulness not proven.

* See page 2 for abbreviations

TABLE 15C: ANTIMICROBIAL PROPHYLAXIS FOR THE PREVENTION OF BACTERIAL ENDOCARDITIS IN PATIENTS WITH UNDERLYING CARDIAC CONDITIONS*
[These are the views of the American Heart Association (JAMA 277:1794, 1997). However, a population-based prospective case-controlled study brings into serious question whether dental procedures predispose to endocarditis and whether antibiotic prophylaxis is of any value (see Ann IM 129:761, 1998; Brit Dent J 189:610, 2000)]

ENDOCARDITIS PROPHYLAXIS RECOMMENDED

Cardiac conditions associated with endocarditis
High-risk conditions:
  Prosthetic valves—bioprosthetic and homograft, as well as mechanical
  Previous bacterial endocarditis
  Complex cyanotic congenital heart disease, e.g., single ventricle, transposition,
    tetralogy of Fallot
  Surgically constructed systemic pulmonic shunts or conduits
Moderate-risk conditions:
  Most other congenital heart abnormalities or acquired valvular disease, hypertrophic
    cardiac myopathy, mitral prolapse with regurgitation

ENDOCARDITIS PROPHYLAXIS NOT RECOMMENDED

Negligible-risk (same as normal population):
  Atrial septal defect (secundum) or repaired ASD/VSD, or PDA (beyond 6 months)
  Previous CABG, mitral prolapse without MI (see discussion JAMA 277:1794, 1997)
  Physiologic, functional, or innocent heart murmurs
  Previous Kawasaki disease or rheumatic fever without valve dysfunction
  Cardiac pacemakers (all) and implanted defibrillators

ENDOCARDITIS PROPHYLAXIS RECOMMENDED

Dental and other procedures where prophylaxis is considered for patients with moderate- or high-risk cardiac conditions
Dental: Extractions, periodontal procedures[1]
  Implants, root canal, subgingival antibiotic fibers/strips
  Initial orthodontic bands (not brackets); intraligamentary local anesthetic
  Cleaning of teeth/implants if bleeding anticipated
Respiratory: T&A surgery on respiratory mucosa, bronchoscopy
GI: Sclerotherapy of esophageal varices; dilation of esophageal stricture; ERCP with
    biliary obstruction
  Biliary tract surgery; surgery on/through intestinal mucosa
GU: Prostate surgery, cystoscopy, urethral dilatation

ENDOCARDITIS PROPHYLAXIS NOT RECOMMENDED

Dental: Filling cavities with local anesthetic
  Placement of rubber dams, suture removal, orthodontic removal
  Orthodontic adjustments, dental x-rays
  Shedding of primary teeth
Respiratory: Intubation, flexible bronchoscopy[2] tympanostomy tube
GI: Transesophageal cardiac echo[2], EGD without biopsy[2]
GU: Vaginal hysterectomy[2] vaginal delivery[2] C-section
  If uninfected, Foley catheter, abortion, tubal ligation, insert/remove IUD
Other: Cardiac cath, balloon angioplasty, implanted pacemaker, defibrillators, coronary stents
  Skin biopsy, circumcision

Abbreviations: T&A = tonsillectomy/adenoidectomy, **ERCP** = endoscopic retrograde cholangiography, **ASD/VSD** = atrial septal defect/ventricular septal defect, **PDA** = patent ductus arteriosus, **EGD** = esophagogastroduodenoscopy, **D&C** = dilation and curettage

PROPHYLACTIC REGIMENS FOR DENTAL, ORAL, RESPIRATORY TRACT, OR ESOPHAGEAL PROCEDURES

SITUATION	AGENT	REGIMEN[3]
Standard general prophylaxis	Amoxicillin	Adults 2 gm, children 50 mg per kg orally 1 hr before procedure
Unable to take oral medications	Ampicillin	Adults 2 gm IM or IV, children 50 mg per kg IM or IV within 30 min. before procedure
Allergic to penicillin	Clindamycin __OR__	Adults 600 mg, children 20 mg per kg orally 1 hr before procedure.
	(Cephalexin* or cefadroxil*), __OR__	Adults 2 gm, children 50 mg per kg orally 1 hr before procedure.
	Azithromycin or clarithromycin	Adults 500 mg, children 15 mg per kg orally 1 hr before procedure.
Allergic to penicillin and unable to take oral medications	Clindamycin __OR__	Adults 600 mg, children 20 mg per kg IV within 30 min. before procedure
	Cefazolin[4]	Adults 1 gm, children 25 mg per kg IM or IV within 30 min. before procedure

[1] Some now recommend that for adults, prophylaxis prior to **extractions** and **gingival surgery** (including implant replacement) and **only** for patients with **prosthetic cardiac valves** or **previous endocarditis** (Ann IM 129:829, 1998). If any of these 4 conditions exist = prophylactic antibiotics according to American Heart Association are recommended.
[2] Prophylaxis optional for high-risk patients
[3] Total children's dose should not exceed adult dose
[4] Cephalosporins should not be used in individuals with immediate-type hypersensitivity reaction (urticaria, angioedema, or anaphylaxis) to penicillins.

* See page 2 for abbreviations

TABLE 15C (2)

PROPHYLACTIC REGIMENS FOR GENITOURINARY/GASTROINTESTINAL (EXCLUDING ESOPHAGEAL) PROCEDURES

SITUATION	AGENT	REGIMEN[1]
High-risk patients	Ampicillin + gentamicin	**Adults: ampicillin** 2 gm IM or IV + **gentamicin** 1.5 mg per kg (not to exceed 120 mg) within 30 min. of starting the procedure, 6 hr later, **ampicillin** 1 gm IM/IV or **amoxicillin** 1 gm orally. **Children: ampicillin** 50 mg per kg IM or IV (not to exceed 2 gm) + **gentamicin** 1.5 mg per kg within 30 min. of starting the procedure; 6 hrs later: **ampicillin** 25 mg per kg IM/IV or **amoxicillin** 25 mg per kg orally
High-risk patients allergic to ampicillin or amoxicillin	Vancomycin + gentamicin	**Adults: vancomycin** 1 gm IV over 1–2 hrs + **gentamicin** 1.5 mg per kg IV/IM (not to exceed 120 mg), complete injection/infusion within 30 min. of starting the procedure **Children: vancomycin** 20 mg per kg IV over 1–2 hrs + **gentamicin** 1.5 mg per kg IV/IM, complete injection/ infusion within 30 min. of starting the procedure
Moderate-risk patients	Amoxicillin or ampicillin	**Adults: amoxicillin** 2 gm orally 1 hr before procedure, or **ampicillin** 2 gm IM/IV within 30 min. of starting the procedure. **Children: amoxicillin** 50 mg per kg orally 1 hr before procedure, or **ampicillin** 50 mg per kg IM/IV within 30 min. of starting the procedure
Moderate-risk patients allergic to ampicillin or amoxicillin	Vancomycin	**Adults: vancomycin** 1 gm IV over 1–2 hrs, complete infusion within 30 min. of starting the procedure **Children: vancomycin** 20 mg per kg IV over 1–2 hrs; complete infusion within 30 min. of starting the procedure[*]

[1] Total children's dose should not exceed adult dose

TABLE 15D: MANAGEMENT OF EXPOSURE TO HIV-1 AND HEPATITIS[*]

OCCUPATIONAL EXPOSURE TO BLOOD, PENILE/VAGINAL SECRETIONS OR OTHER POTENTIALLY INFECTIOUS BODY FLUIDS OR TISSUES WITH RISK OF TRANSMISSION OF HEPATITIS B/C AND/OR HIV-1 (E.G., NEEDLESTICK INJURY)
[Adapted from MMWR 50/RR-11/:1, 2001 and NEJM 348:826, 2003.]
Free consultation for occupational exposures, call (PEPline) 1-888-448-4911.

General steps in management:
1. Wash clean wounds/flush mucous membranes immediately (use of caustic agents or squeezing the wound is discouraged; data lacking regarding antiseptics).
2. Assess risk by doing the following: (a) Characterize exposure; (b) Determine/evaluate source of exposure by medical history, risk behavior, & testing for hepatitis B/C, HIV; (c) Evaluate and test exposed individual for hepatitis B/C & HIV

Hepatitis B Exposure [Adapted from CDC recommendations: MMWR 50/RR-11), 2001]

Exposed Person	Exposure Source		
	HBs Ag+	**HBs Ag–**	**Status Unknown**
Unvaccinated	Give HBIG 0.06 mL per kg IM & initiate HB vaccine	Initiate HB vaccine	Initiate HB vaccine and if possible, check HBs Ag of source person
Vaccinated (antibody status unknown)	Do anti-HBs on exposed person: If titer ≥10 milli-International units per mL, no rx If titer <10 milli-International units per mL, give HBIG + dose HB vaccine[*]	No rx necessary	Do anti-HBs on exposed person: If titer ≥10 milli-International units per mL, no rx If titer <10 milli-International units per mL, give 1 dose of HB vaccine series, **or** re-initiate vaccine series if source high-risk[*]

For known vaccine series responder (titer ≥10 milli-International units per mL), no rx. Known non-responder (<10 milli-International units per mL) to 1st series HB vaccine & exposed to either HBsAg+ source or suspected high-risk source—rx with HBIG & re-initiate vaccine series, **or** give 2 doses HBIG 1 month apart. For non-responders after a 2nd vaccine series, 2 doses HBIG 1 month apart is preferred approach to new exposure [MMWR 40(RR-13):21, 2001].
[*] Follow-up to assess/address vaccine response

Hepatitis C Exposure
Determine antibody to hepatitis C for both exposed person and, if possible, exposure source. If source +, follow-up HCV testing advised. **No recommended prophylaxis**; immune serum globulin not effective. Monitor for early infection, as therapy may ↓ risk of progression to chronic hepatitis. See Table 12 and discussion in Clin Micro Rev 16:546, 2003.

[*] See page 2 for abbreviations

TABLE 15D (2)

HIV: Occupational exposure management

- The decision to initiate post-exposure prophylaxis (PEP) for HIV is a clinical judgment that should be made in concert with the exposed healthcare worker (HCW). It is based on:
  1. Likelihood of the source patient having HIV infection. ↑ with history of high-risk activity—injection drug use, sexual activity with known HIV+ person, unprotected sex with multiple partners (either hetero- or homosexual); receipt of blood products 1978–1985. ↑ with clinical signs suggestive of advanced HIV (unexplained wasting, night sweats, thrush, seborrheic dermatitis, etc.).
     Remember, the vast majority of persons are **not** infected with HIV (1/200 women infected in larger U.S. cities) and likelihood of infection is low if not in above risk groups.
  2. Type of exposure (approx. 1 in 300–400 needlesticks from infected source will transmit HIV).
  3. Limited data regarding efficacy of PEP (PEP with ZDV alone reduced transmission by >80% in 1 retrospective case-controlled study—*NEJM* 337:1485, 1997).
  4. Significant adverse effects of PEP drugs.

- If source person is **known positive for HIV or likely to be infected** and **status of exposure warrants PEP**, antiretroviral drugs should be started **immediately** (ASAP or within hours). If source person is HIV antibody negative, drugs can be stopped **unless source is suspected of having acute HIV infection**. The HCW should be re-tested at **3–4 weeks, 3 & 6 months whether PEP is used or not** (the vast majority of seroconversions will occur by 3 months; delayed conversions after 6 months are exceedingly rare). Tests for HIV RNA should not be used for dx of HIV infection because of false-positives (esp. at low titers) & these tests are only approved for established HIV infection [a possible exception is if pt develops signs of acute HIV (mononucleosis-like) syndrome within the 1st 4–6 wks of exposure when antibody tests might still be negative.]

- PEP for HIV is usually given for **4 weeks** and monitoring of adverse effects recommended: baseline **complete blood count, renal and hepatic panel** to be **repeated at 2 weeks** with repeat CBC at **4 weeks**. Up to ⅓ of HCW on PEP demonstrate mild side-effects (nausea, diarrhea, myalgias, headache, etc.) but in up to ½ severe enough to discontinue PEP *(Antivir Ther 3:195, 2000)*. Consultation with infectious diseases/HIV specialist valuable when questions regarding PEP arise. **Seek help in special situations, such as pregnancy, renal impairment, treatment-experienced source.**

3 Steps to HIV Post-Exposure Prophylaxis (PEP) After Occupational Exposure: *[For latest CDC recommendations, see MMWR 54(RR-9), 2005]*

Step 1: Determine the exposure code (EC)

Step 2: Determine the HIV Status Code (HIV SC)

* Exceptions can be considered when there has been prolonged, high-volume contact.

* See page 2 for abbreviations

TABLE 15D (3)

Step 3: Determine Post-Exposure Prophylaxis (PEP) Recommendation

EC	HIV SC	PEP
1	1	Consider basic regimen [a,b]
1	2	Recommend basic regimen [a,b]
2	1	Recommend basic regimen [a]
2	2	Recommend expanded regimen [c]
3	1 or 2	Recommend expanded regimen [c]
1, 2, 3	Unknown	If exposure setting suggests risks of HIV exposure, consider basic regimen [c]

[a] Based on estimates of ↓ risk of infection after mucous membrane exposure in occupational setting compared with needlestick.

Modification of CDC recommendations:
[b] Or, consider expanded regimen [c].
[c] In high risk circumstances, consider expanded regimen [c] on case-by-case basis.

Around the clock, urgent expert consultation available from:
National Clinicians' Post-Exposure Prophylaxis Hotline
(PEPline) at 1-888-448-4911 (1-888-HIV-4911)

Regimens: (Treat for 4 weeks, monitor for drug side-effects every 2 weeks)
Basic regimen: ZDV + 3TC or FTC + TDF, or possibly d4T + 3TC.
Expanded regimen: Basic regimen + one of the following: lopinavir/ritonavir, nelfinavir, indinavir/ritonavir, fosamprenavir/ritonavir, atazanavir or atazanavir/ritonavir, efavirenz can be considered (except in pregnancy or potential for pregnancy)—**Pregnancy Category D**), but CNS symptoms might be problematic. [**Do not use nevirapine**: serious adverse reactions including hepatic necrosis reported in healthcare workers *(MMWR 49:1153, 2001)*].
Other regimens can be designed. If possible, use 2 antiretroviral drugs that suppress pt (if known) is not currently taking or for which resistance is unlikely based on susceptibility data or treatment history. Seek expert consultation if ARV-experienced source or in pregnancy or potential for pregnancy.

NOTE: Some authorities feel that an expanded regimen should be employed whenever PEP is indicated *(NEJM 349:1091, 2003; Eur J Epidemiol 19:577, 2004; & NY State AIDS Institute, 2004)*. For example, the latter recommends ZDV + 3TC + tenofovir
(www.hivguidelines.org/public_html/center/clinical-guidelines/pep_guidelines/pep_guidelines.htm). Expanded regimens are likely to be advantageous with ↑ numbers of ART-experienced source pts or when there is doubt about exact extent of exposures in decision algorithm. Mathematical model suggests that under some conditions, completion of full course basic regimen is better than prematurely discontinued expanded regimen *(CID 39:395, 2004)*. However, while expanded PEP regimens have ↑ adverse effects, there is not necessarily ↑ discontinuation *(CID 40:205, 2005)*.

POST-EXPOSURE PROPHYLAXIS FOR NON-OCCUPATIONAL EXPOSURES TO HIV
From MMWR 54(RR-2):1, 2005—DHHS recommendations

Because the risk of transmission of HIV via sexual contact or sharing needles by injection drug users may reach or exceed that of occupational needlestick exposure, it is reasonable to consider PEP in persons who have had non-occupational exposure to blood or other potentially infected fluids. (e.g., genital/rectal secretions, breast milk) from an HIV+ source. Risk of HIV acquisition per exposure varies with the act (for needle sharing and receptive anal intercourse, ≥0.5%; approximately 10-fold lower with insertive vaginal or anal intercourse, 0.05–0.07%). Overt or occult traumatic lesions may ↑ risk in survivors of sexual assault.

For pts at risk of HIV acquisition through non-occupational exposure to HIV+ source material having occurred ≤72 hours before evaluation, DHHS recommendation is to treat for 28 days with an antiretroviral **expanded regimen**, using preferred regimens [efavirenz (not in pregnancy or pregnancy risk—**Pregnancy Category D**) + (3TC or FTC) + (ZDV or TDF)] **or** [lopinavir/ritonavir + (3TC or FTC) + ZDV] or one of several alternative regimens [see Table 14C section B & MMWR 54(RR-2):1, 2005].

Areas of uncertainty: (1) expanded regimens are not and proven to be superior to 2-drug regimens, (2) while PEP not recommended for exposures >72 hours before evaluation, it may possibly be effective in some cases, (3) when HIV status of source patient is unknown, decision to treat and regimen selection must be individualized based on assessment of specific circumstances.

Evaluate for exposures to Hep B, Hep C *(see Occupational PEP above)*, and bacterial sexually-transmitted diseases [see Table 15A & MMWR 51(RR-6):1, 2002] and treat as indicated.

---

* See page 2 for abbreviations

TABLE 15E: PREVENTION OF OPPORTUNISTIC INFECTION IN HUMAN STEM CELL TRANSPLANTATION (HSCT) OR SOLID ORGAN TRANSPLANTATION (SOT) FOR ADULTS WITH NORMAL RENAL FUNCTION*

General comments: See Table 15F, page 132 for typical timing of infections post-transplant. References: *MMWR 49(RR-10):1, 2000; CID 33:S26, 2001; COID 17:353, 2004*

OPPORTUNISTIC INFECTION (at risk)	TYPE OF TRANSPLANT	PROPHYLACTIC REGIMENS	COMMENTS/REFERENCES
Herpes simplex (seropositive)	HSCT	Acyclovir 200 mg po 3 times per day from conditioning to engraftment or resolution of mucositis	Do not need acyclovir if receiving CMV prophylaxis
	SOT	Acyclovir 200 mg po 3 times per day—start early post-transplant	
CMV (Recipient + OR Donor +/Recipient –)	HSCT	**Preemptive therapy:** Monitor ≥ once weekly (days 10-100) for CMV-antigenemia or viremia by PCR test (Note: culture alone not sufficiently sensitive) & start rx when positive. [Ganciclovir 5 mg per kg IV q12h for 7-14 days, then 5 mg per kg IV q24h 5 days per week to day 100 or ≥3 wks (whichever is longer) [*MMWR 49(RR-10):1, 2000*]. Some use oral ganciclovir 1 gm q8h after the 7–14 day IV induction phase; however, monitoring tests should be negative before stopping rx (*CID 35:999, 2002*). **OR**	
		Prophylaxis: (for high-risk, see *CID 35:999, 2002*, or where CMV detection tests non-available) From engraftment to day 100, rx with ganciclovir 5 mg per kg q12h for 7 days, then 5 mg per kg q24h 5-6 days per week.	
		General Comments: Review in *CMR 16:647, 2003.* Role of valganciclovir in CMV prevention is under investigation.	
	SOT	**Kidney, kidney/pancreas, heart:** Valganciclovir 900 mg po q24h, start by day 10 & continue through day 100 of transplant.	
		Liver: Ganciclovir 1 gm po q8h, start by day 10 & continue through day 100.	
		Lung: Ganciclovir 5 mg per kg q12h for 5–7 days, then valganciclovir 900 mg po q24h for 6 months (or at least 3 mos.) PLUS consider CMV immune globulin 150 mg per kg within 72 hrs of transplant, then 100 mg per kg at wk 2, 4, 6, 8 & wks post-transplant.	
		Comments: Regimens are evolving & institutional protocols vary. For recommendations by American & Canadian transplantation societies, see *Am J Transpl 4(Suppl):51, 2004 & S:218, 2005.* For lung, see *Transpl 80:157, 2005.* The universal prophylaxis approach (above) is favored by most, but there are proponents of preemptive therapy in liver transplantation (*CID 40:704 & 709, 2005; Transpl 79:85 & 1428, 2005*). Valganciclovir not approved by FDA for liver transplantation, but some use it. Some add CMV Ig for other high-risk SOTs also.	
Hepatitis B-induced cirrhosis	Liver	See *Table 14A, page 107*	
Candida sp. (*CID 38:161, 2004*)	Liver	Fluconazole 200–400 mg IV/po 1 time per day starting before transplant & continuing up to 3 mos. in high-risk pts. Optimal duration unknown. Concerns for ↑ non-albicans candida with fluconazole prophylaxis (*Transpl 75:2023, 2003*).	
	HSCT	Fluconazole 400 mg po 1 time per day from day 0 to engraftment or ANC >1000	
Aspergillus sp.	Lung/Heart-Lung	No controlled trials to determine optimal management, but regimens of an aerosolized ampho B preparation & an oral anti-aspergillus agent have been used [*Am J Transpl 4(Suppl:10):110, 2004*]. Randomized trial suggested nebulized ABLC better tolerated than nebul. ampho B deoxycholate (*Transpl 77:232, 2004*).	
	HSCT	Itraconazole (caution re non-significant ↑ invasive aspergillus (*AnIM 138:705, 2003*) or significant ↓ toxicity/intolerance (*Blood 103:1527, 2003*). Study of voriconazole vs fluconazole in progress (*CID 39:S176, 2004*). Vori assoc. with ↑ risk of zygomycosis (*JID 191:1350, 2005*)	
Coccidioides immitis	All	Reasonable: Fluconazole 400 mg po q24h (*Transpl Inf Dis 5:3, 2003*)	
Pneumocystis carinii (P. jiroveci) & Toxoplasma gondii	All	TMP-SMX-SS or –DS, 1 tab po q24h. Duration: 6 mos.–1 yr renal; 26 mos. for allogenic HSCT; ≥1 yr to lifetime for heart, lung, liver [*Am J Transpl 4(Suppl:10):135, 2004*]. Breakthrough pneumocystis reported with atovaquone doses <1500 mg per day (*CID 38:976, 2004*). For toxo D +/R– heart transplants, 3 mos. pyrimethamine/sulfa prior to lifetime TMP-SMX prophylaxis has been suggested [*see Am J Transpl 4(Suppl:10):142, 2004* for intensive pyri-sulfa regimen & alternatives].	
Trypanosoma cruzi	Heart	If known Chagas' disease in donor or recipient, contact CDC for nifurtimox	

* See page 2 for abbreviations

TABLE 15F

TEMPORAL APPROACH TO DIFFERENTIAL DIAGNOSIS OF INFECTION AFTER ORGAN TRANSPLANTATION*

| USUAL HOSPITAL-ACQUIRED INFECTIONS | OPPORTUNISTIC INFECTIONS | COMMUNITY-ACQUIRED OR CHRONIC INFECTIONS |

VIRAL:
— HSV
— CMV
— Onset of Hepatitis B or C
— EBV, VZV, Influenza, RSV, Adenovirus
— CMV retinitis or colitis.. ‡
— Papillomavirus, PTLD.. ‡

BACTERIAL:
— Pneumonia, IV line, UTI, Wound...
— Nocardia
— Listeria, Tuberculosis

FUNGAL:
— Pneumocystis
— Aspergillus
— Candida
— Cryptococcus
— Coccidioidomycosis, Histoplasmosis
‡

PARASITIC
— Strongyloides
— Toxoplasma
— Trypanosoma cruzi
— Leishmania

MONTHS AFTER TRANSPLANTATION
1   2   3   4   5   6

* Adapted from Fishman and Rubin, *NEJM* 338:1741, 1998. For hematopoietic stem cell transplant recipients, see *MMWR* 49:RR-10, 2000.
‡ Solid lines indicate usual time period for onset of infection; dotted lines indicate risk at reduced level

[1] Symptomatic CMV antigenemia may be delayed in patients receiving 3-mo. ganciclovir prophylaxis (*Transpl Int Dis* 6:3, 2004).

TABLE 16: PEDIATRIC DOSAGES OF SELECTED ANTIBACTERIAL AGENTS*
[Adapted from: (1) Nelson's Pocket Book of Pediatric Antimicrobial Therapy, 2002-2003, 15th Ed., J. Bradley & J. Nelson, eds., Lippincott Williams and Wilkins, and (2) 2003 Red Book, 26th Ed., American Academy of Pediatrics, pages 700–718]

DRUG	DOSES IN MG PER KG PER DAY OR MG PER KG AT FREQUENCY INDICATED[1]				
	BODY WEIGHT <2000 gm		BODY WEIGHT >2000 gm		>28 DAYS OLD
	0–7 days old	8–28 days old	0–7 days old	8–28 days old	
Aminoglycosides, IV or IM (check levels; some dose by gestational age + wks of life; see Nelson's Pocket Book, p. 19)					
Amikacin	7.5 q18–24h	7.5 q12h	10 q12h	10 q12h	10 q8h
Gent/tobra	2.5 q18–24h	2.5 q12h	2.5 q12h	2.5 q12h	2.5 q8h
Aztreonam, IV	30 q12h	30 q8h	30 q8h	30 q6h	30 q6h
Cephalosporins					
Cefaclor					20–40 div tid
Cefadroxil					30 div bid (max 2 gm per day)
Cefazolin	20 q12h	20 q12h	20 q12h	20 q8h	20 q8h
Cefdinir					7 q12h or 14 q24h
Cefepime					150 div q8h
Cefixime					8 as q24h or div bid
Cefotaxime	50 q12h	50 q8h	50 q12h	50 q8h	50 q6h (75 q6h for meningitis)
Cefoxitin				20 q12h	80–160 div q8h
Cefpodoxime					10 div bid (max 400 mg per day)
Cefprozil					15–30 div bid (max 1 gm per day)
Ceftazidime	30 q12h	30 q8h	30 q12h	30 q8h	50 q8h
Ceftibuten					4.5 bid
Ceftizoxime					33–66 q8h
Ceftriaxone	50 q24h	50 q24h	50 q24h	75 q24h	50–75 q24h (meningitis 100)
Cefuroxime IV	50 q12h	50 q8h	50 q8h	50 q8h	50 q8h (80 q8h for meningitis)
po					10–15 bid (max 1 gm per day)
Cephalexin					25–50 div q6h (max 4 gm per day)
Loracarbef					15–30 div bid (max 1 gm per day)
Chloramphenicol IV	25 q24h	25 q24h	25 q24h	15 q12h	12.5–25 q6h (max 2–4 gm per day)
Clindamycin IV	5 q12h	5 q8h	5 q8h	5 q6h	7.5 q6h
po					5–6 q8h
Ciprofloxacin po[2]					20–30 div bid (max 1.5 gm per day)
Ertapenem IV	No data	No data	No data	No data	15 q12h
Imipenem[3] IV			25 q12h	25 q8h	15–25 q6h (max 2 gm per day)
Linezolid	No data	10 q8h	No data	10 q8h	10 q8h to age 12
Macrolides					
Erythro IV & po	10 q12h	10 q8h	10 q12h	13 q8h	10 q6h
Azithro po					10–12 day 1, then 5 per day[4]
Clarithro po					7.5 q12h (max. 1 gm per day)
Meropenem IV	20 q12h	20 q8h	20 q12h	20 q8h	60–120 div q8h (120 for meningitis)
Metro IV & po	7.5 q24h	7.5 q12h	7.5 q12h	15 q12h	7.5 q6h
Penicillins					
Ampicillin	50 q12h	50 q8h	50 q8h	50 q6h	50 q6h
AMP-sulbactam					100–300 div q6h
Amoxicillin po				30 div bid	25–50 div tid
Amox-Clav po	30 div bid	30 div bid	30 div bid	30 div bid	45 or 90 (AM/CL-HD) div bid if over 12 wks of age
Dicloxacillin					12–25 div q6h
Mezlocillin	75 q12h	75 q8h	75 q12h	75 q8h	75 q6h
Nafcillin, oxacillin IV	25 q12h	25 q8h	25 q8h	37 q6h	37 q6h (to max. 8–12 gm per day)
Piperacillin, PIP-tazo IV	75 mg per kg q12h	75 mg per kg q12h	75 mg per kg q8h	75 mg per kg q8h	100–300 div q4–6h
Ticarcillin, T.clav IV	75 q12h	75 q8h	75 q12h	75 q8h	75 q6h
Tinidazole					> Age 3: 50 mg per kg for 1 dose
Penicillin G, U/kg IV	50,000 q12h	75,000 q8h	50,000 q8h	50,000 q6h	50,000 units per kg per day
Penicillin V					25–50 mg per kg per day div q6–8h
Rifampin po		10, single dose	20, single dose		20, single dose (max. 600 mg)
Sulfisoxazole po				120–150	120–150 mg per kg per day div q4–6h
TMP-SMX po, IV; UTI: 8–12 TMP component bid; Pneumocystis: 20 TMP component q6h					
Tetracycline po (age 8 or older)					25–50 div q6h
Doxycycline po, IV (age 8 or older)					2–4 div bid
Vancomycin IV	12.5 q12h	15 q12h	18 q12h	22 q12h	40–60 div q6h

[1] May need higher doses in patients with meningitis: see CID 39:1267, 2004
[2] With exception of cystic fibrosis, not approved for use under age 18.
[3] Not recommended in children with CNS infections due to risk of seizures.
[4] Dose for otitis; for pharyngitis, 12 mg per kg times 5 days
* See page 2 for abbreviations

TABLE 17A: DOSAGE OF ANTIMICROBIAL DRUGS IN ADULT PATIENTS WITH RENAL IMPAIRMENT

Adapted from DRUG PRESCRIBING IN RENAL FAILURE, 4th Ed., Aronoff et al (Eds.), American College of Physicians, 1999 and Berns et al, Renal Aspects of Antimicrobial Therapy for HIV Infection. In: P. Kennimel & J. Berns, Eds. HIV INFECTION AND THE KIDNEY. Wilmington & Livingstone, 1998, pp. 185–236.

UNLESS STATED, ADJUSTED DOSES ARE % OF DOSE FOR NORMAL RENAL FUNCTION.

Drug adjustments are based on the patient's estimated endogenous creatinine clearance (CrCl).

Ideal body weight can be calculated as:

50.0 kg + 2.3 kg per inch over 5 feet for men:

45.5 kg + 2.3 kg per inch over 5 feet for women:

(140−age)(ideal body weight in kg)
─────────────────────────────────
(72)(serum creatinine, mg per dL)

For alternative method to calculate estimated CrCl, see AnIM 130:461, 1999.

NOTE: For summary of drugs requiring NO dosage adjustment with renal insufficiency, see Table 17B, page 139.

ANTIMICROBIAL	HALF-LIFE (NORMAL/ESRD) hr	DOSE FOR NORMAL RENAL FUNCTION[1]	METHOD* (see footnote)	ADJUSTMENT FOR RENAL INSUFFICIENCY: Estimated creatinine clearance (CrCl), mL per min			ADJUSTMENT FOR RENAL FAILURE (CrCl), mL per min		SUPPLEMENT FOR HEMODIALYSIS, CAPD[1] (see footnote)	COMMENTS ± DOSAGE FOR CAVH[1]
				>50–90	10–50	<10	30–40	<10		

ANTIBACTERIAL ANTIBIOTICS

Aminoglycoside Antibiotics

Traditional multiple daily doses—adjustment for renal disease

ANTIMICROBIAL	HALF-LIFE (NORMAL/ESRD) hr	DOSE FOR NORMAL RENAL FUNCTION[1]	METHOD*	>50–90	10–50	<10	SUPPLEMENT FOR HEMODIALYSIS, CAPD[1]	COMMENTS ± DOSAGE FOR CAVH[1]
Amikacin	1.4–2.3/17–150	7.5 mg per kg q12h	D&I	60–90% q12h	30–70% q12–18h **Same dose for CAVH[1]**	20–30% q24–48h	HEMO: Extra ½ of normal renal function dose AD[a] CAPD: 15–20 mg lost per L dialysate per day (see Comment)	High flux hemodialysis membranes lead to unpredictable aminoglycoside clearance, measure post-dialysis drug levels for efficacy and toxicity. With CAPD, pharmacokinetics highly variable— **check serum levels.** Usual method for CAPD: 2 liters of dialysis fluid placed qid & drained: give 8&20 mg lost per day + 160 mg amikacin supplement (V per day)
Gentamicin, Tobramycin	2–3/20–60	1.7 mg per kg q8h	D&I	60–90% q8–12h	30–70% q12h **Same dose for CAVH[1]**	20–30% q24–48h	HEMO: Extra ½ of normal renal function dose AD[a] CAPD: 3–4 mg lost per L dialysate per day	
Netilmicin[NUS]	2–3/35–72	2.0 mg per kg q8h	D&I	50–90% q8–12h	20–60% q12h **Same dose for CAVH[1]**	10–20% q24–48h	HEMO: Extra ½ of normal renal function dose AD[a] CAPD: 3–4 mg lost per L dialysate per day	*Adjust dosing weight for obesity: [ideal body weight + 0.4(actual body weight − ideal body weight)] (CID 25:112, 1997)
Streptomycin	2–3/30–80	15 mg per kg (max. of 1.0 gm) q24h	I	50% q24h	q24–72h **Same dose for CAVH[1]**	q72–96h	HEMO: Extra ½ of normal renal function dose AD[a] CAPD: 20–40 mg lost per L dialysate per day	

ONCE-DAILY AMINOGLYCOSIDE THERAPY: ADJUSTMENT IN RENAL INSUFFICIENCY (see Table 10D for OD dosing/normal renal function)

Creatinine Clearance (mL per min.)		>80	60–80	40–60	30–40	20–30	10–20	<10–0
Drug			Dose q24h (mg per kg)				Dose q48h (mg per kg)	Dose q72h and AD[a]
Gentamicin/Tobramycin		5.1	4		2.5		4	3
Amikacin/Kanamycin/streptomycin		15	12	7.5		7.5	8	3
Isepamicin[NUS]		8	8	4	8 q48h	8 q72h	8 q96h	
Netilmicin[NUS]		6.5	5	3		2.5		

Carbapenem Antibiotics

ANTIMICROBIAL	HALF-LIFE (NORMAL/ESRD) hr	DOSE FOR NORMAL RENAL FUNCTION[1]	METHOD*	>80	60–80	40–60	10	<10	SUPPLEMENT FOR HEMODIALYSIS, CAPD[1]	COMMENTS ± DOSAGE FOR CAVH[1]
Ertapenem	4/>4	1.0 gm q24h	D	1.0 gm q24h	0.5 gm q24h (CrCl <30)		0.5 gm q24h	0.5 gm q24h	HEMO: Dose as for CrCl <10; if dosed <6 hrs prior to HD, give 150 mg supplement AD[a]	
Imipenem (see Comment)	1/4	0.5 gm q6h	D&I	250–500 mg q6–8h	250 mg q6–12h **Dose for CAVH[1]: 0.5–1 gm bid** (AAC 49:2421, 2005)	125–250 mg q12h		HEMO: Dose AD[a] CAPD: Dose for CrCl <10	potential for seizures if recommended doses exceeded in pts with CrCl <20 mL per min. See pkg insert, esp. for pts <70 kg
Meropenem	1/6–8	1.0 gm q8h	D&I	1.0 gm q8h	1.0 gm q12h **Same dose for CAVH[1]**	0.5 gm q24h			HEMO: Dose AD[a] CAPD: Dose for CrCl <10	

* **CAVH** = continuous arteriovenous hemofiltration (NEJM 336:1303, 1997) usually results in CrCl of approx. 30 mL per min.; * **AD** = after dialysis, "**Dose AD**" refers to timing of dose.

See page 2 for abbreviations. **Supplement is to replace drug lost via dialysis; extra drug beyond continuation of regimen used for CrCl <10 mL per min.**

TABLE 17A (2)

ANTIMICROBIAL	HALF-LIFE (NORMAL/ESRD) hr	DOSE FOR NORMAL RENAL FUNCTION†	METHOD* (see footnote)	ADJUSTMENT FOR RENAL FAILURE Estimated creatinine clearance (CrCl), mL per min >50-90	10-50	<10	SUPPLEMENT FOR HEMODIALYSIS, CAPD* (see footnote)	COMMENTS ± DOSAGE FOR CAVH‡ (see footnote)
Cephalosporin Antibiotics: DATA ON SELECTED PARENTERAL CEPHALOSPORINS								
Cefazolin	1.9/40–70	1.0–2.0 gm q8h	I	q8h	q12h **Same dose for CAVH‡**	q24–48h	HEMO: Extra 0.5–1 gm AD* CAPD: 0.5 gm q12h	As for CrCl 10–50
Cefepime	2.2/18	2.0 gm q8h (max. dose)	D&I	2 gm q8h	2 gm q12–24h **Same dose for CAVH‡**	1 gm q24h	HEMO: Extra 1 gm AD* CAPD: 1–2 gm q48h	CAVH‡ dose: As for CrCl 10–50
Cefotaxime, Ceftizoxime	1.7/15–35	2.0 gm q8h	I	q8–12h	q12–24h **Same dose for CAVH‡**	q24h	HEMO: Extra 1 gm AD* CAPD: 1 gm q24h	Active metabolite of cefotaxime in ESRD ↓ dose further for hepatic & renal failure.
Cefotetan	3.5/13–25	1–2 gm q12h	D	100%	50% **Same dose for CAVH‡**	25%	HEMO: Extra 1 gm AD* CAPD: 1 gm q24h	CAVH‡ dose: 750 mg q12h
Cefoxitin	0.8/13–23	2.0 gm q8h	I	q8h	q8–12h **Same dose for CAVH‡**	q24–48h	HEMO: Extra 1 gm AD* CAPD: 1 gm q24h	May falsely increase serum creatinine by interference with assay.
Ceftazidime	1.2/13–25	2 gm q8h	I	q8–12h	q24–48h **Same dose for CAVH‡**	q48h	HEMO: Extra 1 gm AD* CAPD: 0.5 gm q24h	Volume of distribution increases with infection.
Cefuroxime sodium	1.2/17	0.75–1.5 gm q8h	I	q8h	q8–12h **Same dose for CAVH‡**	q24h	HEMO: Dose AD* CAPD: Dose for CrCl <10	CAVH‡ dose: 1.5 gm, then 750 mg IV q24h
Fluoroquinolone Antibiotics								
Ciprofloxacin	4/6–9	500–750 mg po (or 400 mg IV) q12h	D	100%	50–75%	50%	HEMO: 250 mg po or 200 mg IV q12h CAPD: 250 mg po or 200 mg IV q8h	CAVH‡ dose: 200 mg IV q12h
Gatifloxacin	7–14/36	400 mg po/IV q24h	D	400 mg q24h	400 mg q24h, then 200 mg q24h **Same dose for CAVH‡**	400 mg q24h, then 200 mg q24h	HEMO: 200 mg q24h AD* CAPD: 200 mg q24h	CAVH‡ dose: As for CrCl 10–50
Gemifloxacin	7/>7	320 mg q24h	D	320 mg q24h	160 mg q24h **Same dose for CAVH‡**	160 mg q24h	HEMO: 160 mg q24h AD* CAPD: 160 mg q24h	CAVH‡ dose: As for CrCl 10–50
Levofloxacin	6–51/76	750 mg q24h IV, PO	D&I	750 mg q24h	750 mg once, then q48h	750 mg once, then 500 mg q48h	HEMO/CAPD: Dose for CrCl <10	CAVH‡ dose: As for CrCl 10–50
Macrolide Antibiotics								
Clarithromycin	5–7/22	0.5–1.0 gm q12h	D	100%	75%	50–75%	HEMO: Dose AD* CAPD: None	ESRD dosing recommendations based on extrapolation
Erythromycin	1.4/5–6	250–500 mg q6h	D	100%	100%	50–75%	HEMO/CAPD/CAVH‡: None	Ototoxicity with high doses in ESRD
Miscellaneous Antibacterial Antibiotics								
Colistin	<6/=48	80–160 mg q8h	D	160 mg q12h	160 mg q24h	160 mg q36h	HEMO: 80 mg AD*	
Daptomycin	9.4/30	4 mg per kg per day	None	4 mg per kg per day	CrCl <30, 4 mg per kg q48h	4 mg per kg q48h (after dialysis if possible)	HEMO & CAPD: 4 mg per kg q48h	
Linezolid	6.4/7.1	600 mg po/IV q12h	D	600 mg po/IV q12h	600 mg q12h **Same dose for CAVH‡**	600 mg q12h AD*	HEMO: As for CrCl <10 CAPD: No data	CAVH*: Accumulation of 2 metabolites—risk unknown (JAC 56:172, 2005)
Metronidazole	6–14/7–21	7.5 mg per kg q6h	D	100%	100% **Same dose for CAVH‡**	50%	HEMO: Dose AD* CAPD: Dose for CrCl <10	Hemo clears metronidazole and its metabolites (AAC 29:235, 1986)
Nitrofurantoin	0.5/1	50–100 mg q6h	D	100%	Avoid	Avoid	Not applicable	
Sulfamethoxazole	10/20–50	1.0 gm q8h	I	q12h	q18h **Same dose for CAVH‡**	q24h	HEMO: Extra 1 gm AD* CAPD: 1 gm q24h	
Teicoplanin*xtx	45/62–230	6 mg per kg per day	I	q24h	q48h **Same dose for CAVH‡**	q72h	HEMO: Dose for CrCl <10 CAPD: Dose for CrCl <10	
Telithromycin	10/15	800 mg q24h	D	800 mg q24h	600 mg q24h (<30 mL per min) **Same dose for CAVH‡**	600 mg q24h	HEMO: 600 mg AD* CAPD: No data	

* CAVH = continuous arteriovenous hemofiltration (NEJM 336:1303, 1997) usually results in CrCl of approx. 30 mL per min. * AD = after dialysis. † "Dose AD" refers to timing of dose.
See page 138 for other footnotes and page 2 for abbreviations Supplement is to replace drug lost via dialysis; extra drug beyond continuation of regimen used for CrCl <10 mL per min.

TABLE 17A (3)

ANTIMICROBIAL	HALF-LIFE (NORMAL/ESRD) hr	DOSE FOR NORMAL RENAL FUNCTION	METHOD* (see footnote)	ADJUSTMENT FOR RENAL FAILURE Estimated creatinine clearance (CrCl), mL per min >50-90	10-50	<10	SUPPLEMENT FOR HEMODIALYSIS, CAPD* (see footnote)	COMMENTS ± DOSAGE FOR CAVH†
Miscellaneous Antibacterial Antibiotics *(continued)*								
Trimethoprim	11/20-49	100-200 mg q12h	I	q12h	q18h **Same dose for CAVH†**	q24h	HEMO: Dose AD* q24h CAPD: q8h	CAVH† dose: q18h
Trimethoprim-sulfamethoxazole-DS								
Treatment	As above	5 mg per kg IV q8h	D	100% 100%	50% 100%	Not recommended 100%		
Prophylaxis	As above	1 tab po q24h or 3 times per week	No change					
Vancomycin	6/200-250	1 gm q12h	D&I	1 gm q12h	1 gm q24-96h	1 gm q4-7 days	HEMO/CAPD: Dose for CrCl <10	CAVH† 500 mg q24-48h. New hemodialysis membranes ↑ clear. of vanco; **check levels**
Penicillins								
Amoxicillin	1.0/5-20	250-500 mg q8h	I	q8h	q8-12h	q24h	HEMO: Dose AD* CAPD: 250 mg q12h	IV amoxicillin not available in the U.S.
Ampicillin	1.0/7-20	250 mg-2 gm q6h	I	q6h	q6-12h	q12-24h	HEMO: Dose AD* CAPD: 250 mg q12h	
Amoxicillin/Clavulanate	1.3 AM/1.0, 5-20/4.0	500/125 mg q8h	I	500/125 mg q8h	250-500 mg AM component q12h	250-500 mg AM component q24h	HEMO: As for CrCl <10; extra dose after dialysis CAPD: As for CrCl <10	**If CrCl ≤30 mg per mL, do not use 875/125 or 1000/62.5 AM/CL**
Ampicillin/Sulbactam (SB)	1.0 (AM)/1.0 (SB), 9.0 (AM)/10.0 (SB)	2 gm AM + 1.0 gm SB	D&I	q6h	q8-12h	q24h	HEMO: Dose AD* 2 gm AM/1 gm SB q12h CAPD: 2 gm AM/1 gm SB q24h	CAVH† dose: 1.5 AM/0.75 SB q12h
Aztreonam	2.0/6-8	2 gm q8h	D	100%	50-75% **Same dose for CAVH†**	25%	HEMO: Extra 0.5 gm AD* CAPD: Dose for CrCl <10	Technically is a β-lactam antibiotic.
Penicillin G	0.5/6-20	0.5-4 million U q4h	D	100%	75% **Same dose for CAVH†**	20-50%	HEMO: Dose AD* CAPD: Dose for CrCl <10	1.7 mEq potassium per million units. ↑ potential of seizure. 6 million units per day max. dose in ESRD.
Piperacillin	1.0/3.3-5.1	3-4 gm q4-6h	D&I	q4-6h	q6-8h **Same dose for CAVH†**	q8h	HEMO: Dose AD* CAPD: Dose for CrCl <10	1.9 mEq sodium per gm
Pip.(Pi)/Tazo(T)	1.0 P/1.0 T, 3.0 P/4.0 T	3.375 gm q6h	D&I	3.375 gm	2.25 gm q6h	2.25 gm q8h	HEMO: Dose for CrCl <10 + 0.75 gm AD* CAPD: Dose for CrCl <10	
Ticarcillin	1.2/13	3 gm q4h	D&I	1-2 gm q4h	1-2 gm q8h **Same dose for CAVH†**	1-2 gm q12h	HEMO: Extra 3.0 gm AD* CAPD: Dose for CrCl <10	5.2 mEq sodium per gm
Ticarcillin/Clavulanate (CL)	1.0 (TC)/1.0 (CL), 13 (TC)/4.0 (CL)	3.1 gm q4h	D&I	3.1 gm q4h	2.0 gm q4-8h **Same dose for CAVH†**	2.0 gm q12h	HEMO: Extra 3.1 gm AD* CAPD: 3.1 gm q12h	See footnote 2
Tetracycline Antibiotics								
Tetracycline	6-10/57-108	250-500 mg qid	I	q8-12h	q12-24h **Same dose for CAVH†**	q24h	HEMO: None CAPD: None CAVH†: None	Avoid in ESRD
ANTIFUNGAL ANTIBIOTICS								
Amphotericin B & ampho B lipid complex	24/unchanged	Non-lipid: 0.4-1.0 mg per kg per day ABCD: 3-6 mg per kg per day ABLC: 5 mg per kg per day LAB: 3-5 mg per kg per day	I	q24h	q24h **Same dose for CAVH†**	q24h	HEMO: None CAPD: Dose for CrCl <10	For ampho B, toxicity lessened by saline loading; risk amplified by concomitant cyclosporine A, aminoglycosides, or pentamidine
Fluconazole	37/100	200-400 mg q24h	D	200-400 mg q24h	100-200 mg q24h **Same dose for CAVH†**	100-200 mg q24h	HEMO: 100% of recommended dose AD* CAPD: Dose for CrCl <10	
Flucytosine	3-6/75-200	37.5 mg per kg q6h	D&I	q12h	q12-24h **Same dose for CAVH†**	q24h	HEMO: Dose AD* CAPD: 0.5-1.0 gm q24h	Goal is peak serum level > 25 mcg per mL and <100 mcg per mL

† Clavulanate cleared by liver, not kidney. Hence as dose of combination decreased, a deficiency of clavulanate may occur (*JAMA* 285:386, 2001).

‡ **CAVH** = continuous arteriovenous hemofiltration (*NEJM* 336:1303, 1997) usually results in CrCl of approx. 30 mL per min. * **AD** = after dialysis. **"Dose AD" refers to timing of dose.** **Supplement is to replace drug lost via dialysis; extra drug beyond continuation of regimen used for CrCl <10 mL per min.**

See page 1:38 for other footnotes and page 2 for abbreviations.

TABLE 17A (4)

ANTIMICROBIAL	HALF-LIFE (NORMAL/ESRD) hr	DOSE FOR NORMAL RENAL FUNCTION¹	METHOD* (see footnote)	ADJUSTMENT FOR RENAL FAILURE Estimated creatinine clearance (CrCl), mL per min >50-90	10-50	<10	SUPPLEMENT FOR HEMODIALYSIS, CAPD* (see footnote)	COMMENTS ± DOSAGE FOR CAVH¹
ANTIFUNGAL ANTIBIOTICS (continued)								
Itraconazole, po soln	35/–	100-200 mg q12h	–	100%	100%	100%	HEMO/CAPD/CAVH¹ No adjustment with oral solution	
Itraconazole, IV	35/–	200 mg IV q12h	–	200 mg IV q12h			Do not use IV if CrCl <30 due to accumulation of carrier, cyclodextrin	
Terbinafine	36-200/?	250 mg per day	–	q24h			Use has not been studied. Recommend avoidance of drug.	
Voriconazole, IV	Non-linear kinetics	6 mg per kg IV q12h times 2, then 4 mg per kg q12h	–	No change			If CrCl <50 mL per min, accum. of IV vehicle (cyclodextrin). Switch to po or DC	
ANTIPARASITIC ANTIBIOTICS								
Pentamidine		4 mg per kg per day	I	q24h	q24h	q24-36h	HEMO/CAPD/CAVH¹ None	
Quinine	5-16/5-16	650 mg q8h		650 mg q8h	650 mg q8-12h Same dose for CAVH¹	650 mg q24h	HEMO: Dose AD* CAPD: Dose for CrCl <10	Marked tissue accumulation
ANTITUBERCULOUS ANTIBIOTICS (Excellent review: Nephron 64:169, 1993)								
Ethambutol	4/7-15	15-25 mg per kg q24h	I	q24h Same dose for CAVH¹	q24-36h	q48h	HEMO: Dose AD* CAPD: Dose for CrCl <10	25 mg per kg 4-6 hr prior to 3 times per wk dialysis. Streptomycin instead of ethambutol in renal failure.
Ethionamide	2.1/?	250-500 mg q12h	D	100%	100%	50%	HEMO/CAPD/CAVH¹ None	
Isoniazid	0.7-4/8-17	5 mg per kg q24h	D	100%	100%	100%	HEMO: Dose AD* CAPD/CAVH¹: Dose for CrCl <10	
Pyrazinamide	9/26	25 mg per kg q24h (max. dose 2.5 gm q24h)	D	25 mg per kg q24h	25 mg per kg q24h	12-25 mg per kg q24h	HEMO: 25-35 mg per kg after each dialysis CAPD: No reduction; CAVH¹: No data	
Rifampin	1.5-5/1.8-11	600 mg per day	D	600 mg q24h	300-600 mg q24h	300-600 mg q24h	HEMO: None CAPD/CAVH¹: Dose for CrCl <10	Biologically active metabolite
ANTIVIRAL AGENTS								
Acyclovir, IV	2.5/20	5-12.4 mg per kg q8h	D&I	5-12.4 mg per kg q8h	5-12.4 mg per kg q12-24h	2.5 mg per kg q24h	HEMO: Dose AD* CAPD: Dose for CrCl <10	Rapid IV infusion can cause ↑ Ct. CAVH¹ dose: 3.5 mg per kg per day
Adefovir	7.5/–	10 mg q24h	I	10 mg q24h	10 mg q48-72h	No data	HEMO: q7d AD*	
Amantadine	12/500	100 mg po bid	I	q24-48h	q48-72h	q7days	HEMO/CAPD/CAVH¹ None	
Cidofovir: Complicated dosing—see package insert								
Induction	2.5/unknown	5 mg per kg once per wk for 2 wks	–	5 mg per kg once per wk	0.5-2 mg per kg once per wk	0.5 mg per kg once per wk	No data	Major toxicity is renal. No efficacy, safety, or pharmacokinetic data in pts with moderate/severe renal disease.
Maintenance	2.5/unknown	5 mg per kg q2wks	–	5 mg per kg q2wks	0.5-2 mg per kg q2wks	0.5 mg per kg q2wks	No data	
Didanosine tablets¹	0.6-1.6/4.5	125-200 mg q12h buffered tabs	D	200 mg q12h	200 mg q24h	<60 kg: 150 mg q24h >60 kg 100 mg q24h	HEMO: Dose AD* CAPD/CAVH¹: Dose for CrCl <10	Based on incomplete data. Data are estimates.
		400 mg q24h enteric-coated tabs				**Do not use EC tabs**		**If <60 kg & CrCl <10 mL per min, do not use EC tabs**
Emtricitabine	10/>10	200 mg q24h	I	200 mg q24h	200 mg q48-72h	200 mg q96h	HEMO: Dose for CrCl <10	Give after dialysis on dialysis days
Entecavir	128-149/?	0.5 mg q24h	D	0.5 mg q24h	0.15-0.25 mg q24h	0.05 mg q24h	HEMO/CAPD: 0.05 mg q24h	

¹ Ref. for NRTIs and NNRTIs: *Kidney International 60:821, 2001*
CAVH = continuous arteriovenous hemofiltration (*NEJM 336:1303, 1997*) usually results in CrCl of approx. 30 mL per min. * **AD** = after dialysis. **"Dose AD"** refers to timing of dose. **Supplement is to replace drug lost via dialysis; extra drug beyond continuation of regimen used for CrCl <10 mL per min.**
See page 138 for other footnotes and page 2 for abbreviations.

TABLE 17A (5)

ANTIMICROBIAL	HALF-LIFE (NORMAL/ESRD) hr	DOSE FOR NORMAL RENAL FUNCTION[§]	METHOD[*] (see footnote)	ADJUSTMENT FOR RENAL FAILURE Estimated creatinine clearance (CrCl), mL per min >50-90	10-50	<10	SUPPLEMENT FOR HEMODIALYSIS, CAPD (see footnote)	COMMENTS ‡ DOSAGE FOR CAVH[†]
ANTIVIRAL AGENTS (continued)								
Famciclovir	2.3-3.0/10-22	500 mg q8h	D&I	500 mg q8h	500 mg q12-24h	250 mg q24h	HEMO: Dose AD*; CAPD: No data	CAVH dose: As for CrCl 10-50

Foscarnet (CMV dosage) Dosage adjustment based on est. CrCl (mL per min) div. by pt's kg — Half-life: Normal half-life (T½) 3 hrs with terminal T½ of 18-88 hrs. T½ very long with ESRD. Dose for normal renal function: Induction: 60 mg per kg q8h x2-3 wks. Maintenance: 90-120 mg per kg per day IV. Method: D&I. Comments: See package insert for further details.

CrCl as mL per min per kg body weight—ONLY FOR FOSCARNET

Dose	>1.4	>1.0-1.4	>0.8-1.0	>0.6-0.8	>0.4-0.6	<0.4
Induction	60 q8h	45 q8h	50 q12h	40 q12h	60 q24h	Do not use
Maintenance	120 q24h	90 q24h	65 q24h	105 q48h	80 q48h	Do not use

ANTIMICROBIAL	HALF-LIFE (NORMAL/ESRD) hr	DOSE FOR NORMAL RENAL FUNCTION[§]	METHOD[*]	>50-90	10-50	<10	SUPPLEMENT FOR HEMODIALYSIS, CAPD	COMMENTS ‡ DOSAGE FOR CAVH[†]
Ganciclovir — IV: / po:	2.9/30	Induction 5 mg per kg q12h IV Maintenance 5 mg per kg q24h IV 1.0 gm tid po	D&I	5 mg per kg q12h 2.5-5.0 mg per kg q24h 0.5-1 gm tid	1.25-2.5 mg per kg q24h 0.6-1.25 mg per kg q24h 0.5-1.0 gm q24h	1.25 mg per kg 3 times per wk 0.625 mg per kg 3 times per wk 0.5 gm 3 times per week	HEMO: Dose AD*; CAPD: <10 HEMO: 0.6 mg per kg AD*; CAPD: Dose for <10 HEMO: 0.5 gm AD*	As for CrCl 10-50
Lamivudine[†]	5-7/15-35	300 mg po q24h	D&I	300 mg po q24h	50-150 mg q24h	25-50 mg q24h	HEMO: Dose AD*; CAPD/CAVH: No data	
Oseltamivir	1-3/no data	75 mg po bid	D&I	75 mg q12h	75 mg q24h	No data	No data	
Ritonavir	Use with caution in patients with creatinine clearance <10 mL per min.							
Rimantadine	13-65/Prolonged	100 mg bid	I	100%	100 mg q24h-bid	100 mg q24h	HEMO/CAPD: No data	Use with caution, little data
Stavudine, po[†]	1-1.4/5.5-8	30-40 mg q12h	D&I	100%	50% q12h-bid Same dose for CAVH	≥60 kg 20 mg per day; <60 kg 15 mg per day	HEMO: Dose as for CrCl <10 AD*; CAPD: No data	CAVH dose: As for CrCl 10-50
Tenofovir, po		300 mg q24h	D&I	300 mg q24h	300 mg q48h (CrCl 30-50; 2 times per wk (CrCl 10-30)	No data	HEMO: Give 300 mg after every 3rd hemodialysis	
Valacyclovir[†]	2.5-3.3/14	1.0 gm q8h	D&I	1.0 gm q8h	1.0 gm q12-24h Same dose for CAVH	0.5 gm q24h	HEMO: Dose AD*; CAPD: Dose for CrCl <10	CAVH dose: As for CrCl 10-50
Valganciclovir[†]	4/67	900 mg po bid	D&I	900 mg po bid	450 mg q24h to 450 mg every other day Same dose for CAVH	DO NOT USE	HEMO/CAPD: DO NOT USE	CAVH dose: As for CrCl 10-50
Zalcitabine[†]	2.0/>8	0.75 mg q8h	D&I	0.75 mg q8h	0.75 mg q12h Same dose for CAVH	0.75 mg q24h	HEMO: Dose AD*; CAPD: No data	CAVH dose: As for CrCl 10-50
Zidovudine[†]	1.1-1.4/1.4-3	300 mg q12h	D&I	300 mg q12h	300 mg q12h	100 mg q6-8h; if hemo AD*	HEMO: Dose for CrCl <10; CAPD: Dose for CrCl <10	CAVH dose: 100 mg q8h

CrCl as mL per min — usually results in CrCl of approx. 30 mL per min; * AD = after dialysis; * AD* refers to timing of dose. "Dose AD" refers to timing of dose. "Dose AD" refers to timing of dose used for CrCl <10 mL per min. ** Per cent refers to % change from dose for normal renal function.

CAVH = continuous arteriovenous hemofiltration (NEJM 336:1303, 1997). CAVH = continuous arteriovenous hemofiltration (NEJM 336:1303, 1997). Supplement is to replace drug lost via dialysis; extra drug beyond continuation of regimen used for CrCl <10 mL per min. D = Dosage interval.

CAVH = continuous arteriovenous hemofiltration; **D** = Dosage interval; **I** = interval extension; **Supplement is to replace drug lost via dialysis; extra drug beyond continuation of regimen used for CrCl <10 mL per min. "Dose AD" refers to timing of dose.**

§ Dosages are for life-threatening infections.

[†] Ref. for NRTIs and NNRTIs: Kidney International 60:821, 2001
[‡] See page 2 for abbreviations

139

TABLE 17B: NO DOSAGE ADJUSTMENT WITH RENAL INSUFFICIENCY, BY CATEGORY:*

Antibacterials		Antifungals	Anti-TBc	Antivirals	
Azithromycin	Linezolid	Caspofungin	Rifabutin	Abacavir	Lopinavir
Ceftriaxone	Minocycline	Itraconazole oral solution	Rifapentine	Atazanavir	Nelfinavir
Chloramphenicol	Moxifloxacin	Micafungin		Delavirdine	Nevirapine
Ciprofloxacin XL	Nafcillin	Voriconazole, **po only**		Efavirenz	Ribavirin
Clindamycin	Pyrimethamine			Fosamprenavir	Saquinavir
Dirithromycin	Rifaximin			Indinavir	Tipranavir
Doxycycline	Tigecycline				

TABLE 18: ANTIMICROBIALS AND HEPATIC DISEASE DOSAGE ADJUSTMENT*

The following alphabetical list indicates antibacterials excreted/metabolized by the liver **wherein a dosage adjustment may be indicated** in the presence of hepatic disease. Space precludes details; consult the PDR or package inserts for details. List is **not** all-inclusive:

Antibacterials		Antifungals	Antivirals§	
Ceftriaxone	Nafcillin	Caspofungin	Abacavir	Indinavir
Chloramphenicol	Rifabutin	Itraconazole	Atazanavir	Lopinavir/ritonavir
Clindamycin	Rifampin	Voriconazole	Delavirdine	Nelfinavir
Fusidic acid	Synercid**		Efavirenz	Nevirapine
Isoniazid	Tigecycline		Enfuvirtide	Rimantadine
Metronidazole	Tinidazole		Fosamprenavir	Ritonavir

§ Ref. on antiretrovirals: CID 40:174, 2005   ** Quinupristin/dalfopristin

TABLE 19: TREATMENT OF CAPD PERITONITIS IN ADULTS[1]*
(Periton Dial Intl 20:396, 2000)

EMPIRIC Intraperitoneal Therapy:[2] Culture Results Pending

Drug		Residual Urine Output	
		<100 mL per day	>100 mL per day
Cefazolin +	Can mix in same bag	1 gm per bag, q24h	20 mg per kg BW per bag, q24h
Ceftazidime		1 gm per bag, q24h	20 mg per kg BW per bag, q24h

Drug Doses for SPECIFIC Intraperitoneal Therapy—Culture Results Known. NOTE: Few po drugs indicated

Drug	Intermittent Dosing (once per day)		Continuous Dosing (per liter exchange)	
	Anuric	Non-Anuric	Anuric	Non-Anuric
Gentamicin	0.6 mg per kg	↑ dose 25%	MD 8 mg	↑ MD by 25%
Cefazolin	15 mg per kg	20 mg per kg	LD 500 mg, MD 125 mg	LD 500 mg, ↑ MD 25%
Ceftazidime	1000–1500 mg	ND	LD 250 mg, MD 125 mg	ND
Ampicillin	250–500 mg po bid	ND	250–500 mg po bid	ND
Ciprofloxacin	500 mg po bid	ND	LD 50 mg, MD 25 mg	ND
Vancomycin	15–30 mg per kg q5–7 days	↑ dose 25%	MD 30–50 mg per L	↑ MD 25%
Metronidazole	250 mg po bid	ND	250 mg po bid	ND
Amphotericin B	NA	NA	MD 1.5 mg	NA
Fluconazole	200 mg q24h	ND	200 mg q24h	ND
Itraconazole	100 mg q12h	100 mg q12h	100 mg q12h	100 mg q12h
Amp-sulbactam	2 gm q12h	ND	LD 1.0 gm, MD 100 mg	ND
TMP-SMX	320/1600 mg po q1–2 days	ND	LD 320/1600 mg po, MD 80/400 mg po q24h	ND

[1] All doses IP unless indicated otherwise.
  LD = loading dose, MD = maintenance dose, ND = no data; NA = not applicable—dose as normal renal function. **Anuric** = <100 mL per day, **non-anuric** = >100 mL per day
[2] **Does not provide treatment for MRSA.** If Gram-positive cocci on Gram stain, include vancomycin.
* See page 2 for other abbreviations

TABLE 20A: RECOMMENDED CHILDHOOD AND ADOLESCENT IMMUNIZATION SCHEDULE[1]: UNITED STATES, 2005 *(MMWR 54:Q1, 2005) (For overall recommendations, see MMWR 51:RR-2, 2002)*

		Range of recommended ages				Catch-up vaccination				Preadolescent assessment		
VACCINE	Birth	1 mo	2 mos	4 mos	6 mos	12 mos	15 mos	18 mos	24 mos	4-6 yrs	11-12 yrs	13-18 yrs
Hepatitis B[2]	HepB #1 only if mother HBsAg(–)		HepB #2			HepB #3					HepB series	
Diphtheria, Tetanus, Pertussis[3]			DTaP	DTaP	DTaP		DTaP			DTaP	Td	Td
Haemophilus Influenzae Type b[4]			Hib	Hib	Hib[4]	Hib						
Inactivated Poliovirus			IPV	IPV	IPV					IPV		
Measles, Mumps, Rubella[5]						MMR #1				MMR #2	MMR #2	
Varicella[6]						Varicella					Varicella	
Pneumococcal[7]			PCV	PCV	PCV	PCV			PCV		PPV	
Influenza[8]					Influenza (yearly)					Influenza (yearly)		
— — — — — — — — Vaccines below this line are for selected populations — — — —												
Hepatitis A[9]											HepA series	

[1] This schedule indicates the recommended ages for routine administration of currently licensed childhood vaccines, as of Dec. 1, 2004, for children aged ≤18 yrs. Any dose not administered at the recommended age should be administered at any subsequent visit when indicated and feasible. █ indicates age groups that warrant special effort to administer those vaccines not previously administered. Additional vaccines might be licensed & recommended during the year. Licensed combination vaccines may be used whenever any components of the combination are indicated & other components of the vaccine are not contraindicated. Providers should consult package inserts for detailed recommendations. Clinically significant adverse events that follow immunization should be reported to the Vaccine Adverse Event Reporting System; guidance is available at www.vaers.org or by telephone, 800-822-7967.

[2] **Hepatitis B (HepB) vaccine.** All infants should receive the 1st dose of HepB vaccine soon after birth & before hospital discharge; the 1st dose may also be administered by age 2 months if the mother is hepatitis B surface antigen (HBsAg) negative. Only monovalent HepB may be used for the birth dose. Monovalent or combination vaccine containing HepB may be used to complete the series. Four doses of vaccine may be administered when a birth dose is administered. The 2nd dose should be administered at least 4 weeks after the 1st dose, except for combination vaccines, which cannot be administered before age 6 weeks. The 3rd dose should be administered at least 16 weeks after the 1st dose & at least 8 weeks after the 2nd dose. The final dose in the vaccination series (3rd or 4th dose) should not be administered before age 24 weeks. **Infants born to HBsAg-positive mothers** should receive HepB and 0.5 mL of hepatitis B immune globulin (HBIG) at separate sites within 12 hours of birth. The 2nd dose is recommended at age 1–2 months. The final dose in the immunization series should not be administered before age 24 weeks. These infants should be tested for HBsAg and antibody to HBsAg at age 9–15 months. **Infants born to mothers whose HBsAg status is unknown** should receive the 1st dose of the HepB series within 12 hours of birth. Maternal blood should be drawn as soon as possible to determine the mother's HBsAg status; if the HBsAg test is positive, the infant should receive HBIG as soon as possible (no later than 1 week). The 2nd dose is recommended at age 1–2 months. The last dose in the immunization series should not be administered before age 24 weeks.

[3] **Diphtheria and tetanus toxoids and acellular pertussis (DTaP) vaccine.** The 4th dose of DTaP may be administered as early as age 12 months, provided 6 months have elapsed since the 3rd dose and the child is unlikely to return at age 15–18 months. The final dose in the series should be administered at age ≥4 years. **Tetanus and diphtheria toxoids (Td)** is recommended at age 11–12 years if at least 5 years have elapsed since the last dose of tetanus & diphtheria toxoid–containing vaccine. Subsequent routine Td boosters are recommended every 10 years.

[4] **Haemophilus influenzae type b (Hib) conjugate vaccine.** Three Hib conjugate vaccines are licensed for infant use. If PRP-OMP [PedvaxHIB® or ComVax® (Merck)] is administered at ages 2 & 4 months, a dose at age 6 months is not required. DTaP/Hib combination products should not be used for primary immunization in infants at ages 2, 4, or 6 months but can be used as boosters after any Hib vaccine. The final dose in the series should be administered at age ≥12 months.

[5] **Measles, mumps, and rubella vaccine (MMR).** The 2nd dose of MMR is recommended routinely at age 4–6 years but may be administered during any visit, provided at least 4 weeks have elapsed since the 1st dose & both doses are administered beginning at or after age 12 months. Those who have not previously received the 2nd dose should complete the schedule by age 11–12 years.

[6] **Varicella vaccine.** Varicella vaccine is recommended at any visit at or after age 12 months for susceptible children (i.e., those who lack a reliable history of chickenpox). Susceptible persons aged ≥13 years should receive 2 doses administered at least 4 weeks apart.

[7] **Pneumococcal vaccine.** The heptavalent **pneumococcal conjugate vaccine (PCV)** is recommended for all children aged 2–23 months & for certain children aged 24–59 months. The final dose in the series should be administered at age ≥12 months. **Pneumococcal polysaccharide vaccine (PPV)** is recommended in addition to PCV for certain groups at high risk. *See MMWR 49(RR-9), 2000.*

[8] **Influenza vaccine.** Influenza vaccine is recommended annually for children aged ≥6 months with certain risk factors (including, but not limited to, asthma, cardiac disease, sickle cell disease, HIV, & diabetes), health-care workers, & other persons (including household members) in close contact with persons in groups at high risk *[see MMWR 53(R-6), 2004]*. In addition, healthy children aged 6–23 months & close contacts of healthy children aged 0–23 months are recommended to receive influenza vaccine because children in this age group are at substantially increased risk for influenza-related hospitalizations. For healthy persons aged 5–49 years, the intranasally administered, live, attenuated influenza vaccine (LAIV) is an acceptable alternative to the intramuscular trivalent inactivated influenza vaccine (TIV). *See MMWR 53(RR-6), 2004.* Children receiving TIV should be administered a dosage appropriate for their age (0.25 mL if aged 6–35 months or 0.5 mL if aged ≥3 years). Children aged ≤8 years who are receiving influenza vaccine for the first time should receive 2 doses (separated by at least 4 weeks for TIV & at least 6 weeks for LAIV).

[9] **Hepatitis A vaccine.** Hepatitis A vaccine is recommended for children and adolescents in selected states & regions & for certain groups at high risk; consult your local public health authority. Children & adolescents in these states, regions, & groups who have not been immunized against hepatitis A can begin the hepatitis A immunization series during any visit. The 2 doses in the series should be administered at least 6 months apart. *See MMWR 48(RR-12), 1999.*

TABLE 20A (2)

Catch-Up Schedule For Children Aged 4 Months–6 Years

Vaccine	Minimum age for dose 1	Minimum interval between doses			
		Dose 1 to dose 2	Dose 2 to dose 3	Dose 3 to dose 4	Dose 4 to dose 5
DTaP[1]	6 wks	4 wks	4 wks	6 mos.	6 mos.[1]
IPV[2]	6 wks	4 wks	4 wks	4 wks[2]	
HepB[3]	Birth	4 wks	8 wks (& 16 wks after 1st dose)		
MMR[4]	12 mos	4 wks[4]			
Varicella	12 mos				
Hib[5]	6 wks	4 wks: if 1st dose given at age <12 mos 8 wks (as final dose): if 1st dose given at age 12–24 mos No further doses needed if 1st dose given at age ≥15 mos.	4 wks[6]: if current age <12 mos 8 wks (as final dose)[6]: if current age ≥12 mos & 2nd dose given at age <15 mos No further doses needed if previous dose given at age ≥15 mos	8 wks (as final dose): this dose only necessary for children aged 12 mos–5 yrs who received 3 doses before age 12 mos	
PCV[7]	6 wks	4 wks: if 1st dose given at age <12 mos & 2nd dose given at age <24 mos 8 wks (as final dose): if 1st dose given at age ≥12 mos or current age 24–59 mos No further doses needed for healthy children if 1st dose given at age ≥24 mos	4 wks: if current age <12 mos 8 wks (as final dose): if current age ≥12 mos No further doses needed for healthy children if previous dose given at age ≥24 mos	8 wks (as final dose): this dose only necessary for children aged 12 mos–5 yrs who received 3 doses before age 12 mos	

Catch-Up Schedule for Children Aged 7–18 Years

Vaccine	Minimum interval between doses		
	Dose 1 to dose 2	Dose 2 to dose 3	Dose 3 to booster dose
Td[8]	4 wks	6 mos	6 mos[8]: if 1st dose given at age <12 mos & current age <11 yrs 5 yrs[8]: if 1st dose given at age ≥12 mos & 3rd dose given at age <7 yrs & current age ≥11 yrs 10 yrs[8]: if 3rd dose given at age ≥7 yrs
IPV[9]	4 wks	4 wks	IPV[2,9]
HepB	4 wks	8 wks (& 16 wks after 1st dose)	
MMR	4 wks[4]		
Varicella[10]	4 wks		

Note: A vaccine series does not require restarting, regardless of the time that has elapsed between doses.
[1] **Diphtheria and tetanus toxoids and acellular pertussis (DTaP) vaccine:** The 5th dose is not necessary if the 4th dose was given after the 4th birthday.
[2] **Inactivated poliovirus (IPV) vaccine:** For children who received an all-IPV or all-oral poliovirus (OPV) series, a 4th dose is not necessary if 3rd dose was given at age ≥4 yrs. If both OPV and IPV were given as part of a series, a total of doses should be given, regardless of the child's current age.
[3] **Hepatitis B (HepB) vaccine:** All children and adolescents who have not been immunized against hepatitis B should begin the HepB immunization series during any visit. Providers should make special efforts to immunize children who were born in, or whose parents were born in, areas of the world where hepatitis B virus infection is moderately or highly endemic.
[4] **Measles, mumps, and rubella (MMR) vaccine:** The 2nd dose of MMR is recommended routinely at age 4–6 yrs, but may be given earlier if desired.
[5] **Haemophilus influenzae type b (Hib) vaccine:** Vaccine is not generally recommended for children aged ≥5 years.
[6] **Hib vaccine:** If current age is <12 months and the first 2 doses were PRP-OMP [PedVaxHIB® or ComVax (Merck)®], the 3rd (and final) dose should be given at age 12–15 months and at least 8 weeks after the 2nd dose.
[7] **Pneumococcal conjugate (PCV) vaccine:** Vaccine is not generally recommended for children aged ≥5 years.
[8] **Tetanus and diphtheria toxoids (Td):** For children aged 7–10 years, the interval between the 3rd & booster dose is determined by the age when the 1st dose was given. For adolescents aged 11–18 years, the interval is determined by the age when the 3rd dose was administered.
[9] **IPV:** Vaccine is not generally recommended for persons aged ≥18 years.
[10] **Varicella vaccine:** Administer the 2-dose series to all susceptible adolescents aged ≥13 years.

Conjugate pneumococcal vaccine (PCV): For all infants <2 years old & high-risk children (e.g., HIV, asplenia, nephrotic syndrome, sickle cell anemia) between 2 and 5 years of age (Med Lett 42:25, 2000; PIDJ 19:181, 2000; PIDJ 19: 371ff, 2000). Also approved for prevention of otitis media (Med Lett 45:27, 2003) & for cochlear implant recipients (MMWR 52: 739, 2003). Use of vaccine associated with decline in invasive pneumococcal disease (NEJM 348:1737, 2003).

    Immunization schedule: (see Schedule, page 140)

Age at first dose (0.5 mL)	Total number of doses	Timing
Infants	4	2, 4, 6, and 12–15 months
7–11 months	3	2 doses at least 4 wks apart; 3rd dose after 1 year birthday, separated from 2nd dose by at least 2 months
12–23 months	2	2 doses at least 2 months apart
≥24 months	1*	

* For children ≥24 months old who are chronically ill or immunosuppressed, ICIP recommends 2 doses of PCV admin. 2 mos. apart, followed by 1 dose of a 23-valent pneumococcal vaccine 2 or 3 mos. after 2nd PCV dose (MMWR 50:10, 2001).

TABLE 20B: MENINGOCOCCAL VACCINE [MMWR 54(RR-7), 2005]

Population	Age Group (years)				
	<2	2–10	11–19	20–55	>55
General	None	None	Single dose MCV4	None	None
Increased risk groups: College freshmen (in dorms) Traveler's epidemic area Microbiologists/Military recruits	None	Single dose MPSV4	Single dose MCV4	Single dose MCV4	Single dose MCV4
Anatomic/functional asplenia*					
Terminal complement deficiency*					

MCV4 = Meningococcal protein conjugate vaccine (Menactra); **MPSV4** = Meningococcal polysaccharide vaccine (Menomune)
* Revaccinate every 3–5 years.   **NOTE:** 5 cases Guillain-Barré after MCV4; causal relationship unknown

TABLE 20C: ADULT IMMUNIZATION IN THE UNITED STATES (MMWR 53:Q1, 2004)
(Travelers: See Med Lett 38:17, 1996)

Recommended Adult Immunization Schedule—United States, 2004–2005

Vaccine	Age group (years)		
	19–49	50–64	≥65
Tetanus, diphtheria (Td)*	1 dose booster every 10 years[1]		
Influenza	1 dose annually[2]		1 dose annually
Pneumococcal (polysaccharide)	1 dose[3,4]		1 dose[3,4]
Hepatitis B*	3 doses (0, 1–2, 4–6 months)[5]		
Hepatitis A*	2 doses (0, 6–12 months)[6]		
Measles, mumps, rubella (MMR)*	1 or 2 doses[7]		
Varicella*	2 doses (0, 4–8 weeks)[8]		

☐ For all persons in this group   ▨ For persons at risk (i.e., with medical exposure/indications)   ▨▨ For persons lacking documentation of vaccination or evidence of disease

* Covered by the Vaccine Injury Compensation Program.

[1] **Tetanus and diphtheria (Td).** See Table 20D. Adults, including pregnant women with uncertain history of a complete primary vaccination series, should receive a primary series of Td. A primary series for adults is 3 doses: give the 1st 2 doses at least 4 weeks apart & the 3rd dose 6–12 months after the 2nd dose. Give 1 dose if the person received the primary series & if the last vaccination was received ≥10 years previously. The American College of Physicians Task Force on Adult Immunization supports a 2nd option for Td use in adults: a single Td booster at age 50 years for persons who have completed the full pediatric series, including the teenage/young adult booster.

[2] **Influenza vaccination.** Medical indications: chronic disorders of the cardiovascular or pulmonary systems, including asthma; chronic metabolic diseases, including diabetes mellitus, renal dysfunction, hemoglobinopathies, or immunosuppression (including immunosuppression caused by medications or by HIV; and pregnancy during the influenza season. Occupational indications: health-care workers & employees of long-term-care & assisted living facilities. Other indications: residents of nursing homes & other long-term-care facilities; persons likely to transmit influenza to persons at high risk (i.e., in-home caregivers to persons with medical conditions; household/close contacts & out-of-home caregivers of children aged 0–23 months, household members & caregivers of elderly persons & adults with high-risk conditions); & anyone who wishes to be vaccinated. For healthy persons aged 5–49 years without high-risk conditions who are not contacts of severely immunocompromised persons in special care units, either the inactivated vaccine or the intranasally administered influenza vaccine (FluMist®) may be given [see MMWR 53(RR-6), 2004].

[3] **Pneumococcal polysaccharide vaccination.** Medical indications: chronic lung disease (excluding asthma); cardiovascular diseases; diabetes mellitus; chronic liver diseases, including alcohol-induced liver disease; chronic renal failure or nephrotic syndrome; functional or anatomic asplenia; immunosuppression (e.g., congenital immunodeficiency, HIV infection, leukemia/lymphoma/multiple myeloma/Hodgkins disease, or organ or bone marrow transplantation); chemotherapy, long-term systemic corticosteroids; or cochlear implants. Geographic/other indications: Alaska Natives and certain American Indian populations. Other indications: residents of nursing homes & other long-term-care facilities (MMWR 52:739, 2003).

[4] **Revaccination with pneumococcal polysaccharide vaccine.** One-time revaccination after 5 years for persons with chronic renal failure or nephrotic syndrome; functional or anatomic asplenia (e.g., sickle cell disease or splenectomy); immunosuppressive conditions (e.g., congenital immunodeficiency, HIV infection, leukemia/lymphoma/multiple myeloma/Hodgkins disease, generalized malignancy, or organ or bone marrow transplantation); chemotherapy, or long-term systemic corticosteroids. For persons aged ≥65 years, one-time revaccination if they were vaccinated ≥5 years previously & were aged <65 years at the time of primary vaccination [see MMWR 46(RR-8), 1997].

[5] **Hepatitis B vaccination.** Medical indications: hemodialysis or patients who receive clotting factor concentrates. Occupational indications: health-care & public safety workers with exposure to blood, & students of medicine, dentistry, nursing, & other allied health professions. Behavioral indications: injection-drug users; persons with more than 1 sex partner during the previous 6 months; persons with a recent STD; all clients in STD clinics; & men who have sex with men. Other indications: household contacts & sex partners of persons with chronic HBV infection; clients & staff members of institutions for the developmentally disabled; inmates of correctional facilities; or travelers to countries with high prevalence of chronic HBV infection for (www.cdc.gov/travel/diseases/hbv.htm). **If no HBsAb response** (<10 million units per mL), try 0.25 mL of adult vaccine intradermal week 0, repeat 9n 2 wks, & measure HBsAb 2 wks later. If still no response, repeat intradermally.

[6] **Hepatitis A vaccination.** Medical indications: clotting factor disorders or chronic liver disease. Behavioral indications: men who have sex with men & users of illegal drugs. Occupational indications: persons working with hepatitis A virus (HAV)-infected primates. Other indications: persons traveling to or working in countries with high endemic HepA. If the combined HepA & HepB vaccine is used, administer 3 doses at 0, 1, & 6 months (www.cdc.gov/travel/diseases/hav.htm) [see MMWR 48(RR-12), 1999].

[7] **Measles, mumps, rubella (MMR) vaccination.** Measles component: adults born before 1957 are considered immune to measles. Adults born during or after 1957 should receive ≥1 dose of MMR unless they have a medical contraindication, documentation of ≥1 dose, or other acceptable evidence of immunity. A 2nd dose of MMR is recommended for adults who (1) were recently exposed to measles or in an outbreak setting, (2) were previously vaccinated

TABLE 20C (2)

with killed measles vaccine, (3) were vaccinated with an unknown vaccine during 1963-67, (4) are students in post-secondary educational institutions, (5) work in health-care facilities, or (6) plan to travel internationally. <u>Mumps component</u>: 1 dose of MMR vaccine should be adequate for protection. <u>Rubella component</u>: Give 1 dose of MMR vaccine to women whose rubella vaccination history is unreliable & counsel women to avoid becoming pregnant for 4 weeks after vaccination. For women of childbearing age, regardless of birth year, routinely determine rubella immunity & counsel women regarding congenital rubella syndrome. Do not vaccinate pregnant women or those planning to become pregnant during the next 4 weeks. For women who are pregnant & susceptible, vaccinate as early in the postpartum period as possible *[see MMWR 47(RR-8), 1998 & MMWR 50:1117, 2001].*

⁸ **Varicella vaccination.** Recommended for all persons lacking reliable clinical history of varicella infection or serologic evidence of varicella zoster virus (VZV) infection who might be at high risk for exposure or transmission. This includes health-care workers & family contacts of immunocompromised persons; persons who live or work in environments where transmission is likely (e.g., teachers of young children, child care employees, & residents & staff members in institutional settings); persons who live or work in environments where VZV transmission can occur (e.g., college students, inmates, & staff members of correctional institutions, & military personnel); adolescents aged 11-18 years & adults living in households with children; women who are not pregnant but who might become pregnant; & international travelers who are not immune to infection. **Note:** Approx. 95% of U.S.-born adults are immune to VZV. Do not vaccinate pregnant women or those planning to become pregnant during the next 4 weeks. For women who are pregnant & susceptible, vaccinate as early in the postpartum period as possible *[see MMWR 48(RR-6), 1999].*

> This schedule (above) indicates the recommended age groups for routine administration of currently licensed vaccines for persons aged ≥19 years. Licensed combination vaccines may be used whenever any components of the combination are indicated & when the vaccine's other components are not contraindicated. Providers should consult manufacturers' package inserts for detailed recommendations. Report all clinically significant postvaccination reactions to the Vaccine Adverse Event Reporting System (VAERS). Reporting forms & instructions on filing a VAERS report are available by telephone, 800-822-7967, or from www.vaers.org. Additional information about the vaccines listed above & contraindications for immunization is available at www.cdc.gov/nip or from the National Immunization Hotline, 800-232-2522 (English) or 800-232-0233 (Spanish). Approved by the ACIP, the ACOG, & the AAFP.

Recommended Immunizations for Adults with Medical Conditions & Other Indications—U.S., 2004-2005

Indication	Vaccine						
	Tetanus, diphtheria (Td)*,¹	Influenza²	Pneumococcal (polysaccharide)³,⁴	Hepatitis B*,⁵	Hepatitis A*,⁶	Measles, mumps, rubella (MMR)*,⁷	Varicella*,⁸
Pregnancy							
Diabetes, heart disease, chronic pulmonary disease, chronic liver disease (including chronic alcoholism)	A, B		B		I		
Congenital immunodeficiency, cochlear implants, leukemia, lymphoma, generalized malignancy, rx with alkylating agents, antimetabolites, CSF § leaks, radiation, or large amounts of corticosteroids			D				K
Renal failure/endstage renal disease & recipients of hemodialysis or clotting factor concentrates			D	H			
Asplenia including elective splenectomy & terminal complement-component deficiencies		C	D,E,F				
HIV infection			D,G			J	
Health-care workers							

▨ For all persons in this group   ▨ For persons at risk (i.e., with medical/exposure indications)   ▦ For persons lacking documentation of vaccination or evidence of disease   ▓ Contraindicated

¹ Covered by the Vaccine Injury Compensation Program
§ Cerebrospinal fluid

TABLE 20C (3)

Special Notes for Medical and Other Indications
A Although chronic liver disease & alcoholism are not indications for influenza vaccination, administer 1 dose annually if the patient is aged ≥50 years, has other indications for influenza vaccine, or requests vaccination.
B Asthma is an indication for influenza vaccination but not for pneumococcal vaccination.
C No data exist specifically on the risk for severe or complicated influenza infections among persons with asplenia. However, influenza is a risk factor for secondary bacterial infections that can cause severe disease among persons with asplenia.
D For persons aged <65 years, revaccinate once after ≥5 years have elapsed since initial vaccination.
E Administer meningococcal vaccine & consider Haemophilus influenzae type b vaccine (see Table 20B).
F For persons undergoing elective splenectomy, vaccinate ≥2 weeks before surgery.
G Vaccinate as soon after diagnosis as possible.
H For hemodialysis patients, use special formulation of vaccine (40 mcg per mL) or two 20 mcg per mL doses administered at one body site. Vaccinate early in the course of renal disease. Assess antibody titers to hepatitis B surface antigen (anti-HB) levels annually. Administer additional doses if anti-HB levels decline to <10 million units per mL.
I For all persons with chronic liver disease
J Withhold MMR or other measles-containing vaccines from HIV-infected persons with evidence of severe immunosuppression [see MMWR 47(RR-8:21), 1998 & MMWR 51(RR-2):22, 2002].
K Persons with impaired humoral immunity but intact cellular immunity may be vaccinated [see MMWR 48(RR-6), 1999].

Administration schedule for vaccines: Review package insert for specific product being administered

TABLE 20D/1: ANTI-TETANUS PROPHYLAXIS, WOUND CLASSIFICATION, IMMUNIZATION

WOUND CLASSIFICATION			IMMUNIZATION SCHEDULE				
Clinical Features	**Tetanus Prone**	**Non-Tetanus Prone**	**History of Tetanus Immunization**	**Dirty, Tetanus-Prone Wound**		**Clean, Non-Tetanus Prone Wound**	
				Td[1,2]	TIG	Td	TIG
Age of wound	> 6 hours	≤ 6 hours	Unknown or < 3 doses	Yes	Yes	Yes	No
Configuration	Stellate, avulsion	Linear					
Depth	> 1 cm	≤ 1 cm	3 or more doses	No[3]	No	No[4]	No
Mechanism of injury	Missile, crush, burn, frostbite	Sharp surface (glass, knife)					
Devitalized tissue	Present	Absent					
Contaminants (dirt, saliva, etc.)	Present	Absent					

[1] Td = Tetanus & diphtheria toxoids adsorbed (adult)
TIG = Tetanus immune globulin (human)
[2] Yes if wound >24 hours old.
For children <7 years, DPT (DT if pertussis vaccine contraindicated);
For persons ≥7 years, Td preferred to tetanus toxoid alone.
[3] Yes if >5 years since last booster
[4] Yes if >10 years since last booster

(From ACS Bull. 69:22,23, 1984, No. 10)

[From MMWR 39:37, 1990; MMWR 46(SS-2):15, 1997]

TABLE 20D/2: RABIES POST-EXPOSURE PROPHYLAXIS[1]. All wounds should be cleaned immediately and thoroughly with soap and water. This has been shown to protect 90% of experimental animals!
Post-Exposure Prophylaxis Guide, United States, 2000 (CID 30:4, 2000; NEJM 351:2626, 2004)

Animal Type	Evaluation and Disposition of Animal	Recommendations for Prophylaxis
Dogs, cats, ferrets	Healthy and available for 10-day observation	Don't start unless animal develops sx, then immediately begin HRIG + HDCV or RVA
	Rabid or suspected rabid	Immediate vaccination
	Unknown (escaped)	Consult public health officials
Skunks, raccoons, bats,* foxes, coyotes, most carnivores	Regard as rabid	Immediate vaccination
Livestock, rodents, rabbits; includes hares, squirrels, hamsters, guinea pigs, gerbils, chipmunks, rats, mice, woodchucks		Almost never require anti-rabies rx. Consult public health officials.

* Most recent cases of human rabies in U.S. due to contact (not bites) with silver-haired bats or rarely big brown bats (MMWR 46:770, 1997; AnIM 128:922, 1998). For more detail, see CID 30:4, 2000; JAVMA 219:1687, 2001; CID 37:96, 2003 (travel medicine advisory); Ln 363:959, 2004.

Post-Exposure Rabies Immunization Schedule
IF NOT PREVIOUSLY VACCINATED

Treatment	Regimen[2]
Local wound cleaning	All post-exposure treatment should begin with immediate, thorough cleaning of all wounds with soap and water.
Human rabies immune globulin (HRIG)	20 units per kg body weight given once on day 0. If anatomically feasible, the full dose should be infiltrated around the wound(s), the rest should be administered IM in the gluteal area. HRIG should **not** be administered in the **same syringe**, **or** into the **same anatomical site** as vaccine, or more than 7 days after the initiation of vaccine. Because HRIG may partially suppress active production of antibody, no more than the recommended dose should be given.[3]
Vaccine	Human diploid cell vaccine (HDCV), rabies vaccine adsorbed (RVA), or purified chick embryo cell vaccine (PCEC) 1.0 mL **IM** (**deltoid area[4]**), one each on days 0, 3, 7, 14, & 28.

TABLE 20D/2 (2)

IF PREVIOUSLY VACCINATED[5]

Treatment	Regimen[2]
Local wound cleaning	All post-exposure treatment should begin with immediate, thorough cleaning of all wounds with soap and water.
HRIG	HRIG should **not** be administered
Vaccine	HDCV, RVA or PCEC, 1.0 mL **IM** (**deltoid area**[4]), one each on days 0 and 3

CORRECT VACCINE ADMINISTRATION SITES

Age Group	Administration Site
Children and adults	**DELTOID**[4] only (**NEVER** in gluteus)
Infants and young children	Outer aspect of thigh (anterolateral thigh) may be used (**NEVER** in gluteus)

[1] From *MMWR 48:RR-1, 1999; CID 30:4, 2000;* B.T. Matyas, Mass. Dept. of Public Health
[2] These regimens are applicable for all age groups, including children.
[3] In most reported post-exposure treatment failures, only identified deficiency was failure to infiltrate wound(s) with HRIG (*CID 22:228, 1996*). However, several failures reported from SE Asia in patients in whom WHO protocol followed (*CID 28:143, 1999*).
[4] The **deltoid** area is the **only** acceptable site of vaccination for adults and older children. For infants and young children, the outer aspect of the thigh (anterolateral thigh) may be used. Vaccine should **NEVER** be administered in the gluteal area.
[5] Any person with a history of pre-exposure vaccination with HDCV, RVA, PCEC; prior post-exposure prophylaxis with HDCV, RVA, PCEC; or previous vaccination with any other type of rabies vaccine and a documented history of antibody response to the prior vaccination

TABLE 21: SELECTED DIRECTORY OF RESOURCES

ORGANIZATION	PHONE/FAX	WEBSITE(S)
ANTIPARASITIC DRUGS and PARASITOLOGY INFORMATION *(CID 37:694, 2003)*		
CDC	Weekdays: 404-639-3670	www.cdc.gov/ncidod/srp/drugs/drug-service.html
	Evenings, weekends, holidays:	404-639-2888
DPDx: Lab ID of parasites		www.dpd.cdc.gov/dpdx/default.htm
Gorgas Course Tropical Medicine		http://info.dom.uab.edu/gorgas
Panorama Compound. Pharm.	800-247-9767/818-787-7256	www.uniquerx.com
Parasites and Health		www.dpd.cdc.gov/dpdx/HTML/Para_Health.htm
BIOTERRORISM		
Centers for Disease Control & Prevention	770-488-7100	www.bt.cdc.gov
Infectious Diseases Society of America	703-299-0200/	www.idsociety.org
	703-299-0204	
Johns Hopkins Center Civilian Biodefense		www.jhsph.edu
Center for Biosecurity of the Univ. of Pittsburgh Med. Center		www.upmc-biosecurity.org
US Army Medical Research Institute of Inf. Dis.		www.usamriid.army.mil
HEPATITIS C *(CID 35:754, 2002)*		
CDC		www.cdc.gov/ncidod/diseases/hepatitis/C
Individual		http://hepatitis-central.com
Medscape		www.medscape.com
HIV		
General		
HIV InSite		http://hivinsite.ucsf.edu
Johns Hopkins AIDS Service		www.hopkins-aids.edu
Drug Interactions		
Johns Hopkins AIDS Service		www.hopkins-aids.edu
Liverpool HIV Pharm. Group		www.hiv-druginteractions.org
Other		http://AIDS.medscape.com
Prophylaxis/Treatment of Opportunistic Infections; HIV Treatment		www.aidsinfo.nih.gov
IMMUNIZATIONS *(CID 36:355, 2003)*		
CDC, Natl. Immunization Program	404-639-8200	www.cdc.gov/nip
FDA, Vaccine Adverse Events	800-822-7967	www.fda.gov/cber/vaers/vaers.htm
National Network Immunization Info.	877-341-6644/	www.immunizationinfo.org
	703-299-0204	
Influenza vaccine, CDC	404-639-8200	www.cdc.gov/nip/flu
Institute for Vaccine Safety		www.vaccinesafety.edu
OCCUPATIONAL EXPOSURE, BLOOD-BORNE PATHOGENS (HIV, HEPATITIS B & C)		
National Clinicians' Post-Exposure Hotline	888-448-4911	www.ucsf.edu/hivcntr
Q-T$_c$ INTERVAL PROLONGATION BY DRUGS		www.qtdrugs.org
SEXUALLY TRANSMITTED DISEASES		www.cdc.gov/std/treatment/TOC2002TG.htm
		Slides: http://www.phac-aspc.gc.ca/slm-maa/slides/index.html
TRAVELERS' INFO: Immunizations, Malaria Prophylaxis, More		
Amer. Soc. Trop. Med. & Hyg.		www.astmh.org
CDC, general	877-394-8747/888-232-3299	www.cdc.gov/travel/index.htm
CDC, Malaria:		www.cdc.gov/malaria
Prophylaxis	888-232-3228	www.cdc.gov/travel
Treatment	770-488-7788	www.who.int/health topics/malaria
MD Travel Health		www.mdtravelhealth.com
Pan American Health Organization		www.paho.org
World Health Organization (WHO)	(41-22)-791-2122/	www.who.int/home-page
	(00-41-22)-691-0746	
VACCINE AND IMMUNIZATION RESOURCES *(CID 36:355, 2003)*		
American Academy of Pediatrics		www.cispimmunize.org
CDC, National Immunization Program		www.cdc.gov/nip
National Network for Immunization Information		www.immunizationinfo.org

TABLE 22: ANTI-INFECTIVE DRUG-DRUG INTERACTIONS
Significance/Certainty: ± = theory/anecdotal; + = of probable importance; + + = of definite importance

ANTI-INFECTIVE AGENT (A)	OTHER DRUG (B)	EFFECT	SIGNIFICANCE/CERTAINTY
Amantadine (Symmetrel)	Alcohol	↑ CNS effects	+
	Anticholinergic and anti-Parkinson agents (ex. Artane, scopolamine)	↑ effect of B: dry mouth, ataxia, blurred vision, slurred speech, toxic psychosis	+
	Trimethoprim	↑ levels of A & B	+
	Digoxin	↑ levels of B	±
Aminoglycosides—parenteral (amikacin, gentamicin, kanamycin, netilmicin, sisomicin, streptomycin, tobramycin) NOTE: Capreomycin is an aminoglycoside, used as alternative drug to treat mycobacterial infections.	Amphotericin B	↑ nephrotoxicity	+ +
	Cis platinum (Platinol)	↑ nephro & ototoxicity	+
	Cyclosporine	↑ nephrotoxicity	+
	Neuromuscular blocking agents	↑ apnea or respiratory paralysis	+
	Loop diuretics (e.g., furosemide)	↑ ototoxicity	+ +
	NSAIDs	↑ nephrotoxicity	+
	Non-polarizing muscle relaxants	↑ apnea	+
	Radiographic contrast	↑ nephrotoxicity	+
	Vancomycin	↑ nephrotoxicity	+
Aminoglycosides—oral (kanamycin, neomycin)	Oral anticoagulants (dicumarol, phenindione, warfarin)	↑ prothrombin time	+
Amphotericin B and ampho B lipid formulations	Antineoplastic drugs	↑ nephrotoxicity risk	+
	Digitalis	↑ toxicity of B if K+ ↓	+
	Nephrotoxic drugs: aminoglycosides, cidofovir, cyclosporine, foscarnet, pentamidine	↑ nephrotoxicity of A	+ +
Ampicillin, amoxicillin	Allopurinol	↑ frequency of rash	+ +
Amprenavir and fosamprenavir	Antiretrovirals—see Table 22B & C		
	Contraceptives, oral	↓ levels of A; use other contraception	+ +
	Lovastatin/simvastatin	↓ levels of B—avoid	+ +
	Methadone	↓ levels of A & B	+ +
	Rifabutin	↑ levels of B (↓ dose by 50–75%)	+ +
	Rifampin	↓ levels of A—avoid	+ +
Atazanavir	See protease inhibitors and Table 22B & C		
Atovaquone	Rifampin (perhaps rifabutin)	↓ serum levels of A; ↑ levels of B	+
	Metoclopramide	↓ levels of A	+
	Tetracycline	↓ levels of A	+

Azole Antifungal Agents [**Flu** = fluconazole, **Itr** = itraconazole, **Ket** = ketoconazole, **Vor** = voriconazole, + = occurs, **blank space** = either studied & no interaction OR no data found (may be in pharm. co. databases)]

Flu	Itr	Ket	Vor		EFFECT	
+	+	+	+	Amitriptyline	↑ levels of B	+
+	+	+	+	Calcium channel blockers	↑ levels of B	+ +
			+	Carbamazepine (vori contraindicated)	↓ levels of A	+ +
+	+	+	+	Cyclosporine	↑ levels of B, ↑ risk of nephrotoxicity	+
	+	+		Didanosine	↓ absorption of A	+
	+	+	+	Efavirenz	↓ levels of A, ↑ levels of B	+ + (avoid)
+	+	+		H₂ blockers, antacids, sucralfate	↓ absorption of A	+
	+	+	+	Hydantoins (phenytoin, Dilantin)	↑ levels of B, ↓ levels of A	+ +
	+	+		Isoniazid	↓ levels of A	+
	+	+	+	Lovastatin/simvastatin	Rhabdomyolysis reported; ↑ levels of B	+ +
+	+	+	+	Midazolam/triazolam, po	↑ levels of B	+ +
+	+	+	+	Oral anticoagulants	↑ effect of B	+ +
+	+	+	+	Oral hypoglycemics	↑ levels of B	+ +
		+	+	Pimozide	↑ levels of B	+ +
	+	+	+	Protease inhibitors	↑ levels of B	+ +
	+	+	+	Proton pump inhibitors	↓ absorption of A, ↑ levels of B	+ +
+	+	+	+	Rifampin/rifabutin (vori contraindicated)	↓ levels of B, ↓ serum levels of A	+ +
			+	Sirolimus (vori contraindicated)	↑ levels of B	+ +
+	+	+	+	Tacrolimus	↑ levels of B with toxicity	+ +
+		+		Theophyllines	↑ levels of B	+
	+	+	+	Trazodone	↑ levels of B	+ +
		+	+	Zidovudine	↑ levels of B	+
Caspofungin				Cyclosporine	↑ levels of A	+ +
				Tacrolimus	↓ levels of A	+ +
				Carbamazepine, dexamethasone, efavirenz, nevirapine, phenytoin, rifampin	↓ levels of A; ↑ dose of caspofungin to 70 mg/d	+ +
Cephalosporins with methyltetrathiozole-thiol side-chain				Oral anticoagulants (dicumarol, warfarin), heparin, thrombolytic agents, platelet aggregation inhibitors	↑ effects of B, bleeding	+
Chloramphenicol				Hydantoins	↑ toxicity of B, nystagmus, ataxia	+ +
				Iron salts, Vitamin B12	↓ response to B	+ +
				Protease inhibitors—HIV	↑ levels of A & B	+ +

¹ Major interactions given; unusual or minor interactions manifest as toxicity of non-azole drug due to ↑ serum levels: Caffeine (Flu), digoxin (Itr), felodipine (Itr), fluoxetine (Itr), indinavir (Ket), lovastatin/simvastatin (Ket), quinidine (Ket), tricyclics (Flu), vincristine (Itr), and ↓ effectiveness of oral contraceptives.

TABLE 22 (2)

ANTI-INFECTIVE AGENT (A)	OTHER DRUG (B)	EFFECT	SIGNIFICANCE/CERTAINTY
Clindamycin (Cleocin)	Kaolin	↓ absorption of A	+
	Muscle relaxants, e.g., atracurium, baclofen, diazepam	↑ frequency/duration of respiratory paralysis	+
Cycloserine	Ethanol	↑ frequency of seizures	+
	INH, ethionamide	↑ frequency of drowsiness/dizziness	+
Dapsone	Didanosine	↓ absorption of A	+
	Oral contraceptives	↓ effectiveness of B	+
	Pyrimethamine	↑ in marrow toxicity	+
	Rifampin/Rifabutin	↓ serum levels of A	+
	Trimethoprim	↑ levels of A & B (methemoglobinemia)	+
	Zidovudine	May ↑ marrow toxicity	+
Daptomycin	HMG-CoA inhibitors (statins)	DC statin while on dapto	++
Delavirdine (Rescriptor)	*See non-nucleoside reverse transcriptase inhibitors (NNRTIs) and Table 22C*		
Didanosine (ddI) (Videx)	Cisplatin, dapsone, INH, metronidazole, nitrofurantoin, stavudine, vincristine, zalcitabine	↑ risk of peripheral neuropathy	+
	Ethanol, lamivudine, pentamidine	↑ risk of pancreatitis	+
	Fluoroquinolones	↓ absorption 2° to chelation	+
	Drugs that need low pH for absorption: dapsone, indinavir, itra/ketoconazole, pyrimethamine, rifampin, trimethoprim	↓ absorption	+
	Methadone	↓ levels of A	++
	Ribavirin	↑ levels ddI metabolite—**avoid**	++
	Tenofovir	↑ levels of A **(reduce dose of A)**	++
Doxycycline	Aluminum, bismuth, iron, Mg^{++}	↓ absorption of A	+
	Barbiturates, hydantoins	↓ serum t/2 of A	+
	Carbamazepine (Tegretol)	↓ serum t/2 of A	+
	Digoxin	↑ serum levels of B	+
	Warfarin	↑ activity of B	++
Efavirenz (Sustiva)	*See non-nucleoside reverse transcriptase inhibitors (NNRTIs) and Table 22C*		
Ertapenem (Invanz)	Probenecid	↑ levels of A	++
Ethambutol (Myambutol)	Aluminum salts (includes didanosine buffer)	↓ absorption of A & B	+

Fluoroquinolones (*Cipro* = ciprofloxacin; *Gati* = gatifloxacin; *Gemi* = gemifloxacin; *Levo* = levofloxacin; *Lome* = lomefloxacin; *Moxi* = moxifloxacin; *Oflox* = ofloxacin)
NOTE: Blank space = either studied and no interaction OR no data found (pharm. co. may have data)

Cipro	Gati	Gemi	Levo	Lome	Moxi	Oflox	OTHER DRUG (B)	EFFECT	SIG.
	+	+	+	+	+	+	Antiarrhythmics (procainamide, amiodarone)	↑ Q-T interval (torsade)	++
+	+	+	+	+	+	+	Insulin, oral hypoglycemics	↑ & ↓ blood sugar	++
+							Caffeine	↑ levels of B	+
+		+			+		Cimetidine	↑ levels of A	+
+						+	Cyclosporine	↑ levels of B	±
+	+	+	+	+	+	+	Didanosine	↓ absorption of A	++
+	+	+	+	+	+	+	Cations: Al^{+++}, Ca^{++}, Fe^{++}, Mg^{++}, Zn^{++} (antacids, vitamins, dairy products), citrate/citric acid	↓ absorption of A (some variability between drugs)	++
+							Foscarnet	↑ risk of seizures	+
						+	Methadone	↑ levels of B	++
+							NSAIDs	↑ risk CNS stimulation/seizures	++
+							Phenytoin	↑ or ↓ levels of B	+
+	+	+	+		+	+	Probenecid	↓ renal clearance of A	+
+						+	Sucralfate	↓ absorption of A	++
+							Theophylline	↑ levels of B	++
+							Tizanidine	↑ levels of B	++
+		+			+	+	Warfarin	↑ prothrombin time	+

ANTI-INFECTIVE AGENT (A)	OTHER DRUG (B)	EFFECT	SIGNIFICANCE/CERTAINTY
Foscarnet (Foscavir)	Ciprofloxacin	↑ risk of seizures	+
	Nephrotoxic drugs: aminoglycosides, ampho B, cis-platinum, cyclosporine	↑ risk of nephrotoxicity	+
	Pentamidine IV	↑ risk of severe hypocalcemia	++
Ganciclovir (Cytovene)	Imipenem	↑ risk of seizures reported	+
	Probenecid	↑ levels of A	+
	Zidovudine	↓ levels of A, ↑ levels of B	+
Gentamicin	*See Aminoglycosides—parenteral*		
Indinavir	*See protease inhibitors and Table 22B & C*		
Isoniazid	Alcohol, rifampin	↑ risk of hepatic injury	++
	Aluminum salts	↓ absorption (take fasting)	++
	Carbamazepine, phenytoin	↑ levels of B with nausea, vomiting, nystagmus, ataxia	++
	Itraconazole, ketoconazole	↓ levels of B	+
	Oral hypoglycemics	↓ effects of B	+
Lamivudine	Zalcitabine	**Mutual interference—do not combine**	++

TABLE 22 (3)

ANTI-INFECTIVE AGENT (A)	OTHER DRUG (B)	EFFECT	SIGNIFICANCE/ CERTAINTY
Linezolid (Zyvox)	Adrenergic agents	Risk of hypertension	++
	Aged, fermented, pickled or smoked foods — ↑ tyramine	Risk of hypertension	+
	Serotonergic drugs (SSRIs)	Risk of serotonin syndrome	+
Lopinavir	*See protease inhibitors*		

Macrolides *[Ery = erythromycin, Azi = azithromycin, Clr = clarithromycin; Dir = dirithromycin, + = occurs, blank space = either studied and no interaction OR no data (pharm. co. may have data)]*

Ery	Dir	Azi	Clr			
+	+		+	Carbamazepine	↑ serum levels of B, nystagmus, nausea, vomiting, ataxia	++ (avoid with erythro)
+			+	Cimetidine, **ritonavir**	↑ levels of B	+
+			+	Clozapine	↑ serum levels of B, CNS toxicity	+
			+	**Colchicine**	↑ **levels of B (potent, fatal)**	++ (avoid)
+			+	Corticosteroids	↑ effects of B	+
+	+	+	+	Cyclosporine	↑ serum levels of B with toxicity	+
+	+	+	+	Digoxin, digitoxin	↑ serum levels of B (10% of cases)	+
			+	Efavirenz	↓ levels of A	++
+	+		+	Ergot alkaloids	↑ levels of B	++
+			+	Lovastatin/simvastatin	↑ levels of B; rhabdomyolysis	++
+			+	Midazolam, triazolam	↑ levels of B, ↑ sedative effects	+
+			+	Phenytoin	↑ levels of B	+
+	+	+	+	Pimozide	**Q-T interval**	++
+			+	Rifampin, rifabutin	↓ levels of A	+
+			+	Tacrolimus	↑ levels of B	++
+			+	Theophyllines	↑ serum levels of B with nausea, vomiting, seizures, apnea	++
+			+	Valproic acid	↑ levels of B	+
+	+		+	Warfarin	May ↑ prothrombin time	+
			+	Zidovudine	↓ levels of B	+

ANTI-INFECTIVE AGENT (A)	OTHER DRUG (B)	EFFECT	SIGNIFICANCE/ CERTAINTY
Mefloquine	ß-adrenergic blockers, calcium channel blockers, quinidine, quinine	↑ arrhythmias	+
	Divalproex, valproic acid	↓ level of B with seizures	+
	Halofantrine	Q-T prolongation	++ (avoid)
Methenamine mandelate or hippurate	Acetazolamide, sodium bicarbonate, thiazide diuretics	↓ antibacterial effect 2° to ↑ urine pH	++
Metronidazole	Alcohol	Disulfiram-like reaction	+
	Cyclosporin	↑ levels of B	++
	Disulfiram (Antabuse)	Acute toxic psychosis	+
	Lithium	↑ levels of B	++
	Oral anticoagulants	↑ anticoagulant effect	++
	Phenobarbital, hydantoins	↑ levels of B	++
Nelfinavir	*See protease inhibitors and Table 22B & C*		
Nevirapine (Viramune)	*See non-nucleoside reverse transcriptase inhibitors (NNRTIs) and Table 22C*		
Nitrofurantoin	Antacids	↓ absorption of A	+

Non-nucleoside reverse transcriptase inhibitors (NNRTIs): For interactions with protease inhibitors, *see Table 22C.* **Del** = delavirdine, **Efa** = efavirenz, **Nev** = nevirapine

Del	Efa	Nev			
			Co-administration contraindicated:		
+			Anticonvulsants: carbamazepine, phenobarbital, phenytoin		++
+			Antimycobacterials: rifabutin, rifampin		++
+			Antipsychotics: pimozide		++
+	+		Benzodiazepines: alprazolam, midazolam, triazolam		++
+	+		Ergotamine		++
+			HMG-CoA inhibitors (statins): lovastatin, simvastatin, atorvastatin, pravastatin		++
+			St. John's wort		++
			Dose change needed:		
+			Amphetamines	↑ levels of B—**caution**	++
+		+	Antiarrhythmics: amiodarone, lidocaine, others	↓ or ↑ levels of B—**caution**	++
+	+	+	Anticonvulsants: carbamazepine, phenobarbital, phenytoin	↓ levels of A and/or B	++
+	+	+	Antifungals: itraconazole, ketoconazole, voriconazole	Potential ↓ levels of B, ↑ levels of A	++ (avoid)
+			Antipsychotics: pimozide		++
+	+	+	Antirejection drugs: cyclosporine, rapamycin, sirolimus, tacrolimus	↑ levels of B	++
		+	Benzodiazepines: *as above*	↑ levels of B	++
+		+	Calcium channel blockers	↑ levels of B	++
+		+	Clarithromycin	↑ levels of B metabolite	++
+		+	Cyclosporine	↑ levels of B	++
+			Dexamethasone	↓ levels of A	++
+	+	+	Sildenafil, vardenafil, tadalafil	↑ levels of B	++
+		+	Fentanyl, methadone	↑ levels of B	++

TABLE 22 (4)

ANTI-INFECTIVE AGENT (A)	OTHER DRUG (B)	EFFECT	SIGNIFICANCE/ CERTAINTY

Non-nucleoside reverse transcriptase inhibitors (NNRTIs) *(continued)*: For interactions with protease inhibitors, see Table 22B. **Del** = delavirdine, **Efa** = efavirenz, **Nev** = nevirapine

Del	Efa	Nev	Co-administration contraindicated:		
+			Gastric acid suppression: antacids, H-2 blockers, proton pump inhibitors	↓ levels of A	+ +
+			HMG-CoA inhibitors (statins)		
	+	+	Methadone	↓ levels of B	+ +
	+	+	Oral contraceptives	↑ or ↓ levels of B	+ +
+	+	+	Protease inhibitors—see Table 22C		
+	+	+	Rifabutin, rifampin	↑ or ↓ levels of rifabutin; ↓ levels of A—**caution**	+ +
+	+	+	St. John's wort	↓ levels of B	
+			Warfarin	↑ levels of B	+ +
Pentamidine, IV			Amphotericin B	↑ risk of nephrotoxicity	+
			Foscarnet	↑ risk of hypocalcemia	+
			Pancreatitis-associated drugs, e.g., alcohol, valproic acid	↑ risk of pancreatitis	+
Piperacillin			Cefoxitin	Antagonism vs pseudomonas	+ +
Primaquine			Chloroquine, dapsone, INH, probenecid, quinine, sulfon-amides, TMP/SMX, others	↑ risk of hemolysis in G6PD-deficient patients	+ +

Protease Inhibitors—Anti-HIV Drugs. (**Atazan** = atazanavir; **Fosampren** = fosamprenavir; **Indin** = indinavir; **Lopin** = lopinavir; **Nelfin** = nelfinavir; **Riton** = ritonavir; **Saquin** = saquinavir; **Tipran** = tipranavir). For interactions with antiretrovirals, see Table 22B & C

Only a partial list—check package insert

Also see http://aidsinfo.nih.gov

Atazan	Fosampren	Indin	Lopin	Nelfin	Riton	Saquin	Tipran	Analgesics:		
					+		+	1. Alfentanil, fentanyl, hydrocodone, tramadol	↑ levels of B	+
		+		+	+			2. Codeine, hydromorphone, morphine, methadone	↓ levels of B	+
+	+	+	+	+	+	+	+	**Anti-arrhythmics: amiodarone, lidocaine, mexiletine, flecainide**	↑ levels of B; **do not co-administer**	+ +
		+	+	+	+	+		**Anticonvulsants: carbamazepine, clonazepam, phenytoin, phenobarbital**	↓ levels of A, ↑ levels of B	+ +
+	+	+			+		+	Antidepressants, all tricyclic	↑ levels of B	+ +
+							+	Antidepressants, all other	↑ levels of B; do not use pimozide	+ +
					+			**Antihistamine:** Loratadine	↑ levels of B	+ +
	+							Atovaquone	↓ levels of B	+
+	+	+	+	+	+		+	**Benzodiazepines, e.g., diazepam, midazolam, triazolam**	↑ levels of B—do not use	+ +
					+			Beta blockers: Metoprolol, pindolol, propranolol, timolol	↑ levels of B	+
+	+	+	+	+	+	+	+	Calcium channel blockers (all)	↑ levels of B	+ +
+		+	+	+	+			Clarithro, erythro	↑ levels of B if renal impairment	+
+	+		+	+	+	+		Contraceptives, oral	↓ or ↑ levels of B	+ +
		+	+	+	+			Corticosteroids: prednisone, dexamethasone	↓ levels of A, ↑ levels of B	+
+	+	+	+	+	+	+	+	Cyclosporine	↑ levels of B, monitor levels	+
+	+	+	+	+	+	+	+	Ergot derivatives	↑ **levels of B**—do not use	+ +
	+		+	+	+			Erythromycin, clarithromycin	↑ levels of A & B	+
		+			+	+		Grapefruit juice (>200 ml/day)	↑ indinavir & ↑ saquinavir levels	+ +
+	+	+	+	+	+	+	+	H2 receptor antagonists	↓ levels of A	+ +
+	+	+	+	+	+	+	+	**HMG-CoA reductase inhibitors (statins): lovastatin, simvastatin**	↑ **levels of B**—do not use	+ +
+								Irinotecan	↑ **levels of B**—do not use	+ +
	+	+	+	+	+		+	Ketoconazole, itraconazole, ? vori	↓ levels of A, ↑ levels of B	+
+		+			+			Metronidazole	Poss. disulfiram reaction, alcohol	+
+		+		+			+	**Pimozide**	↑ **levels of B**—do not use	+ +
+	+	+	+	+	+	+	+	Proton pump inhibitors	↓ levels of B	+
+	+	+	+	+	+	+	+	Rifampin, rifabutin	↓ levels of A, ↑ levels of B **(avoid)**	+ + **(avoid)**
+	+	+	+	+	+	+	+	Sildenafil (Viagra), tadalafil, vardenafil	Varies, some ↑ & some ↓ levels of B	+ +
+	+	+	+	+	+	+	+	**St. John's wort**	↓ **levels of A**—do not use	+ +
+								Tenofovir	↓ levels of B—add ritonavir	+ +
		+	+	+				Theophylline	↓ levels of B	+
+	+		+		+			Warfarin	↑ levels of B	+

TABLE 22 (5)

ANTI-INFECTIVE AGENT (A)	OTHER DRUG (B)	EFFECT	SIGNIFICANCE/ CERTAINTY
Pyrazinamide	INH, rifampin	May ↑ risk of hepatotoxicity	±
Pyrimethamine	Lorazepam	↑ risk of hepatotoxicity	+
	Sulfonamides, TMP/SMX	↑ risk of marrow suppression	+
	Zidovudine	↑ risk of marrow suppression	+
Quinine	Digoxin	↑ digoxin levels; ↑ toxicity	+ +
	Mefloquine	↑ arrhythmias	+
	Oral anticoagulants	↑ prothrombin time	+ +
Quinupristin-dalfopristin (Synercid)	Anti-HIV drugs: NNRTIs & PIs	↑ levels of B	+ +
	Antineoplastic: vincristine, docetaxel, paclitaxel	↑ levels of B	+ +
	Calcium channel blockers	↑ levels of B	+ +
	Carbamazepine	↑ levels of B	+ +
	Cyclosporine, tacrolimus	↑ levels of B	+ +
	Lidocaine	↑ levels of B	+ +
	Methylprednisolone	↑ levels of B	+ +
	Midazolam, diazepam	↑ levels of B	+ +
	Statins	↑ levels of B	+ +
Ribavirin	Didanosine	↑ levels of B → toxicity—avoid	+ +
	Stavudine	↓ levels of B	+ +
	Zidovudine	↓ levels of B	+ +
Rifamycins (rifampin, rifabutin) See footnote for less severe or less common interactions[1] Ref.: ArIM 162:985, 2002	Al OH, ketoconazole, PZA	↓ levels of A	+
	Atovaquone	↑ levels of A, ↓ levels of B	+
	Beta adrenergic blockers (metoprolol, propranolol)	↓ effect of B	+
	Clarithromycin	↑ levels of A, ↓ levels of B	+ +
	Corticosteroids	↑ replacement requirement of B	+ +
	Cyclosporine	↓ effect of B	+ +
	Delavirdine	↑ levels of A, ↓ levels of B—avoid	+ +
	Digoxin	↓ levels of B	+ +
	Disopyramide	↓ levels of B	+ +
	Fluconazole	↑ levels of A[1]	+
	Amprenavir, indinavir, nelfinavir, ritonavir	↑ levels of A (↓ dose of A), ↓ levels of B	+ +
	INH	Converts INH to toxic hydrazine	+ +
	Itraconazole[e], ketoconazole	↓ levels of B, ↑ levels of A[2]	+ +
	Methadone	↓ serum levels (withdrawal)	+
	Nevirapine	↓ levels of B—avoid	+ +
	Oral anticoagulants	Suboptimal anticoagulation	+ +
	Oral contraceptives	↓ effectiveness; spotting, pregnancy	+
	Phenytoin	↓ levels of B	+
	Protease inhibitors	↑ levels of A, ↓ levels of B—CAUTION	+ +
	Quinidine	↓ effect of B	+
	Sulfonylureas	↓ hypoglycemic effect	+
	Tacrolimus	↓ levels of B	+ +
	Theophylline	↓ levels of B	+
	TMP/SMX	↑ levels of A	+
	Tocainide	↓ effect of B	+
Rimantadine	See Amantadine		
Ritonavir	See protease inhibitors and Table 22B & C		
Saquinavir	See protease inhibitors and Table 22B & C		
Stavudine	Dapsone, INH	May ↑ risk of peripheral neuropathy	±
	Ribavirin	↓ levels of A—avoid	+ +
	Zidovudine	Mutual interference—do not combine	+ +
Sulfonamides	Cyclosporine	↓ cyclosporine levels	+
	Methotrexate	↑ antifolate activity	+
	Oral anticoagulants	↑ prothrombin time; bleeding	+
	Phenobarbital, rifampin	↓ levels of A	+
	Phenytoin	↑ levels of B; nystagmus, ataxia	+
	Sulfonylureas	↑ hypoglycemic effect	+
Telithromycin (Ketek)	Carbamazine	↓ levels of A	+ +
	Digoxin	↑ levels of B—do digoxin levels	+ +
	Ergot alkaloids	↑ levels of B—avoid	+ +
	Itraconazole; ketoconazole	↑ levels of A; no dose change	+
	Metoprolol	↑ levels of B	+ +
	Midazolam	↑ levels of B	+ +
	Oral anticoagulants	↑ prothrombin time	+
	Phenobarb, phenytoin	↓ levels of A	+ +
	Pimozide	↑ levels of B; QT prolongation—AVOID	+ +

[1] The following is a partial list of drugs with rifampin-induced ↑ metabolism and hence lower than anticipated serum levels: ACE inhibitors, dapsone, diazepam, digoxin, diltiazem, doxycycline, fluconazole, fluvastatin, haloperidol, nifedipine, progestins, triazolam, tricyclics, voriconazole, zidovudine
[2] Up to 4 weeks may be required after RIF discontinued to achieve detectable serum itra levels; ↑ levels associated with uveitis or polymyolysis

TABLE 22 (6)

ANTI-INFECTIVE AGENT (A)	OTHER DRUG (B)	EFFECT	SIGNIFICANCE/ CERTAINTY
Telithromycin *(continued)*	Rifampin	↓ **levels of A—avoid**	+ +
	Simvastatin	↑ levels of B (↑ risk of myopathy)	+ +
	Sotalol	↓ levels of B	+ +
	Theophylline	↑ levels of B	+ +
Tenofovir	Atazanavir	↓ levels of B—add ritonavir	+ +
	Didanosine (ddI)	↑ **levels of B (reduce dose)**	+ +
Terbinafine	Cimetidine	↑ levels of A	+
	Phenobarbital, rifampin	↓ levels of A	+
Tetracyclines	*See Doxycycline, plus:*		
	Atovaquone	↓ levels of B	+
	Digoxin	↑ toxicity of B (may persist several months—up to 10% pts)	+ +
	Methoxyflurane	↑ toxicity; polyuria, renal failure	+
	Sucralfate	↓ absorption of A (separate by ≥2 hrs)	+
Thiabendazole	Theophyllines	↑ serum theophylline, nausea	+
Tigecycline	Oral contraceptives	↓ levels of B	+ +
Tinidazole (Tindamax)	*See Metronidazole—similar entity, expect similar interactions*		
Tobramycin	*See Aminoglycosides*		
Trimethoprim	Amantadine, dapsone, digoxin, methotrexate, procainamide, zidovudine	↑ serum levels of B	+ +
	Potassium-sparing diuretics	↑ serum K⁺	+ +
	Thiazide diuretics	↓ serum Na⁺	+
Trimethoprim-Sulfa-methoxazole	Azathioprine	Reports of leukopenia	+
	Cyclosporine	↓ levels of B, ↑ serum creatinine	+
	Loperamide	↑ levels of B	+
	Methotrexate	Enhanced marrow suppression	+ +
	Oral contraceptives, pimozide, and 6-mercaptopurine	↓ effect of B	+
	Phenytoin	↑ levels of B	+
	Rifampin	↑ levels of B	+
	Warfarin	↑ activity of B	+
Vancomycin	Aminoglycosides	↑ frequency of nephrotoxicity	+ +
Zalcitabine (ddC) (HIVID)	Valproic acid, pentamidine (IV), alcohol, lamivudine	↑ pancreatitis risk	+
	Cisplatin, INH, metronidazole, vincristine, nitrofurantoin, d4T, dapsone	↑ risk of peripheral neuropathy	+
Zidovudine (ZDV) (Retrovir)	Atovaquone, fluconazole, metha-done	↑ levels of A	+
	Clarithromycin	↓ levels of A	±
	Indomethacin	↑ levels of ZDV toxic metabolite	+
	Nelfinavir	↓ levels of A	+ +
	Probenecid, TMP/SMX	↑ levels of A	+
	Ribavirin	↓ **levels of A—avoid**	+ +
	Rifampin/rifabutin	↓ levels of A	+ +
	Stavudine	**Interference—DO NOT COMBINE!**	+ +

TABLE 22B: DRUG-DRUG INTERACTIONS BETWEEN PROTEASE INHIBITORS
(Adapted from Guidelines for the Use of Antiretroviral Agents in HIV-Infected Adults & Adolescents; see www.aidsinfo.nih.gov)

NAME (Abbreviation, Trade Name)	Atazanavir (ATV, Reyataz)	Fosamprenavir (FOS-APV, Lexiva)	Indinavir (IDV, Crixivan)	Lopinavir/Ritonavir (LP/R, Kaletra)	Nelfinavir (NFV, Viracept)	Ritonavir (RTV, Norvir)	Saquinavir (SQV, Invirase)	Tipranavir (TPV, Aptivus)
Atazanavir (ATV, Reyataz)		Do not co-administer; risk of additive ↑ in indirect bilirubin	Do not co-administer; risk of additive ↑ in bilirubin	RTV 100 mg ↑ ATV AUC 238%		ATV/RTV 300/100 mg q24h	Combination not recommended	No data
Fosamprenavir (FOS-APV, Lexiva)	Do not co-administer; risk of additive ↑ in indirect bilirubin			Rx-naive: LP/R no dose change. Rx-experienced: LP/R 600/150 mg bid		200 mg RTV q24h + FOS-APV 1400 mg q24h	Insufficient data	Do not combine
Indinavir (IDV, Crixivan)	Do not co-administer; risk of additive ↑ in bilirubin			IDV AUC ↑ IDV 600 mg bid	↑ IDV & NFV levels. Dose: IDV 1200 mg bid, NFV 1250 mg bid	Dose: IDV/RTV ↑ IDV 800/100 mg or 800/200 mg	SQV levels ↑ 4-7 fold. Dose: Insufficient data	Do not combine
Lopinavir/Ritonavir (LP/R, Kaletra)	RTV 100 mg ↑ ATV AUC 238%	Rx-naive: LP/R no dose change. Rx-experienced: LP/R 600/150 mg bid	IDV AUC ↑ IDV 600 mg bid		Rx-naive: LP/R no dose change. Rx-experienced: LP/R 600/150 mg bid	LP is co-formulated with RTV	SQV levels ↑. Dose: SQV 1000 mg bid; LP/R standard	Do not combine
Nelfinavir (NFV, Viracept)			↑ IDV & NFV levels. Dose: IDV 1200 mg bid, NFV 1250 mg bid	Rx-naive: LP/R no dose change. Rx-experienced: LP/R 600/150 mg bid		Dose: RTV 400 mg bid + NFV 500-750 mg bid	Dose: NFV standard; SQV 800 mg tid or 1200 mg bid	Do not combine
Ritonavir (RTV, Norvir)	ATV/RTV 300/100 mg q24h	200 mg RTV q24h + FOS-APV 1400 mg q24h	Dose: IDV/RTV ↑ IDV 800/100 mg or 800/200 mg	LP is co-formulated with RTV	Dose: RTV 400 mg bid + NFV 500-750 mg bid		Dose: 1000 mg, SQV/100 mg RTV bid or 400/400 mg bid	TPV 500 mg bid + RTV 200 mg bid
Saquinavir (SQV, Invirase)	Combination not recommended	Insufficient data	SQV levels ↑ 4-7 fold. Dose: Insufficient data	SQV levels ↑. Dose: SQV 1000 mg bid; LP/R standard	Dose: NFV standard; SQV 800 mg tid or 1200 mg bid	Dose: 1000 mg, SQV/100 mg RTV bid or 400/400 mg bid		Do not combine
Tipranavir (TPV, Aptivus)	No data	Do not combine	Do not combine	Do not combine	Do not combine	TPV 500 mg bid + RTV 200 mg bid	Do not combine	

TABLE 22C: DRUG-DRUG INTERACTIONS BETWEEN NON-NUCLEOSIDE REVERSE TRANSCRIPTASE INHIBITORS (NNRTIs) AND PROTEASE INHIBITORS.
(Adapted from Guidelines for the Use of Antiretroviral Agents in HIV-Infected Adults & Adolescents; see www.aidsinfo.nih.gov)

NAME (Abbreviation, Trade Name)	Atazanavir (ATV, Reyataz)	Fosamprenavir (FOS-APV, Lexiva)	Indinavir (IDV, Crixivan)	Lopinavir/Ritonavir (LP/R, Kaletra)	Nelfinavir (NFV, Viracept)	Ritonavir (RTV, Norvir)	Saquinavir (SQV, Invirase)	Tipranavir (TPV, Aptivus)
Delavirdine (DLV, Rescriptor)	No data	Co-administration not recommended	IDV levels ↑ 40%. Dose: IDV 600 mg bid. DLV standard	Expect LP levels to ↑. No dose data	NFV levels ↑ 2X; DLV levels ↓ 50%. Dose: No data	Levels of RTV ↑ 70%. Dose: DLV standard, RTV no data	SQV levels ↑ 5X. Dose: SQV 800 mg tid. DLV standard	No data
Efavirenz (EFZ, Sustiva)	ATV AUC ↓ 74%. Dose: EFZ standard; ATA/RTV 300/100 mg q24h with food	FOS-APV levels ↓. Dose: EFZ standard; FOS-APV 1400 mg + RTV 300 mg q24h or 700 mg FOS-APV + RTV 100 mg bid	Levels: IDV ↓ 31%. Dose: IDV 1000 mg q8h; EFV standard	Rx-naive: LP/R no dose change. Rx-experienced: LP/R 600/150 mg bid	NFV levels ↑ 20%. Dose: Standard doses	Levels of RTV ↑ 18%. Dose: Standard doses	Level ↓ 62%. Dose: SQV softgel 400 mg + RTV 400 mg bid	No data
Nevirapine (NVP, Viramune)	No data	No data	IDV levels ↓ 28%. Dose: IDV 1000 mg q8h or combine with RTV. NVP standard	Rx-naive: LP/R no dose change. Rx-experienced: LP/R 600/150 mg bid	Standard doses	Standard doses	Dose: SQV softgel + RTV 400/400 mg both bid	No data

TABLE 23: LIST OF GENERIC AND COMMON TRADE NAMES

GENERIC NAME: TRADE NAMES	GENERIC NAME: TRADE NAMES	GENERIC NAME: TRADE NAMES
Abacavir: Ziagen	Drotrecogin alfa: Xigris	Nitroxanide: Alinia
Acyclovir: Zovirax	Efavirenz: Sustiva	Nystatin: Mycostatin, Macrobid, Macrodantin
Adefovir: Hepsera	Emtricitabine: Emtriva	Ofloxacin: Floxin
Albendazole: Albenza	Emtricitabine + tenofovir: Truvada	Oseltamivir: Tamiflu
Amantadine: Symmetrel	Enfuvirtide (T-20): Fuzeon	Oxacillin: Prostaphlin
Amikacin: Amikin	Entecavir: Baraclude	Palivizumab: Synagis
Amoxicillin: Amoxil, Polymox	Ertapenem: Invanz	Paromomycin: Humatin
Amox./clav.: Augmentin, Augmentin ES-600; Augmentin XR	Erythromycin(s): Ilotycin	Pentamidine: NebuPent, Pentam 300
	Ethyl succinate: Pediamycin	Piperacillin: Pipracil
Amphotericin B: Fungizone	*Glucoheptonate:* Erythrocin	Piperacillin/tazobactam: Zosyn
Ampho B-liposomal: AmBisome	*Estolate:* Ilosone	Piperazine: Antepar
Ampho B-cholesteryl complex: Amphotec	Erythro/sulfisoxazole: Pediazole	Podophyllotoxin: Condylox
Ampho B-lipid complex: Abelcet	Ethambutol: Myambutol	Posaconazole: Noxafil
Ampicillin: Omnipen, Polycillin	Ethionamide: Trecator	Praziquantel: Biltricide
Ampicillin/sulbactam: Unasyn	Famciclovir: Famvir	Primaquine: Primachine
Atazanavir: Reyataz	Fluconazole: Diflucan	Proguanil: Paludrine
Atovaquone: Mepron	Flucytosine: Ancobon	Pyrantel pamoate: Antiminth
Atovaquone + proguanil: Malarone	Fosamprenavir: Lexiva	Pyrimethamine: Daraprim
Azithromycin: Zithromax	Foscarnet: Foscavir	Pyrimethamine/sulfadoxine: Fansidar
Azithromycin ER: Zmax	Fosfomycin: Monurol	Quinupristin/dalfopristin: Synercid
Aztreonam: Azactam	Ganciclovir: Cytovene	Ribavirin: Virazole, Rebetol
Caspofungin: Cancidas	Gatifloxacin: Tequin	Rifabutin: Mycobutin
Cefaclor: Ceclor, Ceclor CD	Gemifloxacin: Factive	Rifampin: Rifadin, Rimactane
Cefadroxil: Duricef	Gentamicin: Garamycin	Rifapentine: Priftin
Cefazolin: Ancef, Kefzol	Griseofulvin: Fulvicin	Rifaximin: Xifaxan
Cefdinir: Omnicef	Halofantrine: Halfan	Rimantadine: Flumadine
Cefditoren pivoxil: Spectracef	Idoxuridine: Dendrid, Stoxil	Ritonavir: Norvir
Cefepime: Maxipime	INH + RIF: Rifamate	Saquinavir: Invirase, Fortovase
Cefixime[NUS]: Suprax	INH + RIF + PZA: Rifater	Spectinomycin: Trobicin
Cefoperazone-sulbactam: Sulperazon[NUS]	Interferon alfa: Roferon-A, Intron A	Stavudine: Zerit
	Interferon, pegylated: PEG-Intron, Pegasys	Stibogluconate: Pentostam
Cefotaxime: Claforan	Interferon + ribavirin: Rebetron	Silver sulfadiazine: Silvadene
Cefotetan: Cefotan	Imipenem + cilastatin: Primaxin	Sulfamethoxazole: Gantanol
Cefoxitin: Mefoxin	Imiquimod: Aldara	Sulfasalazine: Azulfidine
Cefpodoxime proxetil: Vantin	Indinavir: Crixivan	Sulfisoxazole: Gantrisin
Cefprozil: Cefzil	Itraconazole: Sporanox	Telithromycin: Ketek
Ceftazidime: Fortaz, Tazicef, Tazidime	Iodoquinol: Yodoxin	Tenofovir: Viread
Ceftibuten: Cedax	Ivermectin: Stromectol	Terbinafine: Lamisil
Ceftizoxime: Cefizox	Kanamycin: Kantrex	Thalidomide: Thalomid
Ceftriaxone: Rocephin	Ketoconazole: Nizoral	Thiabendazole: Mintezol
Cefuroxime: Zinacef, Kefurox, Ceftin	Lamivudine: Epivir, Epivir-HBV	Ticarcillin: Ticar
Cephalexin: Keflex	Lamivudine + abacavir: Epzicom	Tigecycline: Tygacil
Cephradine: Anspor, Velosef	Levofloxacin: Levaquin	Tinidazole: Tindamax
Chloroquine: Aralen	Linezolid: Zyvox	Tipranavir: Aptivus
Cidofovir: Vistide	Lomefloxacin: Maxaquin	Tobramycin: Nebcin
Ciprofloxacin: Cipro, Cipro XR	Lopinavir/ritonavir: Kaletra	Tretinoin: Retin A
Clarithromycin: Biaxin, Biaxin XL	Loracarbef: Lorabid	Trifluridine: Viroptic
Clindamycin: Cleocin	Mafenide: Sulfamylon	Trimethoprim: Proloprim, Trimpex
Clofazimine: Lamprene	Mebendazole: Vermox	Trimethoprim/sulfamethoxazole: Bactrim, Septra
Clotrimazole: Lotrimin, Mycelex	Mefloquine: Lariam	
Cloxacillin: Tegopen	Meropenem: Merrem	Valacyclovir: Valtrex
Colistimethate: Coly-Mycin M	Mesalamine: Asacol, Pentasa	Valganciclovir: Valcyte
Cycloserine: Seromycin	Methenamine: Hiprex, Mandelamine	Vancomycin: Vancocin
Daptomycin: Cubicin	Metronidazole: Flagyl	Voriconazole: Vfend
Delavirdine: Rescriptor	Micafungin: Mycamine	Zalcitabine: HIVID
Dicloxacillin: Dynapen	Minocycline: Minocin	Zanamivir: Relenza
Didanosine: Videx	Moxifloxacin: Avelox	Zidovudine (ZDV): Retrovir
Diethylcarbamazine: Hetrazan	Mupirocin: Bactroban	Zidovudine + 3TC: Combivir
Diloxanide furoate: Furamide	Nafcillin: Unipen	Zidovudine + 3TC + abacavir: Trizivir
Dirithromycin: Dynabac	Nelfinavir: Viracept	
Doxycycline: Vibramycin	Nevirapine: Viramune	

LE 23 (2)
TRADE AND GENERIC NAMES
LIST OF CO...

TRADE NAME: GENERIC NAME	TRADE NAME: GENERIC NAME	TRADE NAME: GENERIC NAME
Abelcet: Ampho B-lipid complex	Garamycin: Gentamicin	Retin A: Tretinoin
Albenza: Albendazole	Halfan: Halofantrine	Retrovir: Zidovudine (ZDV)
Aldara: Imiquimod	Hepsera: Adefovir	Reyataz: Atazanavir
Alinia: Nitazoxanide	Herplex: Idoxuridine	Rifadin: Rifampin
AmBisome: Ampho B-liposomal	Hiprex: Methenamine hippurate	Rifamate: INH + RIF
Amikin: Amikacin	HIVID: Zalcitabine	Rifater: INH + RIF + PZA
Amoxil: Amoxicillin	Humatin: Paromomycin	Rimactane: Rifampin
Amphotec: Ampho B-cholesteryl complex	Ilosone: Erythromycin estolate	Rocephin: Ceftriaxone
Ancef: Cefazolin	Ilotycin: Erythromycin	Roferon-A: Interferon alfa
Ancobon: Flucytosine	Intron A: Interferon alfa	Septra: Trimethoprim/sulfa
Anspor: Cephradine	Invanz: Ertapenem	Seromycin: Cycloserine
Antepar: Piperazine	Invirase: Saquinavir	Silvadene: Silver sulfadiazine
Antiminth: Pyrantel pamoate	Kantrex: Kanamycin	Spectracef: Cefditoren pivoxil
Aptivus: Tipranavir	Kaletra: Lopinavir/ritonavir	Sporanox: Itraconazole
Aralen: Chloroquine	Keflex: Cephalexin	Stoxil: Idoxuridine
Asacol: Mesalamine	Kefurox: Cefuroxime	Stromectol: Ivermectin
Augmentin, Augmentin ES-600	Ketek: Telithromycin	Sulfamylon: Mafenide
Augmentin XR: Amox./clav.	Lamisil: Terbinafine	Sulperazon[NUS]: Cefoperazone-sulbactam
Avelox: Moxifloxacin	Lamprene: Clofazimine	Suprax: Cefixime[NUS]
Azactam: Aztreonam	Lariam: Mefloquine	Sustiva: Efavirenz
Azulfidine: Sulfasalazine	Levaquin: Levofloxacin	Symmetrel: Amantadine
Bactroban: Mupirocin	Lexiva: Fosamprenavir	Synagis: Palivizumab
Bactrim: Trimethoprim/sulfamethoxazole	Lorabid: Loracarbef	Synercid: Quinupristin/dalfopristin
Baraclude: Entecavir	Macrodantin, Macrobid: Nitrofurantoin	Tamiflu: Oseltamivir
Biaxin, Biaxin XL: Clarithromycin	Malarone: Atovaquone + proguanil	Tazicef: Ceftazidime
Biltricide: Praziquantel	Mandelamine: Methenamine mandel.	Tegopen: Cloxacillin
Cancidas: Caspofungin	Maxaquin: Lomefloxacin	Tequin: Gatifloxacin
Ceclor, Ceclor CD: Cefaclor	Maxipime: Cefepime	Thalomid: Thalidomide
Cedax: Ceftibuten	Mefoxin: Cefoxitin	Ticar: Ticarcillin
Cefizox: Ceftizoxime	Mepron: Atovaquone	Timentin: Ticarcillin-clavulanic acid
Cefotan: Cefotetan	Merrem: Meropenem	Tinactin: Tolnaftate
Ceftin: Cefuroxime axetil	Minocin: Minocycline	Tindamax: Tinidazole
Cefzil: Cefprozil	Mintezol: Thiabendazole	Trecator SC: Ethionamide
Cipro, Cipro XR: Ciprofloxacin & extended release	Monocid: Cefonicid	Trizivir: Abacavir + ZDV + 3TC
Claforan: Cefotaxime	Monurol: Fosfomycin	Trobicin: Spectinomycin
Coly-Mycin M: Colistimethate	Myambutol: Ethambutol	Truvada: Emtricitabine + tenofovir
Combivir: ZDV + 3TC	Mycamine: Micafungin	Tygacil: Tigecycline
Crixivan: Indinavir	Mycobutin: Rifabutin	Unasyn: Ampicillin/sulbactam
Cubicin: Daptomycin	Mycostatin: Nystatin	Unipen: Nafcillin
Cytovene: Ganciclovir	Nafcil: Nafcillin	Valcyte: Valganciclovir
Daraprim: Pyrimethamine	Nebcin: Tobramycin	Valtrex: Valacyclovir
Diflucan: Fluconazole	NebuPent: Pentamidine	Vancocin: Vancomycin
Duricef: Cefadroxil	Nizoral: Ketoconazole	Vantin: Cefpodoxime proxetil
Dynapen: Dicloxacillin	Norvir: Ritonavir	Velosef: Cephradine
Emtriva: Emtricitabine	Noxafil: Posaconazole	Vermox: Mebendazole
Epivir, Epivir-HBV: Lamivudine	Omnicef: Cefdinir	Vfend: Voriconazole
Epzicom: Lamivudine + abacavir	Omnipen: Ampicillin	Vibramycin: Doxycycline
Factive: Gemifloxacin	Pediamycin: Erythro. ethyl succinate	Videx: Didanosine
Famvir: Famciclovir	Pediazole: Erythro. ethyl succinate + sulfisoxazole	Viracept: Nelfinavir
Fansidar: Pyrimethamine + sulfadoxine	Pegasys, PEG-Intron: Interferon, pegylated	Viramune: Nevirapine
Flagyl: Metronidazole	Pentam 300: Pentamidine	Virazole: Ribavirin
Floxin: Ofloxacin	Pentasa: Mesalamine	Vread: Tenofovir
Flumadine: Rimantadine	Pipracil: Piperacillin	Vistide: Cidofovir
Fortaz: Ceftazidime	Polycillin: Ampicillin	Xifaxan: Rifaximin
Fortovase: Saquinavir	Polymox: Amoxicillin	Xigris: Drotrecogin alfa
Fulvicin: Griseofulvin	Priftin: Rifapentine	Yodoxin: Iodoquinol
Fungizone: Amphotericin B	Primaxin: Imipenem + cilastatin	Zerit: Stavudine
Furadantin: Nitrofurantoin	Proloprim: Trimethoprim	Ziagen: Abacavir
Fuzeon: Enfuvirtide (T-20)	Prostaphlin: Oxacillin	Zinacef: Cefuroxime
Gantanol: Sulfamethoxazole	Rebetol: Ribavirin	Zithromax: Azithromycin
Gantrisin: Sulfisoxazole	Rebetron: Interferon + ribavirin	Zmax: Azithromycin ER
	Relenza: Zanamivir	Zovirax: Acyclovir
	Rescriptor: Delavirdine	Zosyn: Piperacillin/tazobactam
		Zyvox: Linezolid

INDEX TO MAJOR ENTITIES

Bold numbers indicate major considerations. *Recommendations in Table 1 not indexed; antibiotic selection often depends on modifying circumstances and alternative agents.*